Intelligent Technologies for Bridging the Grey Digital Divide

Jeffrey Soar
University of Southern Queensland, Australia

Rick Swindell
Griffith University, Australia

Philip Tsang
Caritas Francis Hsu College, Hong Kong

Information Science REFERENCE

INFORMATION SCIENCE REFERENCE
Hershey · New York

Director of Editorial Content: Kristin Klinger
Director of Book Publications: Julia Mosemann
Acquisitions Editor: Lindsay Johnston
Development Editor: Christine Bufton
Publishing Assistant: Milan Vracarich Jr.
Typesetter: Michael Brehm
Production Editor: Jamie Snavely
Cover Design: Lisa Tosheff

Published in the United States of America by
Information Science Reference (an imprint of IGI Global)
701 E. Chocolate Avenue
Hershey PA 17033
Tel: 717-533-8845
Fax: 717-533-8661
E-mail: cust@igi-global.com
Web site: http://www.igi-global.com

Library of Congress Cataloging-in-Publication Data

Intelligent technologies for bridging the grey digital divide / Jeffrey Soar, Rick Swindell, and Philip Tsang, editors.
p. cm.
Includes bibliographical references and index. Summary: "The main focus of the book is to provide insights into current innovation, issues to be resolved and approaches for widespread adoption to enable seniors and their families to enjoy the promised benefits of technology"--Provided by publisher. ISBN 978-1-61520-825-8 (hardcover) -- ISBN 978-1-61520-826-5 (ebook) 1. Technological innovations--Social aspects. 2. Internet and older people. 3. Computers and older people. I. Soar, Jeffrey. II. Swindell, Rick. III. Tsang, Philip. HM846.I58 2010
303.48'340846--dc22

British Cataloguing in Publication Data
A Cataloguing in Publication record for this book is available from the British Library.

Mehryar Nooriafshar, *University of Southern Queensland, Australia*
Nancy Pachana, *The University of Queensland, Australia*
Jeffrey Soar, *University of Southern Queensland, Australia*
Rick Swindell, *Griffith University, Australia*
Judith Symonds, *Auckland University of Technology, New Zealand*
Man-Wo Tsang, *United Christian Hospital, Hong Kong*
Philip Tsang, *Caritas Francis Hsu College, Hong Kong*
Trudy Yuginovich, *University of Southern Queensland, Australia*
Zoe Wang, Australian *Catholic University, Australia*
Ian Yip, *UCLA, USA*
Hong Zhou, *University of Southern Queensland, Australia*

Table of Contents

Detailed Table of Contents

Ubiquitous computing technology (ICT) shows great potential in supporting the infirm elderly, and others managing complex health issues, to live independently in their own home. While these technologies have great promise, their adoption level is low in Australia. It is suggested that two concurrent strategies are needed to improve the penetration of ICT-based assistive technology in the community. Firstly, significant trials are needed to verify that such systems can provide improved health outcomes and reduce health system costs for suitably targeted patients. Secondly, research in security and privacy, open standards, human-computer interfaces and new models of care driving software specifications is needed, so that these health system benefits can be achieved at a reasonable cost, and with adequate consideration of the needs of clients and carers.

This chapter explores ageing, chronic disease, technology and social change. Healthcare has been transformed through medical technology but there is much still to be done to enable seamless exchanges between all carers, which is expected to improve safety, quality and efficiency. There is massive potential for technology to transform the experience of ageing including assisting with the management of chronic disease, coordinated care and guided self-care for consumers. Innovative technologies are increasingly available to assist in maintaining health and independent living. This includes telecare,

This chapter presents the research, results and lessons learned from a project to evaluate currently available assisted living technologies for elderly people with mild to severe memory impairments who want to age in place. During the project a number of households were equipped with assistive technology to enable the end users to better cope with the barriers and problems associated with their forgetfulness. End users were involved in different phases, starting with a problem and needs analysis and ending with an evaluation of the technology installed in their homes. It seemed that technology did have a positive impact on their lives as well as on the lives of the informal caregivers who often live with those who suffer from amnesia. This project gives insight into how we are coming closer to optimizing the positive effects which assistive technology holds for the elderly with memory impairments. Key insights are presented.

"Pluggable user interfaces" is a software concept that facilitates adaptation and substitution of user interfaces and their components due to separation of the user interface from backend devices and services. Technically, the concept derives from abstract user interfaces, mainly in the context of device and service control. Abstract user interfaces have been claimed to support benefits such as ease of implementation, support for User Centered Design, seamless user interfaces, and ease of use. This paper reports on experiences in employing pluggable user interfaces in the European project i2home, based on the Universal Remote Console framework, and the Universal Control Hub architecture. In summary, our anecdotal evidence supports the claims on the benefits, but also identifies significant costs. The experience reports also include some hints as to how to mitigate the costs.

This chapter describes the mechanical design, manufacture and performance of a three-degree-of-freedom manipulator arm and gripper that can be attached to a mobile vehicle or electric scooter. This

The rapid ageing of South Korea's population requires expanded opportunities for older Koreans to continue to participate in society. Digital literacy is a critical element of Active Ageing. By promoting increased digital literacy, Korea's Research Institute of Science for the Better Living of the Elderly (RISBLE) aims to increase Korean elders' access to information and their opportunities for communication and participation. RISBLE's programs - Cyber Family, Internet Navigator, and the 1080 Family Online Game Festival - help elders master new technology, strengthen intergenerational relations, gain leadership roles, and contribute as community teachers. This chapter reviews the Korean situation of ageing, outlines our commitment to Active Ageing with Digital Ageing, and presents information on three RISBLE programs. These "best practices" are shared in hopes that other communities can learn from RISBLE's work to reduce the ageing digital divide and promote digital life for older persons.

This chapter covers current and future technologies relevant to older drivers. It begins with a review of salient characteristics of older drivers, before discussing current and future technologies at each level of the adopted framework: the road user, the road, and the vehicle. While most Intelligent Transportation Systems currently exist at the level of the vehicle (technologies such as satellite navigation, collision avoidance, and hazard alerting systems), research and development at the infrastructure level also holds promise of significant improvements in automotive safety through the exchange and coordination of digital information between vehicles and the roads upon which they are driven. At the individual level, there are also increasingly sophisticated technologies being developed that aim to accurately identify potentially unsafe drivers, and to maintain and even enhance cognitive capacities that are critically important to safe driving.

Contrary to expectations, assistive technology (AT) usage by the elderly has not increased in proportion to availability and ease of access. This is despite a belief that technology can contribute significantly towards improving their quality-of-life. Our Rehabilitation Mechatronics research group is developing a "unified neuro-physio platform", taking a cue from Eastern philosophies which emphasize that the "internal environment" of the users strongly affects how they interact with the "external environment". This chapter highlights the need to bridge these two environments meaningfully through "sensitive" technologies which address the mindsets and learning mechanisms of users. The technology platform we propose helps the elderly to understand and enhance their internal environment in order to interact at various levels with AT in their external environment. It provides a fresh approach to understanding and minimizing the persistent "digital divide" between the elderly and high technology.

Efficient and cost-effective solutions are needed to meet the demands for services required by an ever increasing number of users. We discuss the characteristics of Ambient Assisted Living (AAL) as a new approach that promises to address the needs of elderly people. We propose combining social aspects with technology to build a community of mutual care which, among other things, can serve as a platform to effectively organize the social resources, promote social connection, and introduce intergenerational activities. Our research analyzes the characteristics of a mutual assistance community to help elderly people age well. The needed technologies are investigated, challenges of building such a community are reviewed, and the design of some prototypic solutions and preliminary research on organizing services inside the community are discussed.

Australia's ageing population has escalated the demand for current health services and the trend could compound to unsustainable levels under the current health system. This chapter proposes a preventative healthcare model based on assistive technology to strengthen wellbeing at the individual and community level. The proposed model could minimise premature and inappropriate admission of Australians to care facilities while enhancing their independence and self care. It could also present a cost effective approach for policy makers by helping to alleviate the escalating costs of the health system. Importantly, this program offers an effective and sustainable alternative for delivering future health services.

Nursing homes provide long-term care services and can help preserve the quality of life of elderly people subject to physical and cognitive impairments. In this chapter, we explore the role of intelligent technologies as a supplement to human care-giving and the potential to improve quality of life for both older adults and their caregivers in nursing homes. A study was conducted on elderly people's and caregivers' attitudes toward the use of intelligent technologies in nursing homes, with the aim of understanding in which domains of everyday activities the application of intelligent technologies can be more suitable. Results showed that attitude toward the application of intelligent technologies in nursing homes is positive, although multifaceted. Elderly people and caregivers considered intelligent technologies as relevant devices for the improvement of quality of life in different domains. Nonetheless, differences related to the role that technologies played in nursing homes clearly emerged.

Chapter 16
Supporting Family-Based Care for Aged Patients with Chronic Illness.. 254
Lemai Nguyen, Deakin University, Australia

Family carers play an important role in care for aged patients with chronic illness, particularly in home and community settings. The information needs of these family carers and their patients are poorly understood and current health information systems do not adequately support their needs. This chapter describes current models in understanding patient and family carer information needs and analyses technology solutions in a new field of consumer health informatics. The analysis shows that current technology solutions in consumer health informatics fail to effectively support aged people in their own management of chronic illness and as well fail to support their family carers. The chapter also identifies key research issues in developing technologies that support aged patients and family carers in chronic illness management.

Chapter 17
Telenursing in Aged-Care: Systematic Evidence of Practice.. 270
Sisira Edirippulige, University of Queensland, Australia
Rohana Basil Marasinghe, University of Sri Jayewardenepura, Sri Lanka

Global ageing, combined with other challenges, has compelled health systems to explore new methods for providing health care. Telenursing, providing nursing care at a distance using new technologies, is identified as one alternative. The lack of evidence for the effectiveness of telenursing in aged care is a drawback for its wider use. The aim of this chapter is to review the evidence of randomised controlled trials (RCT) in geriatric telenursing practices. We performed a systematic literature review using the Ovid Medline and Pubmed databases on telenursing. A total of 62 articles were retrieved and 18 studies were selected for comprehensive analysis. The review found that the RCTs were conducted in different areas of geriatric telenursing and various information and communication technologies (ICT) were used in the interventions. Although robust evidence based on RCTs in aged care telenursing is yet to emerge, the majority of current studies suggest that telenursing is an effective tool.

This chapter looks into the systems and institutions for the elderly population covered by long-term care insurance in Japan and the Republic of Korea. It discusses the historical changes in policies in these two nations. The Health Care and Welfare Complex elements that make up a single business model for the Health Care and Social Services of the aged in Japan and Korea are also discussed. Serious competition between medical facilities for patients occurred following considerable changes in the management environment for medical facilities adjustments brought about by population and social structure change. Medical facilities in Japan and Korea showed a rapid increase in comprehensive medical and welfare management. Consequently, there were provisions in both health care and social services through affiliation, chain affiliation and multiplication, before and after the enforcement of long-term care insurance.

More aged care services are needed in Taiwan. Research has demonstrated that nursing home placement of older adults in need of advanced care is the most cost effective option for family caregivers. However, filial piety, which entails looking after older parents at home, is one of the core tenets of Chinese society. Placing older parents into nursing homes can lead to family conflict and can continue to evoke deep emotional responses in some former family caregivers. This chapter draws on findings from two case studies to illustrate the dilemmas facing Taiwanese families who must cope with changing social conditions and customary filial expectations. The use of assistive technologies as solutions to these dilemmas is outlined. These technologies are argued to be a cost effective way to assist adult caregivers, their charges, and staff in nursing homes. Their use may apply to other Asian countries with similar cultural beliefs and values.increasingly available to assist in maintaining health and independent living. This includes telecare, telehealth, assistive technologies, robots and smart homes. A challenge is in providing access to and support in the use of technologies where there are clear benefits to consumers, carers, providers and funders of healthcare. The chapter also reports on the Queensland Smart Home Initiative which is one of several organisations internationally that share a mission of assisting people to be supported through these technologies.

Foreword

It is almost an axiom to say that the world population is ageing. 'Everybody' knows this. By the year 2050 it is projected that more than one in every six persons throughout the world will be at least sixty five years old (UN, 2002) and people in this cohort will exceed the number of children in the world. By 2050 around 22% will be over 65 years old and the fastest growing group, the over 85s, will account for 2 in 10 of the world population. Disability affects a large number of older people – and their carers. Dementia is considered to be one of the major contributors to disease burden. Other conditions that often result in social isolation, reduce quality of life and have a significant impact on health care costs include: arthritis, hearing loss, depression and incontinence.

Figures suggest at least 32-42% of people over 70 fall each year and falls are a factor in 40% of injury related deaths.

There are many causes and types of disability but I want to focus on these here to provide some human faces to the rather dry statistics.

Elly is aged 94; she lives alone in the home she shared with her husband of 70 years. She is determined to live out her days and die in this house where she raised six of her eight children and has so many memories – good and bad – but special to her. Elly's children, like many these days, have moved to various parts of the country and Jim, the eldest lives in the UK. Most of the family members generally try to get home for Christmas. Her daughter Emma, who lives in Tokyo, calls Elly on the phone every Sunday.

Before Jack died, he was very reluctant to leave the house unless he knew there would be a convenient toilet and people to assist him to access venues. He was incontinent of urine but too embarrassed to discuss this with anyone. His incontinence restricted his social activity. In addition he had fairly debilitating arthritis. Public transport was not an option and he could no longer drive so he depended on local service clubs for any social outings.

When Emma had her first child Elly travelled to Japan alone to spend a couple of weeks with her. When she returned home she found Jack dead, on the bathroom floor – he had fallen and died alone. This was desperately upsetting for Elly; not only did she feel guilty for leaving him alone but she also developed a dreadful fear of falling and went from being a very social community member to socially isolated. When her family and local doctor tried to suggest perhaps it was time to think about moving into a hostel, Elly just became more determined to stay put. Gradually her mood changed and she appeared to her local doctor to be developing depression. She was also having some difficulty hearing Emma on the phone and so many times did not bother to talk to her when she rang.

It was too difficult now for her to do many of her usual household chores but her determination to be independent meant she refused most community services. She ate less as getting to the shops was too much of an effort. Her younger sister Kate, who recently was widowed, moved in with Elly. Sadly, within a few months, it became obvious to neighbours that Kate had dementia and was becoming more of a burden to Elly than a help. Kate would forget to take her medications, wander off to do the shopping and forget either to buy the food and/or to come home. Elly hated to worry the neighbours so she would sit for hours just wondering if Kate was okay. She worried if she tried to find her she might fall – she worried maybe Kate had fallen. The neighbours tried to check in on them and called the police when Kate was missing. They usually found her quite quickly, until on one occasion it took several days before she was found drowned in a lake six kilometres from the house.

Tim, the son living in the UK, knew if he could interact more with his mum and she could see the grandchildren that would help but he could not afford to come home. Emma arrived from Tokyo and found Elly was sleeping on the couch and washing in the sink because she could not get up the stairs to the bedrooms and shower. The garden, once her pride and joy, was a mess. Mum could not get down the stairs and consequently she was also suffering Vitamin D deficiency from lack of exposure to sunlight and poor nutrition.

You can see what we have here is a complex and degenerating situation – not uncommonly experienced by older people. Assistive technology could have improved the quality of life for all concerned and probably prevented Kate's drowning.

Alongside the ageing of the population we have a shrinking labour-force. The movement of women into the employment market is increasing the need for paid support for older people both at home and in nursing homes. Internationally, governments and other health care providers are exploring ways in which to cope with fewer doctors, nurses and allied health professionals. A potential contributor is of course workforce redesign taking account of the growing acceptance and uses of assistive technology.

This book demonstrates how Smart Houses and intelligent devices can improve social participation, reduce fear of falling, facilitate access within and external to houses and negotiation of stairs, and generally allow older people to remain 'in touch' with loved ones and their communities.

There are of course ethical issues that must be considered, for example, are tracking devices an abuse of privacy? I would argue that assistive technology should be embraced provided it meets the principles of person-centred care. Does the technology improve quality of life for the older person and is it acceptable to them, individualized and safe – or is it simply making life easier for staff and family? If the former I would support it.

This book opens up many possibilities for using assistive technology to ensure older people continue to enjoy independence, dignity of risk and harm minimization. I recommend it to practitioners, policy makers, researchers and students.

Rhonda Nay
Professor of Interdisciplinary Aged Care
Director ISP / ACEBAC / TIME for dementia / AIPC
Australian Centre for Evidence Based Aged Care
La Trobe University, Australia

REFERENCES

Alzheimer's Disease International (2008) 'the prevalence of dementia worldwide'. Available from http://www.alz.co.uk/adi/pdf/prevalence.pdf

Murray, C.J., & Lopez, A.D. (Eds.). (1996) The Global Burden of Disease. A comprehensive assessment of mortality and disability from diseases, injuries and risk factors in 1990 and projected to 2020. Boston: Harvard School of Public Health, Harvard University Press.

Sousa, R.M., Ferri, C.P., Acosta, D., Albanese, E., Guerra, M., Huang, Y., Jacob, K.S., Jotheeswaran, A.T., Juan, J., Libre Rodriguez, J., Rodriguez Pichardo, G., Rodriquez, M.C.,

Salas, A., Sosa, A.L., Williams, J., Zuniga, T. & Prince, M. (2009). Contribution of chronic disease to disability in elderly people in countries with low and middle incomes: 10/66 Dementia Research Group population-based survey. Lancet, 374, 1821-30

United Nations (2007) World Population Ageing. Executive Summary. Retrieved from http://www.un.org/esa/population/publications/WPA2007/ES-English.pdf

United Nations (2007). World Population Ageing. Summary Tables. Retrieved from http://www.un.org/esa/population/publications/WPA2007/SummaryTables_new.pdf

World Health Organisation (2007) WHO Global Report on Falls Prevention in Older Age, France. Retrieved from http://www.stopfalls.org/files/WHO_Report.pdf

World House Organization (2008) The Global Burden of Disease. 2004 update, Switzerland. Retrieved from http://www.who.int/healthinfo/global_burden_disease/GBD_report_2004update_full.pdf

Rhonda Nay *is Foundation Professor of Interdisciplinary Aged Care and Director of the Institute for Social Participation (ISP); TIME –the Victorian and Tasmanian Dementia Training Studies Centre; the Australian Centre for Evidence Based Aged Care (ACEBAC) and the Australian Institute for Primary Care (AIPC) at La Trobe University. She also leads the Victorian hub of the Dementia Collaborative Research Centre. Rhonda has chaired the Minister's Awards for Excellence in Aged Care and has been a judge for the Aged and Community Services Awards. Her research is focused on getting evidence based, interdisciplinary, person-centred care into practice. Rhonda is a Director of the Aged Care Standards and Accreditation Agency Ltd.*

Preface

Welcome to this book of research into ageing and technology. This book covers a broad range of related topics by leading and emerging researchers in the new field of technology innovation for ageing. Chapter authors are from Canada, Germany, UK, Greece, Czech Republic, Korea, Singapore, the USA, Ireland, Spain, the Netherlands, Belgium, Italy, Sri Lanka, Japan, Taiwan and Australia. The topic is an important one, that is, how to enrich the experience of ageing and relieve some of the pressures and stresses associated with an ageing population through intelligent technology and the intelligent use of technology.

There is a movement towards an agenda of active ageing, so the support for older people goes beyond traditional models of "care" to models that promote social participation and active independent lives. Technology is a potentially powerful medium for facilitating this.

The aim of compiling this book was to provide high-quality academic, industry and practice articles in research on intelligent technologies for seniors. The main focus is to provide insights from current research and innovations, to discuss issues to be resolved and approaches for widespread adoption to enable seniors, their families and carers, and wider society to benefit from the many advantages that technology can contribute towards ageing societies.

BACKGROUND

Information and communications technology and the widespread adoption of the Internet have transformed industries, and enabled new services and delivery at the convenience of the consumer. There is a plethora of new sophisticated technologies with the potential to transform ageing and aged care, enable independent living and provide access to care at the convenience of the consumer. There are also exciting projects in many countries involving telecare, telehealth and other technologies that might assist seniors. Demonstrator smart homes can be found in many countries. Governments are beginning to develop strategies and policies to reduce barriers to the adoption of technologies for ageing and promote their adoption. Some of the large-rollouts of intelligent home care technologies are providing confirmation of the anticipated benefits. Researchers have a responsibility to contribute to and disseminate results of the findings of quality research so as to guide policy development, resource allocation and evidence-based decision making.

The technologies promise to alleviate some of the challenges of ageing. These include adverse events such as falls, risks involved in wandering by people with cognitive decline, workforce participation by seniors, maintaining physical activity, maintaining social contacts and involvement, addressing the shortages of professional and family carers, and providing reminders of activities of daily living and medications.

That there is a great need for these technologies is demonstrated by the high rates of adverse events. There are as yet few people living in smart home environments and the adoption of intelligent technology for ageing is slow compared to the adoption of technologies in many other sectors. There are many issues to be resolved before the adoption of intelligent technologies for ageing becomes mainstream and there is much to learn from current research and project experience. Issues include design, acceptance by seniors, design agreement and standards by manufacturers, equipment funding, service funding, business models, maintenance, monitoring, education and training, awareness raising, standards, prioritisation of resources more towards home and community care, confirmation of the benefits and national strategy and policy.

AGEING

The context for this book is the global surge in the percentages of older people in the populations of almost all countries and the imperative to find creative ways to manage growing demand for services, to manage costs and better support people – consumers, families and carers. Older age confronts all of us in different ways throughout life from the experience of ageing grandparents, the move of our own parents into later stages of life and ultimately our own transition into society's senior citizens. Few people would not want the ageing experience to be better for themselves and subsequent generations than it might have been for our grandparents and parents.

Many will be aware of the way technology has transformed our lives in almost every field. It may come as a surprise to people drawn into arrangements to support elderly parents to find out how little technology is used by the current generation of seniors and many of the aged care providers. Technology has the potential to assist in maintaining active, productive and independent lives, support the care workforce, provide access to health and medical services, facilitate social connectivity and assist in countless other ways such as those explained in this book. For this to happen, researchers may have to look at ageing and at people from a fresh perspective.

Exciting innovations in intelligent assistive technologies, smart home environments and information systems to support care in home and community settings have been undertaken internationally. Some of these are presented in this book. Much of these approaches are yet to be mainstreamed, that is to be made available to a broader community beyond projects, pilots or limited roll-outs. To achieve this there is still much to be done in research. Issues that need further development include awareness raising, promotion, improving availability and support, developing systems for responding appropriately to the signals from the technology, funding arrangements and new models for providing care that optimise the potential benefits.

DEVELOPMENT OF THE BOOK

Researchers and practitioners were invited to submit chapter proposals clearly explaining the mission and concerns of their proposed chapters. From these a number were selected on the basis of likely interest to readers, innovation, quality, balance and the research standing of the authors. Authors of accepted proposals were provided with organizational guidelines to assist in the development of full chapters. All submitted chapters were reviewed by at least two reviewers on a blind review basis.

This book of research brings together a range of complementary ideas. It is aimed at contributing to the further development and adoption of assistive technology through quality research. We were delighted with the diversity of chapter proposals submitted for publication and regret that not all could be included.

CONTRIBUTIONS

The book is divided into three thematic sections. Section 1: Innovations supporting ageing in place opens with a chapter on the potential of Ubiquitous Computing for Independent Living from Neil Bergmann. Bergmann suggests that two concurrent strategies are needed to improve the penetration of ICT-based assistive technology in the community. Firstly, significant trials are needed to verify that such systems can provide improved health outcomes and reduce health system costs for suitably targeted patients. Secondly, research in security and privacy, open standards, human-computer interfaces and new models of care driving software specifications is needed, so that these health system benefits can be achieved at a reasonable cost, and with adequate consideration of the needs of clients and carers.

Jeffrey Soar in the chapter, "Ageing, Chronic Disease, Technology and Smart Homes: An Australian Perspective," explores issues of ageing, chronic disease, technology and social change. He suggests a challenge is in providing access to and support for the use of technologies where there are clear benefits to consumers, carers, providers and funders of healthcare. The chapter also reports on the Queensland Smart Home Initiative which is one of several organisations internationally that share a mission of assisting people to be supported through these technologies.

A leading European project on Ambient Assisted Living systems for older people, The SOPRANO Project, is reported on by Andrew Sixsmith and co-authors. The chapter, "A user-driven approach to developing Ambient Assisted Living systems for older people: The SOPRANO Project," outlines SOPRANO's experience and application research approach to ensure that end-users are involved in all stages of the research and development. The chapter reports that in the SOPRANO project a number of key areas for application development were identified and developed as a set of use cases (or descriptive models), for example for medication reminding, and to support exercise. These use cases were further refined through visualization and iterative prototyping techniques with end-users to ensure usability, usefulness and acceptability for users. The SOPRANO prototype system is described together with future plans for deployment in demonstration sites and field trials.

One in three people over the age of 65 experience falls each year, consequently falls prevention is a major issue and is discussed in the book in the chapter "Falls prevention in the home: Challenges for new technologies" by Rose A Kenny, Cliodhna Ni Scanaill and Michael McGrath. They review the latest best practices for the identification of falls risk including the technology available and the challenges of using technology for in-home falls prevention, risk assessment and falls detection. Recommendations and suggestions for future research directions are discussed.

Claire Huijnen presents the research, results and lessons learned from a project to evaluate currently available assisted living technologies for older people with mild to severe memory impairments who want to age in place, in her chapter "The use of assistive technology to support the wellbeing and independence of people with memory impairments." She found that technology did have a positive impact on their lives as well as on the lives of the informal caregivers who often live with those who suffer from amnesia. This chapter gives insight into how we are coming closer to optimizing the positive effects which assistive technology holds for older people with memory impairments.

"Pluggable user interfaces" is a software concept that facilitates adaptation and substitution of user interfaces and their components due to separation of the user interface from backend devices and services. In their chapter, "Meeting the Needs of Diverse User Groups: Benefits and Costs of Pluggable User Interfaces in Designing for Older People and People with Cognitive Impairments."

Gottfried Zimmerman and co-authors report on experiences in employing pluggable user interfaces in the European project i2home. Their anecdotal evidence supports the claims on the benefits, the costs and some hints as to how to mitigate the costs.

Samuel Cubero describes the mechanical design, manufacture and performance of a three-degree-of-freedom manipulator arm and gripper that can be attached to a mobile vehicle or electric scooter in the chapter "A robotic arm for electric scooters." This reports on a device that can be remotely or automatically controlled to pick up and retrieve heavy objects, such as books or grocery products, from high shelves or difficult-to-reach locations. Such tasks are often considered to be arduous or even impossible for the frail elderly and people with disabilities. A brief overview of existing "state of the art" robotic and machine vision technologies, and how these can be used to perform many everyday domestic or household chores, is also provided.

Section 2: contains chapters on the theme of Innovations supporting engagement with daily life. In the first chapter in this section Nancy Pachana and Emma Poulsen aim to examine the adoption of technology by older adults within a framework of current gerontological theories and research in their chapter "Thinking Outside the Box: Novel Uses of Technology to Promote Well-being in Older Populations." Cognitive, physical, mental and interpersonal development and change later in life are described. Two main psychological frameworks for understanding successful ageing are briefly outlined and within these frameworks, the role of technology in enhancing the lives of older adults, regardless of the level at which they incorporate it into their lives, are discussed. The chapter concludes with suggestions for removing barriers and enhancing uptake of technology for older adults, helping to bridge the grey digital divide.

Richard Swindell, Peter Grimbeek and Jan Heffernan in their chapter, "U3A Online and successful aging: A smart way to help bridge the grey digital divide," set three aims: 1) to outline the elements of the successful aging model; 2) to explain the worldwide, self-help University of the Third Age (U3A) program and 3) to discuss findings from two related studies of older adults who were members of the first virtual U3A called U3A Online. Their focus group research examined the characteristics of older people who are attracted to online learning. Results supported a conclusion that electronic communication can reduce feelings of isolation and provide stimulating and enjoyable pastimes with the potential to assist older people in aging successfully.

Donghee Han and Kathryn L. Braun examined "Promoting Active Ageing through Technology Training in Korea." Their chapter reviews the Korean situation of ageing, outlines commitment to Active Ageing with Digital Ageing, and presents information on three "best practices" for expanding digital literacy and involvement of older adults. Internet Navigators are older adults trained to train other older adults in the use of computers, the Internet, and various software programs. Cyber-Family links older adults and youth as online pen-pals. The annual1080 Online Game Festival brings three-generation families together for a day of internet play, which has led the Korean IT industry to expand computer and software options for older adults.

Being able to continue to drive a car is of great concern to older people in many societies and Christopher G. Hatherly in his chapter "Intelligent Transportation Systems for Older Drivers: A Systems Approach to Improving Safety and Extending Driving Longevity" covers current and future technologies relevant to older drivers. It begins with a review of salient characteristics of older drivers, before discussing current and future technologies at the levels of the vehicle, the infrastructure and the individual.

Assistive technology (AT) usage by older people has not increased in proportion to availability and ease of access. This is the finding of John Heng and Subhasis Banerji in their chapter "Low Usage of Intelligent Technologies by the Aged: New Initiatives to Bridge the Digital Divide." This is despite a belief that technology can contribute significantly towards improving their quality-of-life. Their Rehabilitation Mechatronics research group is developing a "unified neuro-physio platform", taking a cue from Eastern philosophies which emphasize that the "internal environment" of the users strongly affects how they interact with the "external environment". They propose a technology platform to help older people to understand and enhance the internal environment in order to interact at various levels with AT in their external environment.

Hong Sun and co-authors discuss the characteristics of Ambient Assisted Living (AAL) to address the needs of older people in the chapter "Building a Mutual Assistance Community for Older Elderly pPeople." They propose combining social aspects with technology to build a community of mutual care which, among other things, can serve as a platform to effectively organize the social resources, promote social connection, and introduce intergenerational activities. Technical issues of building their community through service orientation and web services are discussed. Their research also analyzes the characteristics of a mutual assistance community to help older people age well.

The last chapter in Section 2 is an industry perspective: "Preventative Healthcare: A Proposed Holistic Assistive Technology Model based on Industry Practice" from James Barrientos and Michele Barry. This chapter proposes a preventative healthcare model based on assistive technology to strengthen wellbeing at the individual and community level. The proposed model could minimise premature and inappropriate admission of Australians to care facilities while enhancing their independence and self care. It could also present a cost effective approach for policy makers by helping to alleviate the escalating costs of the health system. Importantly, this program offers an effective and sustainable alternative for delivering future health services.

The last of the three sections of the book contains chapters on the theme of Innovations supporting the frail elderly and aged care providers. Lorenza Tiberio and co-authors begin this section with a chapter on "Attitudes toward intelligent technologies: Older people and caregivers in nursing homes." They explore the role of intelligent technologies as a supplement to human care-giving and the potential to improve quality of life for both older adults and their caregivers in nursing homes. The chapter reports on a study on older people's and caregivers' attitudes toward the use of intelligent technologies in nursing homes, with the aim of understanding in which domains of everyday activities the application of intelligent technologies can be more suitable. Their results showed that attitudes of older people and care-givers toward the application of intelligent technologies in nursing homes is positive, although multifaceted.

José Luis Jorge Marrasé describes the approach followed to create a new communications platform that can support a citizen centric home care service in the chapter Citizen centric care: A Telecom perspective based on Integrated Video Assistance for Elders (IVAE). This strategy is based on offering application enablers to care providers to simplify the use of the capacity of telecom networks. The chapter also discusses the required supporting changes in the care provider systems and procedures to deliver the outcomes needed in healthcare.

Lemai Nguyen in the chapter "Supporting Family-based Care for Aged Patients with Chronic Illness" describes current models in understanding patient and family carer information needs and analyses technology solutions in a new field of consumer health informatics. Her analysis shows that current technology solutions in consumer health informatics fail to effectively support aged people in their own management of chronic illness and as well fail to support family carers. She also identifies key research issues in developing technologies to support aged patients and family carers in chronic illness management.

Sisira Edirippulige and Rohana Basil Marasinghe undertook a systematic review of randomised controlled trials (RCT) in geriatric telenursing practices telenursing in aged care that is reported in "Telenursing in aged-care: Systematic evidence of practice." They found that robust evidence based on RCTs in aged care telenursing is yet to emerge however the majority of current studies suggest that telenursing is an effective tool.

Seungwon Jeong and Yusuke Inoue in Health insurance systems as models for managing the increasing elderly populations of Japan and Korea report on research into the systems and institutions for older people covered by long-term care insurance in Japan and the Republic of Korea. They discuss the historical changes in policies in these two nations. They found changes occurred in competition between medical facilities for patients and changes in the management and organisational environment of medical facilities.

The book ends with an interesting chapter "Assistive Technologies as aids to family caregivers in Taiwan" by Szu-Yao (Zoe) Wang. She discusses filial piety, the obligation to care for older parents at home, as one of the core tenets of Chinese societies across Asia. Placing older parents into nursing homes can lead to family conflict and can continue to evoke deep emotional responses in some former family caregivers. This chapter draws on findings from two case studies to illustrate the dilemmas facing Taiwanese families who must cope with changing social conditions and customary filial expectations, and potential solution for these dilemmas by using assistive technologies.

Jeffrey Soar
University of Southern Queensland, Australia

Rick Swindell
Griffith University, Australia

Philip Tsang
Caritas Francis Hsu College, Hong Kong

Acknowledgment

Particular thanks are due to Dr Rick Swindell; without his involvement this book would not have been completed in time and would not be of such high quality. Rick worked with several authors to guide them in polishing their chapters and assisted speakers of other languages with some of the challenges of writing in English. He undertook most of the day-to-day liaison with the publishers and with each of the authors to keep us all on track with deadlines and quality standards.

Particular thanks are also due to Jan Heffernan who worked tirelessly on helping us to enhance the overall quality of the book.

Philip would like to give special thanks to his wife Dr Sandy Tse for her support during the project activities in the past 12 months. As his writing and editing project comes to completion, Philip promises to catch up on his share of babysitting Jenny who recently turned 18 months old. Jenny is a joy and a gift to us. This project has also benefited from the research grants (06/21) (R189-2)(ST-08/09-2) from The Open University of Hong Kong and (HK-R1209) from the Johnson & Johnson. For these, Philip wants to thank both the OUHK & Johnson and Johnson research committees.

Jeffrey Soar
University of Southern Queensland, Australia

Rick Swindell
Griffith University, Australia

Philip Tsang
Caritas Francis Hsu College, Hong Kong

Section 1
Innovations Supporting Ageing in Place

Chapter 1
Ubiquitous Computing for Independent Living

Neil W. Bergmann
University of Queensland, Australia

ABSTRACT

Ubiquitous computing technology (ICT) shows great potential in supporting the infirm elderly, and others managing complex health issues, to live independently in their own home. While these technologies have great promise, their adoption level is low in Australia. It is suggested that two concurrent strategies are needed to improve the penetration of ICT-based assistive technology in the community. Firstly, significant trials are needed to verify that such systems can provide improved health outcomes and reduce health system costs for suitably targeted patients. Secondly, research in security and privacy, open standards, human-computer interfaces and new models of care driving software specifications is needed, so that these health system benefits can be achieved at a reasonable cost, and with adequate consideration of the needs of clients and carers.

INTRODUCTION

A defining characteristic of humans is that they are inventive and habitual tool users. We all use tools to enhance our physical, cognitive and communicative capabilities. Assistive technologies are one class of tools which aim to improve the quality of life of those faced with particular medical, physical, or cognitive challenges. An important class of assistive technologies is enabled by Information and Communication Technologies (ICT). This chapter looks at a subset of ICT called ubiquitous computing. It investigates how such devices and systems can be best used to develop assistive technologies that can help the ageing and infirm to live more independently in their own homes, rather than in institutional settings.

The chapter will first look in some detail at the characteristics of modern ubiquitous computing systems and then the requirements for independent living, before bringing the two topics together to investigate ways in which ubiquitous computing

DOI: 10.4018/978-1-61520-825-8.ch001

systems can be better designed to enhance living independently.

BACKGROUND

Ubiquitous Computing

Ubiquitous Computing has emerged in the past two decades as a term meaning computers everywhere. Much of the early thinking around this topic was due to the late Mark Weiser of Xerox PARC, and his idea of the disappearing computer (Weiser, 1991). There are many different views on what ubiquitous computing means, but it can be summarised as computers everywhere, communications everywhere and information everywhere. It is useful to explore trends of the near past and the envisioned future, to give more meaning to this domain of research.

Firstly, we have already seen computers becoming a key component of both simple and complex devices and systems. Of course, it depends what we mean by a computer. For the purposes of this discussion, we can consider a device whose function is programmable by software as a computer. In particular, the small microcontrollers which one finds in televisions, cameras, digital watches, and the like are certainly considered here as computers. One of the first signs of "computers everywhere" has been the rapid adoption of microcontrollers as key components in almost every electrical and electronic device.

Such devices exhibit a key characteristic of ubiquitous computing, that of the disappearing computer. The embedded computer in an appliance is often not obvious in either the function or user interface to a device. For example, it may be more economical to put a small microprocessor in a toaster to calculate the average toasting time given the "darkness setting" than it is to design a mechanical device for achieving the same function. Once the microcontroller is there, it is then easy to add additional features, such as a "defrost" button, or an asymmetric "crumpet" toasting setting. The computers in such devices are usually called embedded computers, since they are not directly programmable by the user, but rather are embedded as part of the core function of the device. Analysts suggest at least 99% of all computers sold annually are embedded computers, and in many cases their presence is not immediately obvious to the purchaser (Zurawski, 2006).

Computers Everywhere

When I was an undergraduate student, our first year electrical engineering professor asked us to go home and count how many electric motors we could find in our home, to motivate us in how important electric engineering was in our daily lives. Most people managed totals of around 20 or 30 motors. Nowadays, a similar exercise of asking how many computers are in our house would yield a total closer to 100.

A modern automobile is a good example of a complex device whose function now depends critically on embedded computers. Modern luxury cars may contain up to 70 micro-controllers, and electronics contribute almost 50% of the car's cost, up from around 20% a decade ago (Sangiovanni-Vincentelli, 2007). Almost every "power" device such as power windows, mirrors, or seats has its own controller, as well as controllers for audio entertainment, navigation systems, braking and stability programs (ABS, traction control), and multiple controllers for engine components such as ignition and fuel injection.

A modern car also provides a valuable lesson in what can go wrong with such a ubiquitous computing approach. For today's car, it is not enough for each microcontroller to be a separate subsystem – rather the microcontrollers are now integrated onto high-speed data buses. This allows programmed coordination of multiple microcontrollers, for example resetting mirror and seat positions on the basis of individual drivers recognised automatically from their car keys. It also means easy diagnostic analysis of equipment failures and more customised maintenance schedules. However, it has also led to spiralling development and verification times because of the complex interactions between multiple devices from multiple component suppliers. In response to this problem, automotive manufacturers have established large consortia (such as AutoSAR) to develop rigorous and complex specifications for the ways in which devices can reliably and efficiently communicate (Sangiovanni-Vincentelli, 2007).

Communications Everywhere

This naturally brings us to the next theme of ubiquitous computing which is communications everywhere, or ubiquitous communications (Committee on Networked Systems of Embedded Computers, 2001). The real power of ubiquitous computing occurs when the computers inside individual appliances and subsystems are able to communicate with each other to allow new corporate behaviours and capabilities to be provided. Every set of modern traffic lights in a city is controlled by its own microcontroller; however, when all of these controllers are linked together, one has a much more powerful traffic control system. The timing of traffic light cycles can be adjusted according to predictable (e.g. daily peak) and unpredictable (e.g. traffic accident) changes in traffic density. Light sequences can be synchronised along primary traffic routes to improve traffic flow. Lights can respond appropriately to emergency vehicles. In the near future, individual cars may be able to communicate with traffic system to identify better routes to take, and in return provide the system with feedback on upstream traffic densities (Vaa, Penttinen & Spyropoulou, 2007).

However, communicating subsystems bring with them a whole range of associated problems, the most pressing of which are security and privacy. Take, for example, a system which allows me to switch my home air conditioner on or off when I am away from the house, using either the Internet or a mobile phone. I want this to be a relatively easy and perhaps even a semi-automatic process for me and my family members. However, I also want it to be impossible for others to remotely operate the air conditioner without my permission. I also want the "state" of my house to be a secret – I do not want it generally known when my house is occupied and when it is empty.

Privacy and security in embedded systems are significant challenges, and not well addressed by many current systems (Jurjens, 2007). The computing requirements for many appliance control functions are quite modest. Adding communications introduces some complexity, but there has been considerable research into low-cost wired and wireless communications systems for embedded systems. However, adding secure communications, with state-of-the-art encryption and authentication adds significantly to the cost and complexity of many embedded systems (Bergstrom, Driscoll, & Kimball, 2001).

Information Everywhere

Ubiquitous computing and ubiquitous communications mean that we can sense and control appliances intelligently and remotely. In addition to computing everywhere and communications everywhere, we also desire information everywhere. Much of the developed world economy depends upon the capture, storage and manipulation of information. Even in our daily lives, we depend on the availability of information. We have address books, diaries, documents, bank accounts, medical records, photographs, music and video collections and much more. We all have our own information environment, and we use a wide range of different interface devices and methodologies to access our information environment. The goal of ubiquitous information is to be able to access our information environments any "where", any "when" and any "how". We are currently a long way from this goal, not least because of some fundamental challenges of ubiquitous information environments.

Ubiquitous information needs to be stored in (at least) one place, and accessed using some other device, often in another location. In some cases, the data access is easy – my music is stored in the flash memory on my MP3 player, and accessed using that same device. However, there is typically no access to the music stored on my MP3 player anywhere else. I need to carry the data with me whenever I wish to access this information.

My weekly schedule and my emails are stored on a central university server, which is accessed efficiently and effectively when I am on campus and my computer is connected via the backbone network. It is accessible more slowly, and less flexibly, by a web-based interface away from the campus, and is also accessible via mobile phone with significantly higher communication costs and lower performance. Many other parts of my information environment suffer from similar problems. The more widely available my data is, generally the slower and more cumbersome it is to access. The Internet seems to continually struggle along at a barely acceptable level of performance and convenience, and each new improvement in speed seems to be consumed by new applications which more aggressively consume bandwidth.

Of course security and privacy are equally significant problems with ubiquitous information. Health informatics deals with some very private information in terms of medical histories and treatments, and it is still fully to come to terms with how to provide high security and privacy, but also adequate access to the information for medical professionals. Online commerce faces many of the same problems, when sensitive information needs to be provided to relatively unknown vendors. Reliability also becomes a significant concern when information environments become mission-critical. Most people who have suffered a hard-disk failure on their desktop machine quickly realise the difficulty of reconstructing this part of their information environment, even with the best backup plans and technologies.

Another issue is in accessing information environments – the human-computer interface, or perhaps it is better to call it the human-information interface. There are certainly issues about the physical way in which we access information – the size of the screen, the number of buttons, the format of menus, and the way we search and navigate. These are relatively straightforward, with a large body of knowledge on how to design good interfaces, at least for mainstream computer users (Sears & Jacko, 2007).

However, a larger issue is how we can present a unified interface to our whole information environment which is appropriate to the particular interface devices we might currently have available without having to write a separate interface program for every device and every data repository.

Challenges in Ubiquitous Computing

When we examine the progress that has been made in ubiquitous computing, we can be both amazed and disappointed at the results. On the one hand, computers have become part of almost all electrical and electronic devices that we come in contact with. They have reduced the cost, and increased the flexibility of many common appliances and systems. Most devices (at least those successful in the marketplace) are relatively intuitive to use.

When we come to ubiquitous communications, progress in much less advanced. Reductions in the cost of computing have been much more rapid than cost reductions in communications, and so in many cases the cost of providing communications outweighs the benefits. If I wished, it would be relatively easy to broadcast my position (or at least the position of my phone) continuously on a webpage to authorised viewers, using suitable satellite navigation outdoors, or WiFi localisation indoors. However, 3G mobile data costs would be prohibitive.

In addition to bandwidth cost, security and privacy concerns also reduce the spread of ubiquitous communications. Secure communications and appropriate user authentication are not just a small impost on top of the cost of communications between embedded devices; rather, they are a significant burden. Adding even moderate security could increase the computational requirements of devices by orders of magnitude (Zurawski, 2006).

Ubiquitous information suffers from similar problems to ubiquitous communications. This is not surprising since data storage is relatively cheap, but secure high speed communications is expensive. It is often still the case that it is easier to carry our data with us, than to access it remotely.

In the next section, we will imagine, at least for a short while, that the problems of low-cost, easy-to-use and secure communications have been solved, and we will investigate the potential applications that ubiquitous computing, ubiquitous communication, and ubiquitous information have in assistive technologies for independent living. We will then return to the real world, to outline research needed to achieve some of these applications.

Assistive Technologies

Assistive technologies are generally taken to mean technologies which allow those with a disability to live more normally. Assistive technologies can be thought of as those which help to compensate for some deficiency, and so can be thought of as being in the same class of devices as prosthetics and orthotics. However, it should also be acknowledged that naming equipment as an assistive technology is a rather arbitrary process. Our everyday life is filled with technologies which are required to assist us with our modern style of living. Whether we think of these technologies as mainstream technologies, or as assistive technologies that make up for some acquired deficits, is largely a matter of choice. For example, we probably wouldn't consider a room light as an assistive technology, yet its purpose is to compensate for our poor night vision. A telephone compensates for our inability to communicate over long distances. A refrigerator compensates for our intolerance of decaying food. Winter clothes could be considered an assistive technology to compensate for our lack of fur. We normally define assistive technologies as those extra technologies over and above what "normal" or "average" or "healthy" people require, but such definitions of people are themselves arbitrary and discriminatory.

In this chapter, we will talk about assistive technologies for independent living as those technologies which support people to stay in their homes, who would otherwise need to move to institutional care. We think particularly of the elderly, who are managing chronic health conditions, including physical and cognitive impairment. We are looking specifically at new assistive technologies based on ubiquitous computing technologies. We'll refer to these as Ubicomp-AT (Ubiquitous computing for Assistive Technologies). We are not looking here at purely mechanical devices such as walking frames or mobility scooters.

To motivate our Ubicomp-AT discussions, we will first present one typical scenario for use of these technologies.

Mary: An Assistive Technology Scenario

Mary suffers from several chronic conditions which limit her balance, mobility and physical strength. These conditions also put her at risk from a fall in her home. She is also managing a heart condition. She could benefit in the following ways from Ubicomp-AT.

Firstly, a medical alert pendant will allow her to call for help if she falls, and is conscious. The pendant has a voice communications capability, so she can talk to a call centre without needing to get to the phone. The pendant is waterproof, so she can wear it in the shower, one of the places she is most likely to fall. The pendant also provides her with the ability to call for help if she feels that her personal safety is at risk.

Her bed has an occupancy sensor, which triggers a call centre alarm in the case of unusual behaviour, such as a prolonged bed absence during the night, or a prolonged occupancy during the day.

Mary has a recommended daily activity plan. A pedometer integrated with the pendant is able to track her mobility and recommend more activity.

An entry-phone system in Mary's apartment complex, with terminals in the lounge, bedroom and kitchen, allows Mary to more easily deal with visitors. The system includes a remote lock for her front door, which she can operate while seated.

Mary likes to cook, but finds shopping difficult. The local supermarket provides an on-line and telephone shopping service, including a delivery service. Groceries are delivered via a service pantry, which has a door external to the apartment which can be unlocked with a one-time code. The service pantry has separate pantry, refrigerator and freezer sections.

A robot vacuum cleaner helps with cleaning, and also includes a camera. In response to an alarm, the robot can be guided by the call centre to investigate the alarm (Jardón, Gonzáles, Stoelen, Martinez, & Balaguer, 2009).

Smoke alarms automatically switch off appliances such as heaters, stoves and irons.

In order to monitor her heart condition, as well as her general health, Mary has physiological monitoring equipment in her apartment. Each day she measures her weight, temperature, blood pressure, pulse, and oxygen saturation. Records are monitored regularly by her care-givers, including automatic triggering of alarm conditions for readings outside acceptable bounds.

Within a moderate set of bounds, the monitoring system may recommend small changes in medication doses or timing. An automated medication dispensing system ensures that the correct medication is provided at the correct intervals.

Video conferencing facilities, accessed through a television, allow Mary to talk to her community carer every week, reducing her regular face-to-face visits to monthly. Her carer has access to her current medication history and current medications.

Mary also uses the video-conferencing facility to (remotely) have dinner with her daughter's family who live interstate, and she also has a weekly book club that meets on-line.

The Ubicomp-AT services for Mary's house are coordinated by a health-authority service centre. The service centre also manages Mary's medical records. These include her medical history, case notes from her GP, her community care worker, her medications, and her daily physiological readings. Her medical records also record a number of response plans for some possible incidents. For example, in the case of a minor fall where the call centre has made contact with Mary and established that there is not a need for hospitalisation, a community care nurse may be sent to provide care for Mary in her home for the next day or two, avoiding an expensive paramedic visit and hospital admission.

If an after-hours consultation is required, the after-hours GP is provided with a full copy of Mary's medical history, and current medications directly to their laptop.

The automated medication dispensing system monitors medication use, and can initiate procedures to restock or reorder medication.

Each month, Mary's GP reviews her records, and sends a message by email or telephone if she thinks Mary needs a consultation.

With the help of her Ubicomp-AT, Mary has not had any hospital admissions in the past year.

CLASSIFYING ASSISTIVE TECHNOLOGIES

How Can We Catalogue the Range of Available Ubicomp-AT?

There are many different taxonomies which could be developed. We could develop a taxonomy based on the technical characteristics of the technology, such as which other systems it connects to, what information it accesses, and its human-computer interface modalities. We could develop taxonomies based on devices' functional characteristics – whether they are sensors (input information in some form from the environment), actuators (produce effects into the environment), storage devices (record and access information from system storage), transformers (change information in one form to another form) or controllers (use sensed and stored information to command actuators), and we could then define Ubicomp-AT systems, based on the devices they use.

In the chapter, we will instead present a rather informal taxonomy based on human-oriented capabilities and affordances. In other words, we will look, from a resident's point of view, at what capabilities are enhanced by the particular Ubicomp-AT systems.

Assisting with Mobility Issues

Reduced mobility makes it harder to reach typical fixed-location devices and controls in a house such as lighting, telephones and entry doors. Reduced mobility also makes it harder to undertake activities outside the house, such as shopping, visiting friends and family, and medical appointments.

Ubicomp-AT can assist with mobility issues in two ways. Inside the house, smart wiring and control can make it easier to control lighting, curtains, and appliances. Room occupancy sensors can provide default lighting conditions based on time of day and who is present in a room. Similar control for air conditioning can appropriately direct heating and cooling in a house based on patterns of activity, rather than on active control (Helal, Mokhtari, & Abdulrazack, 2009). Active lighting is especially useful for situations where a resident wakes at night, say for a bathroom visit. These activities have a high risk of a fall in the infirm elderly. Here, active lighting can be switched on to provide a clear path to and from the bedroom. Entry-phone systems can reduce the need to walk to the door to answer a caller. Personal communicators, perhaps linked to an alarm pendant, can reduce the need to find a fixed or even mobile handset to answer a call.Domestic robotics potentially has much to offer in this area, although currently available products are rather meagre (Jardón et al., 2009).

Outside the house, telecommunications can replace some travel needs. Grocery shopping can be conducted over the Internet, although appropriate delivery systems have not advanced with the purchasing technology. The availability of delivery systems with appropriately accessible external pantry systems is still some years off (Hsu et al., 2006). The Smart Fridge can take advantage of RFID tags on foods which include use-by date information to suggest items for weekly shopping (Park, Won, Lee, & Kim, 2003). In terms of medical appointments, the combination of home physiological monitoring equipment, plus videoconferencing can reduce the number of visits to a GP or specialist, replacing those with video consultations.

Cognitive Problems

Even moderate failures in memory and situational awareness abilities can be problematic in maintaining independence (Greiner, Snowdon, & Schmitt, 1996). Often these patients have complex medication needs, in addition to other problems. Ubicomp-AT systems can help with situation awareness, such as providing date, time and calendar information which is easily accessible, replacing a wall calendar. These can be linked with automated medication assistance, perhaps providing information about what medications need to be taken when, or even automatically dispensing medication, and checking the medication has been taken. Wandering is a problem with some patients with cognitive impairment. Entry sensors, perhaps keyed to alarm pendants or similar devices, can monitor patient location and trigger alarms if absences are unexpected and extended (Wherton & Monk, 2008). Sensors for smoke, heat, gas or flooding can help with taps or stoves that have been turned on and forgotten about (Grossi, Matrella, De Munrai, & Ciampolini, 2007).

Medical Conditions

Community care nurses will continue to be needed to assist patients in their homes. However, current workforce predictions show a large increase in the number of patients likely to need such care, without a corresponding increase in the available workforce (Armstrong, Gillespie, Leeder, Rubin, & Russell, 2007).

The use of home physiological monitoring will allow more regular measurements to be taken, and better use to be made of visiting nurses (Rialle, Duchene, Noury, Bajolle, & Demongeot, 2002). Nurses can be scheduled to visit earlier in the case of emerging problems, such as post-operative infections, fluid retention, or similar. Patients who are monitoring their own conditions can adjust their activities to deal with their immediate conditions, such as delaying excursions if measurements indicate temporary high blood pressure or low blood oxygenation.

Home-based medical care suggests the notion of an Electronic Community of Care, which is enabled by ICT (Soar & Seo, 2007). This is based around appropriate and accurate access to relevant information about a patient's condition and management plan by carers. It also enables appropriate communications between all those involved in the care, including the patient. Issues such as hospital discharge reports, electronic referrals, remote patient monitoring, and electronic medical records are all part of this community of care. There are still many issues to be addressed with such a system, especially in the areas of data security and privacy, data location and ownership, data formatting, data quality and workforce training.

Social Issues

Loneliness and depression are major issues in the aged, especially those living alone (Mirowsky & Ross, 1992). Relatives and friends also worry about those living alone, often feeling guilt at their inability to provide greater levels of personal attention. Ubicomp-AT has significant potential to assist in these social issues.

For the family of an elderly relative living alone, they wish to know that the person is "OK", that is, not in need of emergency assistance from them. Home-based monitoring equipment can provide information about resident's apparent health. If a resident can be located within a house, then movement about the house can be monitored to indicate the resident's state of health. Lack of movement from a fixed position could be an indicator of a potential problem. Monitoring of the operation of devices such a kettle, opening of a refrigerator door, flushing of a toilet, changing of a television channel may all be indicators of activity. Lack of such indicators can trigger alarms which, as a first step in a care protocol, might simply seek to establish communications with the resident.

For housebound residents, Ubicomp-AT can assist with maintaining social networks. Many residents enjoy visits from community care nurses, and the social contact can be as important as the medical care. Technologies such as video conferencing can replace some of the need for carers (or residents) to travel, while still maintaining some level of social contact. On-line social groups (e.g. book clubs, bridge clubs) meeting via videoconferencing or similar may reduce loneliness and social isolation, and can also provide an informal support and monitoring network (Wright, 2000).

In information linked communities, Ubicomp-AT can also assist with informal organisation of social activities. For example, within a community of co-located acquaintances, one could send a query such as "Does anybody want to go for a walk to the park between 3 and 4pm this afternoon?"

Social networking systems (Facebook, Twitter) also have potential to reduce social isolation.

Personal safety is often a concern of the elderly living alone (Jones, 1987). Their fear of crime is often disproportionate to their risk. Devices such as personal emergency alarms have been demonstrated to provide benefits in reducing the effect of both medical emergency and personal safety and crime issues (Hyer & Rudick, 1994). Entry-phone systems provide residents with the ability to more safely screen visitors (Bowes & McColgan, 2006).

OBSTACLES OF UBICOMP AND AT

Having briefly described the issues and challenges in modern ubiquitous computing, and having also briefly explained the potential of such technologies to impact assistive technologies, this section now aims to identify problems which need to be solved to enable more widespread adoption of these technologies.

Available Technologies

The availability of Ubicomp-AT devices is not a problem. Smart house wiring and control systems, which allow computer control of lighting, entry doors, etc., are readily available. Sensors such as room occupancy sensors, bed and chair sensors, gas detectors, flood detectors, heat detectors and smoke detectors are all available. Home-based physiological monitoring devices are also readily available. Home-based videoconferencing, especially via systems such as Skype, is convenient and inexpensive. Medical alert systems, with appropriate call-centre response systems are available.

Some of the above systems (such as Smart House wiring and control systems) are relatively expensive and difficult to retrofit to existing housing stock. However, this is more an artefact of relatively small market size, the perceived "luxury" market for such systems, and the fragmented nature of the current market. There do not appear to be any significant technical reasons why widespread deployment of such technologies for support of independent living needs to be unreasonably expensive.

Available Systems

Whilst devices and technologies are readily available, integrated systems for Ubicomp-AT are not. Components such as telecommunications, smart house wiring and control, physiological monitoring, medical alert systems, and community-based nursing services are all relatively discrete market segments, with only limited understanding of how to build holistic Ubicomp-AT solutions (Chan, Estève, Escriba & Campo, 2008).

It is relatively easy to describe some scenarios, as outlined in the previous section, and to explain potential benefits. It is relatively easy to find the available devices and technologies which could implement such scenarios. It is much harder to implement the social and commercial systems that allow such scenarios to be successful. Each new Ubicomp-AT deployment needs to be largely designed from scratch, and many of the system issues still need to be better understood before meaningful systems can be implemented. Some of these issues are discussed below.

Open Standards

A key issue in the adoption of new technologies is the issue of open versus proprietary standards. Vendor-based standards protect a particular vendor's investment in technology development, and can lead to useful innovation. Vendors protect their IP, in order to maintain a market share, and to "lock-in" customers to their system. Prices often remain high, and market sizes are often limited.

Open standards allow systems to be built from many different vendors' products, promote competition and often lead to lower prices and wider adoption of technologies. They also encourage innovation and experimentation (Chesbrough, Vanhaverbecke, & West, 2006).

Many Ubicomp-AT devices and systems fall into the proprietary standards camp, and are expensive and incompatible with other systems components. Smart House wiring systems, with the exception of the hobbyist-level X.10 standard, are largely proprietary and closed standards. Programming such systems is difficult, and more general interfacing to computer-based Smart House control is problematic.

Available home physiological monitoring devices similarly tend to be closed standards, with proprietary back-end software and systems for collection, storage and analysis of data.

It is argued here that open-standards interfaces to Ubicomp-AT devices would significantly enhance the ability of systems designers to provide low-cost, well-integrated systems. Open-standards do not preclude the use of parallel proprietary standards. They simply require that devices provide a gateway that speaks an open-standards protocol in addition to any of their own communications methods.

Software Support for Community Care

Health care in general is a field which has long struggled to make effective use of Information Technology. Despite decades of work, universal electronic health records have yet to be effectively deployed in Australia, and in many other countries. As a result, health care systems are often poorly coordinated, and patient care is compromised.

Effective community health care would benefit from integrated patient information systems, which allow on-line review of a patient's treatment and condition, and coordination of services between care providers, including with informal carers (Soar & Seo, 2007). Such a system also encourages integrated care plans to be developed between all the carers involved with a patient, including GPs, after-hours GPs, specialists, community nurses, allied health professionals, pharmacists, medical-alert call centre staff, paramedics, and hospital staff, as well as family and friends.

Such integrated management plans, or models of care, need to drive the specification and implementation of their supporting software systems. Development of such software systems is seen as a critical step in providing effective Ubicomp-AT support.

Privacy and Security

Any universal computer-based medical records system obviously requires strict controls on privacy and security of that information, while allowing such information to be effectively used. The same principles apply to many aspects of Ubicomp-AT. Many home automation systems have had sensing and control information restricted to an internal home network. Without external network access, security is relatively easy to maintain by appropriate restrictions on physical access to the home and the internal network. Home monitoring systems which connect directly via a telephone modem to an external database are also relatively easy to secure.

However, external networking of Ubicomp-AT systems is key to providing much of the enhanced functionality described above. As soon as sensors, actuators and data are networked, the problems of privacy and security become critical. Security and privacy issues have inhibited the widespread networking of Ubicomp-AT systems. A more thorough investigation of the security and privacy needs of such systems, plus research into how such privacy and security can be effectively provided at an economical cost, is needed.

User Interfaces and Programming

Many of us have difficulty managing relatively simple ICT devices in our homes. There is a very apparent grey divide between generations in their use of information-based technologies. Bosman &

Charness (1996) describe links between reduced dexterity and motor skills and difficulty with seniors using interface devices such as keyboards and mice. Rogers & Frisk (1991) noted that elderly technology users find it more difficulty to learn new processes and procedures, and are more affected by distracting clutter. Kaufmann et al. (2003) find that these and other similar factors can reduce the ability of seniors to make best use of ICT-based technologies in the home, and proposes that any such assistive technologies need to undergo rigorous usability testing with their intended audience. In addition, such systems must address the attitudes of elderly users towards assistive technology, which is often to delay use until it is necessary and not merely convenient (Mynatt, Melenhorst, Fisk, & Rogers, 2004).

The task of managing a Smart Home by a patient with mobility, sensory or cognitive impairment presents many potential problems. By the same token, good user interface design can aid the problems of managing a household, managing one's health and maintaining social networks. User-interface modalities such as speech and gesture interfaces have substantial potential. Appropriate, intuitive and efficient user-interface design for Ubicomp-AT, especially for those with mobility, sensory and cognitive impairment, is another area that would benefit from additional research.

Who Pays?

Providing infirm elderly patients with the option of living independently in their own home, supported by appropriate models of care has many advantages. It provides enhanced quality of life for patients who do not wish to be in institutional care. It can provide improved health outcomes by improving the management of chronic conditions, reducing unexpected hospital admissions, allowing earlier discharges from hospital, and delaying entry to longer-term institutional care (Bowes & McGolgan, 2006).

Appropriate models of care supported by Ubicomp-AT should be able to provide enhanced health outcomes at a reduced cost, especially in terms of staffing costs. Projected shortfalls in future health workforce levels mean that the efficient use of staff time needs to be maximised.

A major issue with assistive technologies at present is who pays for the technology, and the systems which use that technology. Should it be governments who pay for the costs of public hospital care and who have a more general mandate to improve quality of life for their constituents? Should it be private health insurers who will see a reduction in hospital costs? Should it be the consumer who sees a benefit in quality of life?

So far, none of these groups have been sufficiently convinced of the efficacy of Ubicomp-AT to heavily invest in the technology in Australia.

Technology Trials

There is still much work to do before Ubicomp-AT becomes widespread in the community. Having identified the obstacles to its current adoption, what is needed to overcome these? I'd suggest that there are two areas to be addressed.

Firstly, some larger trials of the technology in an Australian setting are needed to establish the efficacy of new models of care, based on Ubicomp-AT. These need to be rigorously conducted, with quantitative output measures, just like any other clinical trial of new treatment regimes. These trials need to evaluate both the health outcomes, and the financial cost/benefits of these technologies. Such trials can be conducted with existing technologies as a starting point, even if current systems are not ideal. However, the trials cannot be simply technology demonstrators: They need to be sufficiently large in sample size and duration to draw meaningful conclusions. The trials will also highlight practical shortcomings of existing systems and technologies. Such trials are now being undertaken in overseas contexts, and shown useful results (Bowes & McColgan, 2006; "SO-

PRANO", 2009). However, these results need to be replicated in an Australian context to identify potential benefits as well as potential obstacles to adoption in this specific national health-care context.

The second requirement is to undertake research and development into the technical and structural problems with current Ubicomp-AT. As described above, security and privacy, open standards, human-computer interfaces and new models of care-driving software specifications are all areas that require significant research input. One would expect that large-scale trials will unearth additional areas for research.

CONCLUSION

Ubiquitous computing is an area of significant commercial and research interest at the moment. Ubicomp-AT has great potential in supporting the infirm elderly and others managing complex health issues, to live independently in their own homes. While these technologies have great promise, their adoption level is low in Australia. The elderly are traditionally late adopters of new technology, and yet they are amongst those who could benefit most from ubiquitous computing. Ways are needed to overcome this grey divide in ICT-based assistive technologies.

This chapter has suggested that two concurrent strategies are needed to improve the penetration of Ubicomp-AT in the community. Firstly, significant trials are needed to determine to what extent such systems can provide improved health outcomes and reduce health system costs for suitably targeted patients. Secondly, research in security and privacy, open standards, human-computer interfaces and new models of care driving software specifications is needed to determine whether observable health system benefits can be achieved at a reasonable cost, and with adequate consideration of the needs of clients and carers.

REFERENCES

Armstrong, B. K., Gillespie, J. A., Leeder, S. R., Rubin, G. L., & Russell, L. M. (2007). Challenges in health and health care for Australia. *The Medical Journal of Australia, 187*(9), 485–489.

Bergstrom, P., Driscoll, K., & Kimball, J. (2001). Making home automation communications secure. *IEEE Computer, 34*(10), 50–56.

Bosman, E. A., & Charness, N. (1996). Age-related differences in skilled performance and skill acquisition. In Blanchard-Fields, S., & Hess, T. (Eds.), *Perspectives on cognition in adulthood and aging*. New York: McGraw-Hill.

Bowes, A., & McColgan, G. (2006). *Smart technology and community care for older people: innovation in West Lothian, Scotland*. Edinburgh, UK: Age Concern Scotland.

Chan, M., Estève, D., Escriba, C., & Campo, E. (2008). A review of smart homes - present state and future challenges. *Computer Methods and Programs in Biomedicine, 91*(1), 55–81. doi:10.1016/j.cmpb.2008.02.001

Chesbrough, H., Vanhaverbeke, W., & West, J. (Eds.). (2006). *Open innovation: Researching a new paradigm*. Oxford, UK: Oxford University Press.

Committee on Networked Systems of Embedded Computers, National Research Council. (2001). *Embedded, Everywhere: A research agenda for networked systems of embedded computers*. Washington, DC, USA: National Academy of Sciences.

Greiner, P. A., Snowdon, D. A., & Schmitt, F. A. (1996). The loss of independence in activities of daily living: the role of low normal cognitive function in elderly nuns. *American Journal of Public Health, 86*, 62–66.

Grossi, F., Matrella, G., De Munrai, I., & Ciampolini, P. (2007). A flexible home automation system applied to elderly care. *International Conference on Consumer Electronics,* 1-2.

Helal, A., Mokhtari, M., & Abdulrazak, B. (2009). *The engineering handbook on smart technology for aging, disability and independence*. Hoboken, NJ: John Wiley & Sons.

Hsu, C. F., Liao, H. Y. M., Hsiu, P. C., Lin, Y. S., Shin, C. S., Kuo, T. W., & Liu, W. S. (2006). Smart pantries for homes. *IEEE International Conference on Systems, Man and Cybernetics* (pp. 4276-4283).

Hyer, K., & Rudick, L. (1994). The effectiveness of personal emergency response systems in meeting the safety monitoring needs of home care clients. *The Journal of Nursing Administration*, *24*(6), 39–43. doi:10.1097/00005110-199406000-00010

Jardón, A., González, J. C., Stoelen, M., Martínez, S., & Balaguer, C. (2009). ASIBOT Assistive robot in a domestic environment. In *Proceedings of the 2nd ACM International Conference on Pervasive Technologies Related to Assistive Environments.* New York: ACM.

Jones, G. M. (1987). Elderly people and domestic crime: Reflections on ageism, sexism, victimology. *The British Journal of Criminology*, *27*(2), 191–201.

Jurjens, J. (2007). Developing secure embedded systems: pitfalls and how to avoid them. *29th International Conference on Software Engineering - ICSE 2007* (pp. 182-183).

Kaufman, D. R., Patel, V. L., Hilliman, C., Morin, P. C., Pevzner, J., & Weinstock, R. S. (2003). Usability in the real world: Assessing medical information technologies in patients' homes. *Journal of Biomedical Informatics*, *36*(1-2), 45–60. doi:10.1016/S1532-0464(03)00056-X

Koch, S. (2006). Home telehealth - current state and future trends. *International Journal of Medical Informatics*, *75*(8), 565–576. doi:10.1016/j.ijmedinf.2005.09.002

Mirowsky, J., & Ross, C. E. (1992). Age and depression. *Journal of Health and Social Behavior*, *33*(3), 187–205. doi:10.2307/2137349

Mynatt, E. D., Melenhorst, A.-S., Fisk, A.-D., & Rogers, W. A. (2004). Aware technologies for aging in place: understanding user needs and attitudes. *IEEE Pervasive Computing / IEEE Computer Society [and] IEEE Communications Society*, *3*(2), 36–41. doi:10.1109/MPRV.2004.1316816

Park, S. H., Won, S. H., Lee, J. B., & Kim, S. W. (2003). Smart home-digitally engineered domestic life. *Personal and Ubiquitous Computing*, *7*(3–4), 189–196. doi:10.1007/s00779-003-0228-9

Rialle, V., Duchene, F., Noury, N., Bajolle, L., & Demongeot, J. (2002). Health "smart" home: Information technology for patients at home. *Telemedicine Journal and e-Health*, *8*(4), 395–409. doi:10.1089/15305620260507530

Rogers, W. A., & Fisk, A. D. (1991). Age-related differences in the maintenance and modification of automatic processes: arithmetic stroop interference. *Human Factors*, *33*, 45–56.

Sangiovanni-Vincentelli, A., & Di Natale, M. (2007). Embedded system design for automotive applications. *IEEE Computer*, *40*(10), 42–51.

Sears, A., & Jacko, J. A. (Eds) (2007). *The Human-Computer Interaction handbook: Fundamentals, evolving technologies and emerging applications* (2nd ed.). New York: CRC Press.

Soar, J., & Seo, Y. (2007). Health and aged care enabled by information technology. *Third international conference on healthy ageing and longevity. Annals of the New York Academy of Sciences*, *1114*, 154–161. doi:10.1196/annals.1396.040

SOPRANO. (2009). *Service-oriented Programmable Smart Environments for Older Europeans*. Retrieved August 31, 2009 from http://www.soprano-ip.org

Vaa, T., Penttinen, M., & Spyropoulou, I. (2007). Intelligent transport systems and effects on road traffic accidents: State of the art. *IET Intelligent Transport Systems*, *1*(2), 81–88. doi:10.1049/iet-its:20060081

Weiser, M. (1991). The computer for the twenty-first century. *Scientific American*, (September): 94–100. doi:10.1038/scientificamerican0991-94

Wherton, J. P., & Monk, A. F. (2008). Technological opportunities for supporting people with dementia who are living at home. *International Journal of Human-Computer Studies*, *66*(8), 571–586. doi:10.1016/j.ijhcs.2008.03.001

Wright, K. (2000). Computer-mediated social support, older adults, and coping. *The Journal of Communication*, *50*, 100–118. doi:10.1111/j.1460-2466.2000.tb02855.x

Zurawski, R. (Ed.). (2006). *Embedded systems handbook*. Boca Raton: Taylor & Francis.

ADDITIONAL READING

AAL. (2009). The Ambient Assisted Living (AAL) Joint Programme. Retrieved August 31, 2009, from: http://www.aal-europe.eu/

European Commission and the Economic Policy Committee. (2009). *The 2009 Ageing Report: Economic and budgetary projections for the EU-27 Member States (2008-2060)*. Retrieved August 31, 2009, from http://ec.europa.eu/economy_finance/publications/publication_summary14911_en.htm

Van den Broek, G., Cavallo, F., Odetti, L., & Wehrmann, C. (2009). *Ambient Assisted Living Roadmap*. Retrieved September 8, 2009, from http://www.aaliance.eu/public/documents/aaliance-roadmap/aaliance-roadmap-document-august-2009.pdf

Wolf, W. (2007). Special issue on Embedded Systems, *IEEE Computer, 40*(10).

KEY TERMS AND DEFINITIONS

Assistive Technologies: Devices and systems (including software systems) which assist those with physical and cognitive impairments to compensate for those impairments.

Embedded Systems: Computer based appliances and systems where the computer is an integrated part of the device.

Information Security: The ability to restrict access to information systems to authorised users, and to ensure that information in a system has not been accessed or tampered with by third parties.

Open Standards: Specifications for devices and systems which are freely available, rather than being held privately by a particular vendor.

Privacy: The ability for individuals to restrict access to private information, and to control the use and access to information provided to others.

Smart Home: A home equipped with ICT-based assistive technologies.

Ubiquitous Computing: The trend for computers to be located throughout the environment. Also known as computers everywhere, communications everywhere, and information everywhere.

Chapter 2
Ageing, Chronic Disease, Technology, and Smart Homes:
An Australian Perspective

Jeffrey Soar
University of Southern Queensland, Australia

ABSTRACT

This chapter explores ageing, chronic disease, technology and social change. Healthcare has been transformed through medical technology but there is much still to be done to enable seamless exchanges between all carers, which is expected to improve safety, quality and efficiency. There is massive potential for technology to transform the experience of ageing including assisting with the management of chronic disease, coordinated care and guided self-care for consumers. Innovative technologies are increasingly available to assist in maintaining health and independent living. This includes telecare, telehealth, assistive technologies, robots and smart homes. A challenge is in providing access to and support in the use of technologies where there are clear benefits to consumers, carers, providers and funders of healthcare. The chapter also reports on the Queensland Smart Home Initiative which is one of several organisations internationally that share a mission of assisting people to be supported through these technologies.

INTRODUCTION

An aspect of the grey digital divide is the difference between the support that older people currently receive and the potential that technology has for enabling independent living and better access to care. That there are opportunities for the support that smart homes and assistive technology can provide is evident in the rates of events such as falls, medication difficulties and social isolation. Technology can help to maintain social connections, provide access to information for self-care, enhance access to professional services, and it can also help to ensure people are safe, receiving needed support and participating in activities of daily living.

Over the subsequent sections of this chapter we will explore technology and social change, healthcare technology, ageing, chronic illness and disability, coordinated care and self-management,

DOI: 10.4018/978-1-61520-825-8.ch002

guided self-care, ageing and technology, robots, adoption issues, smart homes and the experiences of the QSHI (Queensland Smart Home Initiative).

Technology has the potential to transform ageing, aged care and healthcare just as it has other industries. Technology is highlighted in the healthcare reform agendas of Australian and other governments. It has the potential to overcome the digital divide and provide the elderly with better access to support arrangements, information, care and other services; technology can also reduce travel of patients and carers across often vast distances and sometimes just for routine checks which could be provided more safely and conveniently through telecare and telehealth systems. There is increasing interest and attention given to the unprecedented ageing of populations which has captured the attention of the public and policy-makers. The phenomenon of ageing is discussed along with associated issues of increasing chronic illness and disability. Recent strategy around chronic illness self-management is explored along with the needs to ensure the availability of quality, relevant and timely sources of consumer health information.

The technology itself is developing at a dramatic rate and there are prototype robots that are expected to be our carers of the future. The robot may be a mechanical device or it may take the form of software that interacts through other devices, or it may be a combination of both. Given how pervasive robots are in automobile production and other manufacture it is reasonable to expect they will be available in people's homes. There are smart homes as demonstrators in many countries and some of these are discussed. An exciting development has been the large-scale deployment of some of this technology into people's homes in some countries and localities.

The QSHI is discussed as one of a number of industry-government research consortia around the world that promotes the adoption of smart home and assistive technology. The QSHI does this through research evaluating the benefits of technology for consumers, families, carers, provider organisations, funders and governments.

TECHNOLOGY AND SOCIAL CHANGE

There are many aspects to the grey digital divide that will be explored in this paper. These include a lower level of use of ICT (Information and Communication Technologies) by older people (Madden & Savage, 2000), the unequal availability of ICT across sectors of healthcare and aged care, the need for ICT infrastructure and applications for home and community care, the need for technology to assist with chronic illness and the need to help consumers and carers with access to information.

That our lives have been and continue to be transformed by technology is a given. It has liberated people from drudgery and has been the key to social transformation over millennia. Where modern technology is applied, there are many-fold increases in productivity, higher quality, greater convenience, lower costs and lower prices. Technology usually results in a range of changes including simplification of work processes and disintermediation as whole steps in the production process are eliminated; it also provides for both greater standardisation and individual customisation.

There are endless examples of this including banking, e-commerce. e-procurement and supply-chain management, freight and shipping, hotels and airline bookings. Subject to Internet access and payment of fees, students from around the world have access to some of the best universities. Through on-line learning systems lecturers can provide a rich educational experience to ten or more times as many students as they might have in a physical class-room. Learning is shifting from instructor-centered to learner-centered, and is undertaken anywhere, from classrooms to homes and offices. E-Learning, referring to learning via the Internet, provides people with a flexible and personalised way to learn. It offers learning-on-demand opportunities and reduces learning cost (Zhang & Nunamaker, 2004, 204). Students can interact on-line with instructors and other students, review on-line lectures and use interactive learning tools. Many of the world's knowledge repositories are freely accessible, and in most cases the lowest prices for goods and services are available through the Internet. People on the wrong side of the digital divide and without access to the Internet miss out on the convenience and the ready access to current information; in most cases they will pay more for purchases.

This change is not without conflict going back as far as the Industrial Revolution which transformed society from an agricultural base to the beginnings of a modern capitalist society. In more recent years technology has transformed shipping and stevedoring with massive reductions in labour demand and huge increases in productivity (Duras, 2007). The introduction of automation in newspaper production in the mid-1980s saw the protracted strikes around the world. Newspaper production changed forever with the introduction of electronic processes and the abolition of a range of trades and skills.

Transformation of business and commerce through technology is a continual process. This has been accelerated since the advent of information and communication technology (Friedman, 2005). Industries have been transformed or lost and new ones created and many industries are now totally dependent upon new information technologies.

HEALTHCARE TECHNOLOGY

Healthcare technology is linked to our better health and longevity. Lives can now be saved that would previously have been lost and people are enabled to lead fulfilling lives through life-critical technologies such as cardiac pacemakers, renal dialysis and new medications. The healthcare industry is generally not as good at using technology for sharing patient information between provider organisations. In many cases a person's health history is likely to be spread across the computer systems or filing cabinets of all the providers they have received services from including primary care practitioners, retail pharmacies, hospitals, and diagnostic laboratories. In only very few countries are there centralised repositories of patient information.

Healthcare consumers still have little access to or control over their own information (Eysenbach & Jadad, 2001). Few health professionals exchange emails with their consumers or allow consumers to access their computer systems in the way, for example, that airline passengers can access their airline flight bookings, personal profiles and preferences, or travel histories.

In many countries there are now strategies aimed at providing electronic personal health records, electronic referrals between care providers, better linking of clinical practice systems with research evidence databases, and decision-support tools to assist busy clinicians. Healthcare around the world has shared a common agenda for reform for several decades (Giaimo, 2002). This includes moving from an episodic focus to a more holistic approach; from fragmentation to better coordinated care; moving from end-stage intervention focus to more prevention; from an acute care focus to more public health and primary care, and from provider-driven care to a more consumer focus.

Enabling access to hospital patient records may be some time away. The author is involved in a research project in Australia which aims to link professional carers in community settings, particularly General Practice physicians and community aged-care providers, with hospital records for sharing of patient data. Achieving this is not without challenge. The project will be a first in this region in sharing data electronically between primary and secondary providers. Currently, a common practice of hospitals in Australia is to use fax machines to send patient data to community-based providers; however to have this information sent electronically raises issues of processes, security, confidentiality and control. If it is a challenge for professional carers to access their patients' data held by other providers, then it is likely to be even more of a challenge to enable consumer access.

The majority of the investment in health ICT (Information and Communication Technology) in Australia has been in hospital-based applications, and there is still little technology infrastructure for managing patient information between carers outside of hospital settings as well as between carers across hospitals. That may change with the report of the National Health and Hospitals Reform Commission (2009). This is likely to require providers to better facilitate access to patient data by other providers and by patients themselves.

AGEING

The future sustainability of public funding for social and health services is a major policy concern for many counties as it is clear that the need for publicly provided services will increase with the ageing of the populations and the shrinking of the work force (Marin, Leichsenring, Rodrigues & Huber, 2009, 5). The ageing of Australia's population, already evident in the current age structure, is expected to increase rapidly. This is the result of sustained low levels of fertility combined with increasing life expectancy at birth. The age composition of Australia's population is projected to change considerably as a result of population ageing. By 2056 there will be a greater proportion of people aged 65 years and a lower proportion of people under the age of 15 years. In 2007 people aged 65 years and over made up 13% of Australia's population. This proportion is projected to increase to between 23% and 25% in 2056 and to between 25% and 28% in 2101 (ABS, 2009). There are similar demographic changes and predicted increases in the percentages of the elderly in the populations of most countries (Cohen, 2003; Kinsella & Velkoff, 2001).

The prevalence of chronic illness and disability usually increases with age. About one-quarter (23%) of all people aged 65 years and over in Australia have a profound or severe core activity limitation, and chronic illnesses such as dementia, hypertension, asthma and diabetes are common conditions (AIHW, 2006a). However, Rice and Fineman (2004) found the prevalence of disability among the elderly in the USA is declining, and expenditures for their care are increasingly concentrated at the end of life rather than during extra years of relatively healthy life. The same relative decline in disability could well occur in Australia, which has a similar standard of living to the USA. Nevertheless, health care costs will undoubtedly increase during the next 30 years, if only as a result of the large numbers of Babyboomers entering late life.

At any time older people occupy more than half of the hospital beds in Australia and have a longer average length of stay than younger patients (AIHW, 2008a). The media, as in many other countries, carries frequent reports of healthcare systems that are struggling to cope with an ageing population. Whether these are occasional slip-ups in otherwise reasonably well-functioning systems or whether they reflect profoundly dysfunctional systems is debatable. Regardless, health systems are under pressure and ageing is yet to fully impact on these systems. The Australian Government's Intergenerational Report indicates that much of the pressure in the growth of healthcare costs is due to medications and medical technologies (Australian Government Treasury, 2007). The first of the Babyboomers are now moving into their mid 60s and this is likely to herald the beginning of an upward spiral in demand for healthcare services.

In many countries governments have recently renewed their interest in healthcare reform. A notable example of this is several attempts which have been made to introduce reforms to the health system in the USA. In Australia the 2009 National Health and Hospitals Reform Commission report advocated for greater prevention, individual responsibility, e-health and use of technology (NHHRC, 2009). Prior to that report the Australian Health Ministers' Council (AHMC, 2005) had already developed a national strategic policy approach to chronic disease prevention and care. This approach included the National Chronic Disease Strategy and supporting National Service Improvement Frameworks, which cover the national health priority areas of asthma, cancer, diabetes, heart, stroke and vascular disease, osteoarthritis, rheumatoid arthritis and osteoporosis.

The current ageing population and increasing incidence of long term conditions presents the health sector with a major challenge because many older people, who may be living with more than one long term condition, often have both clinical and social problems. Caring for these people consumes a large proportion of health and social care resources. Better coordination in community settings aided by technology can be expected to improve the effectiveness and safety of care for the frail aged population in particular, and for people generally who need support (Bowes & McColgan, 2005). The spectre of a "tsunami" of ageing Babyboomers is likely to compel governments and other healthcare funders to more fully explore the potential of assistive technology for independent living and home-care.

CHRONIC ILLNESS AND DISABILITY

The digital divide will also impact on how chronic illness sufferers and their carers are equipped to best manage their conditions. Associated with increasing life-expectancy is an increase in the incidence of chronic disease. Chronic illnesses such as asthma, dementia and coronary heart disease are the leading causes of disability and mortality (Australian Institute of Health and Welfare, 2008). Chronic diseases disproportionately affect older adults and are associated with disability, diminished quality of life, and increased costs for health care and long-term care. In the USA about 80% of older adults have at least one chronic condition, and 50% have at least two (CDC, 2009). These conditions can cause years of pain, loss of function and lead to depression. More than fifteen million Australians are directly affected by at least one chronic disease (Australian Institute of Health and Welfare, 2006). One third of problems presented in primary care general practice are chronic in nature (ACT GP Taskforce, 2009). Older people commonly present to hospitals with multiple, complex conditions. It may also be the case that some elderly people are admitted to hospital because adequate facilities for their care are not available in the community (Siggins Miller, 2003).

Gains in life expectancy have been accompanied by an increase in expected years of life lived with disability, including severe or profound limitations. People who identify as having a disability account for almost 20 per cent of the Australian population (ABS, 2004). Today on average, people can expect to live with a disability for almost 20 years (AIHW, 2006b, 210). This will rise as the percentage of older people in the population increases resulting in increasing demands for support (AIHW, 2008b).

The unprecedented increase in dementia around the world is of particular concern for the quality of life of individuals and their families as well as the associated surge in demands for support and care. More than 35 million people worldwide will have dementia in 2010 (ADI, 2009, 2). This is a 10% increase over previous global dementia prevalence reported in 2005 (Ferri et al, 2005). The ADI report predicts that dementia prevalence will nearly double every 20 years, to 65.7 million in 2030 and 115.4 million in 2050.

If chronic conditions are not managed effectively in primary and community care, they can progress to produce acute care episodes with impacts and cost implications. Poorly managed chronic illness can progress to severe episodes resulting in premature death or permanent disability. There has been growing interest over several decades in CDM (Chronic Disease Management) (National Health Priority Action Council, 2006), and more recent attention to patient self-management (Australian Department of Health and Ageing, 2008). The interest is associated with expectations of the likelihood of benefits including better partnerships between patients, their carers and clinicians in the management of their conditions, better guidance for patients to ensure the right information is provided at the right time and place to guide self-management, clinical outcomes including a slowing of the advance of chronic conditions, earlier and more timely interventions with clinical and economic benefits, reduction in unplanned hospital attendances and admissions and reductions in health expenditure on patients with chronic illness (Soar & Wang, 2009). Indications are that successful self-management is dependent on the engagement of health care professionals, particularly General Practitioners (Jordan & Osbourne, 2007). Assistive technology can greatly improve the independence and quality of life for people with a disability and/or chronic disease through enhancing self-care. It can provide quality and relevant information at the point of care and help reduce or reverse the progression of disease.

COORDINATED CARE AND SELF-MANAGEMENT

A further aspect of the digital divide is the difference in availability of technology support and integrated information management between sectors of care. Hospitals have long been the focus of much of the investment in healthcare ICT. The health sector historically has had an episodic approach and an acute care focus and has been not been well structured to provide coordinated care in community settings. Coordination of care is difficult in countries such as Australia with fragmentation of funding and payment systems, a mix of public and private funding and care provision, and a complexity of reporting lines and accountability (Dwyer & Eager, 2008, 5). Consequently care providers are rarely financially rewarded nor equipped to provide coordinated care.

There are increasing pressures on home care services as governments explore strategies to provide more healthcare for the aged and chronic ill in their homes (CSCI, 2006). Home care is generally presumed to be a less costly alternative to institutional care and is usually preferred by patients.

Disease-specific associations and programmes such as for asthma, diabetes, stroke and many others provide information and other services for sufferers of chronic disease. CDM programmes are also provided by community health services, Divisions of General Practice and others to better manage conditions and slow the progress of disease. There is however no common approach to providing this information and it is often provider rather than consumer-driven. Social marketing is also used by health departments to encourage behaviour change and current media programmes address diabetes, obesity, alcohol abuse, smoking and gastric reflux. Some evidence suggests that patients with effective self-management skills make better use of health care professionals' time and have enhanced self-care (Jordan and Osborne, 2007).

The concept of self-management and its practice is changing (Kralik, Koch, Price and Howard, 2004; Newman, Steed & Mulligan, 2004; NIH, 2000). The availability of health information on the Internet is an indication of the interest people have in independently searching for information to help them understand and cope with their health conditions. A more proactive self-management role is being promoted rather than a health care provider giving instructions and hoping the patient will adhere to them. The UK has introduced the Expert Patients Program that recognises this change (NHS, 2007). The Expert Patients Programme is a lay-led self-management programme that has been specifically developed for people living with long-term conditions. The aim of the programme is to support people to increase their confidence, improve their quality of life and better manage their condition.

GUIDED SELF-CARE

A grey digital divide also exists between the elderly who have good access to technology and are skilled in its use, and those people without either the access or skills. In 2009, 44% of Australians over the age of 65 had never used the Internet (ACMA, 2009). By contrast, many Babyboomers routinely use the Internet and as this technology-savvy group moves through retirement the disparity between elderly Internet users and non users should drop sharply. Self-management has been an expectation for individuals with a chronic disease for much of the past century although the dominant model of care is one where the clinician, particularly the physician, provides advice for patients to follow. Community-based associations for many of the chronic illnesses assist patients in accessing quality information for self-care. There are also CDM programmes provided by community health providers, General Practice and others to better manage conditions and to slow the progress of disease.

For some time it has been recognised that people living with a long term illness develop expertise and wisdom about their condition and want to play a part in making decisions about their own health care (Wilson, 1999). There is encouragement or perhaps recognition that care often involves partnerships between individual patients and healthcare professionals and between consumer disease organisations and the healthcare system. The latter can be effective at influencing government policy development and resource allocation. A successful use of consumer health information has been the social marketing used by health departments to encourage behaviour change through media campaigns addressing smoking, obesity, alcohol abuse and gastric reflux.

The World Health Organisation's framework for innovative care of chronic diseases identifies self-management support as part of the building blocks for effective health care organisations (World Health Organisation, 2002). Self-management needs to be guided to be most effective and to guard against patients being mis-informed or influenced by the poor quality information that is also available through the Internet. Successful self-management is related to the engagement of health care professionals (Jordan and Osborne, 2007). Technology offers the means to link consumers, family carers and professional carers, to provide timely access to quality information and to enhance the patient-clinician partnership (Coye, Haselkorn & DeMello, 2009).

Telecare may involve consumer health information. It can be simply passive involving the use of devices that collect data for professional carers to view or alternatively it may help people to better manage their own conditions through providing information back to consumers. In the latter case consumers will require telecare services to provide them with quality information in addition to feedback from the devices involved. Telehealth links can be between patients and their clinicians or between clinicians such as between a remote or general practice clinician and a specialist for advice. This can provide guidance and quality information to assist consumers and enhance the partnership between the consumer and healthcare professionals. The technology can be of particular value for isolated communities (Weinert, 2008).

An essential component for addressing this aspect of the grey digital divide that has not as yet been provided for is in developing a model for the information that patients need and a model for capturing, managing and transmitting quality and timely information. Most self-management support has been for specific conditions although many people, particularly as they age, suffer from multiple co-morbidities. Many of the technology developers have focused on the technology itself and there is an ever more sophisticated range of products can be found through an Internet search for Assistive Technology.

AGEING AND TECHNOLOGY

Assistive technology (AT) can be defined as 'any item, piece of equipment, product or system that is used to increase, maintain or improve the functional capabilities of individuals and independence of people with cognitive, physical or communication difficulties' (UK Audit Commission 2004). AT aims to increase the ability of a person to remain independent, reduce risk and maintain engagement in meaningful activities, and includes a wide range of products from simple, low tech and low cost to very technologically complex.

Technology is expected to offer significant potential for equipping societies to respond to pressures of ageing populations. Provided that successful efforts are made to bridge many aspects of the digital divide which were addressed earlier, technology will assist aged people in extending active and independent lives, maintaining productivity and in delivering care in home and community settings. Globally there is an increasing level of activities, strategy development, research projects, and adoptions of telecare, telehealth, smart homes and assistive technologies by consumers and care provider organisations (Soar, 2008). Several of these are discussed in different chapters of this book.

The application of these technologies has an array of added benefits including a reduction in the level of incidence of adverse events, providing support and new service interventions for conditions amongst the elderly such as chronic illness, falls, dementia, medication problems, wandering and social isolation (Horner, Soar & Koch, 2009).

There is recognition of the potential for technology to enhance the safety and independence of frail older people, enable access to quality care services and to extend their ability to remain in their own homes. Intelligent monitors can keep a continuous watch on older people's vital signs, activity patterns and their safety and security (Soar & Croll, 2007). Technology can monitor indicators of their state of health, provide alerts to events such as falls, and give early warnings of potential problems. The technology can detect changes in activities and alert a carer. Monitoring devices can be more accurate guides to the health risks such as a heart attack than are the patient's symptoms, providing advance warnings and reducing unnecessary emergency callouts. Home automation can enhance security, safety and independence at home. This helps to maintain quality of life and decrease the demand for carer support hours. Communication technologies provide important benefits for people whose mobility is limited, or who live alone.

Richards (2006) was commissioned by the Scottish Executive Development Department to review housing for older people. The review reported that AT projects in Scotland were considered to be helping people to continue living in their own homes, and that users had become accustomed to the technology and appreciated the benefits it afforded them. Some older people had fears about whether the technology might go wrong and that carers and relatives would be bothered in that event. Some people also had concerns about the pace of technological change leading to rapid obsolescence and issues with upgrading. Bowes and McColgan (2003) found that a control group without the technology were more likely to have received increasing hours of home care, been admitted to care homes or hospitals, or visited their GP more frequently than those using the assistive technology care package.

The largest known study of the benefits of home telehealth implementation was undertaken amongst clients of the Veterans' Health Administration in the USA (Darkins et al., 2008). This involved 17,025 home telecare and telehealth installations. The results included a 19% reduction in numbers of hospital admissions and a 25% reduction in numbers of hospital bed days. Clients reported a high level of satisfaction with the telecare/telehealth service with a satisfaction score of 86%.

Technology can also assist in directing people to the most appropriate form and place for care delivery, which is not always admission to hospital. The author is involved in a project to evaluate the benefits of integration of patient information in community settings including reductions in hospital admissions. An Internet search using the term "hospital avoidance" reveals a number of pilots and projects with similar aims around most Australian health jurisdictions as well as in other countries.

Technology has the potential to extend older persons' physical independence and thus enable them to remain living in their own homes for longer. This has the dual benefit of affording individuals a more dignified life while potentially leading to savings of public and private money. In geographically diverse countries like Australia, technology has great potential for bringing services into communities as well as to individuals. There are reports of reductions in health service use associated with the availability of home telecare (Barlow, Singh, Bayer & Curry, 2007). In circumstances when patients do present, the emergency department staff may be more confident of them returning to their technology equipped homes.

ROBOTS

Robots have for many years performed much of the work in manufacturing, have made some inroads into medicine and particularly surgery, but have yet to impact home and aged care. There is a report of a robot to assist stroke victims with limb movement (Cox, 2005). Work is underway to build a humanoid robot personal assistant or carer, and developments in this field suggest that a robot assistant in homes may not be far off. The robot may be a mechanical device or it may take the form of software that interacts through other devices, or it may be a combination of both. Some robotic devices are already available to provide support for a range of basic activities, including eating, bathing, dressing, and toileting (Forlizzi, DiSalvo & Gemperle, 2004); and evidence suggests that available robotic pets provide pleasure and interest to people with dementia (Filan & Llewellyn-Jones, 2006).

There is work on a humanoid robot assistant and even a robot dog carer. In France, the Alcatel-Lucent research laboratory enhanced a robot dog to become a personal carer (Alcatel-Lucent, 2008). The dog has a camera, microphone and wireless connection. It can provide reminders and alerts and through pattern recognition it will know its owner and can continuously monitor his/her safety and well-being. If, for example, a carer was unable to contact an older person, the dog could be contacted and could search for its owner. The carer could see though the dog's camera "eyes". The dog was originally designed as a robot companion for children in hospital and particularly for those in isolation rooms. The robot dog would provide a companion to an isolated child patient as well as a multimedia terminal complete with camera, microphone, loudspeaker, gaming and links the child could use to clinicians, friends and family. The potential for similar use in care of older people is obvious.

Given the pace of automation in industries such as vehicle production or newspaper printing it is reasonable to expect that robots will play a role in healthcare in the future, both in home and institutional settings. This is likely to include robots as personal home carers.

ADOPTION ISSUES

High levels of assistive technology abandonment are well documented (Wessels, 2003). Approaches to reduce abandonment include processes for the selection of assistive technology that involve the end-user, access to expert advice, making the right choice and social factors. The latter includes whether the device might stigmatise the user and remind them of their disability.

If assistive technologies are to meet their intended purposes with older users they must be user friendly (Livingstone, Soar & Wang, 2009). Technology is often developed by young people who may not always be aware of age-related difficulties that afflict many older people, for example fading eye-sight or poor dexterity. If the intended users cannot easily see or operate the devices, they will not persevere with these. At the person-to-person interface older people are not always treated with respect and as partners in their own care. Indications are that if older people are involved in decisions such as selection of assistive technologies then there is a higher rate of successful adoption.

SMART HOMES

Terms such as 'intelligent home', 'smart home', 'digital home' and 'connected home' describe the convergence of a range of technologies and their increased use (Essen & Conrick, 2007). There has also been increasing use of intelligent controls engineered into modern buildings (Horner, Soar and Koch, 2009). Examples include smoke detectors linked to the building fire sprinkler systems and elevators that are remotely monitored. CCTV (Closed Circuit Television) for security is now ubiquitous in commercial and public places. In Queensland, Australia the Department of Health has begun installing intelligent controls with remote monitoring for some of its hospitals. These control, for example, hot water systems that can monitor use and then reduce energy-consumption according to demand. Knowing the periods of peak demand allows advance scheduling of the boilers. These kinds of controls applied to heating, lighting, air-conditioning and other services can learn patterns of use and reduce energy consumption at quiet times and build up in preparation to periods of peak demand.

QUEENSLAND SMART HOME INITIATIVE

The interest internationally in the promotion of ambient living and wellness models of health care through the utilisation of Smart Homes particularly for the frail elderly is shared in Australia. In 2006 a consortium of stakeholders, the Queensland Smart Home Initiative (QSHI), was established with the aim of investigating new models of care delivery based on supporting independent living, improving quality of life and enabling new models of home care particularly for the frail elderly, chronically ill, and people with disabilities (see http://www.qshi.org.au/) The QSHI aims to enhance the national and regional capacity for research and development, commercialisation and adoption of assistive technologies. The focus is, through research, to encourage the wide-scale adoption of assistive technologies where there are demonstrable social, clinical, environmental and economic benefits. The QSHI aims to demonstrate those benefits through the quality of its research.

The first phase of the project involved building the research consortium based upon a shared high-level vision of the potential ICT and assistive technologies for care in home and community settings. The selection of organisations for invitation to participate in the QSHI was based upon whether an organisation was considered to share a common interest in the field as well as on its capacity to contribute a unique perspective. Selection of organisations was also based upon an assessment of complementary skills and interests, and avoidance of duplication. Organisations that committed to support the initiative included a department of health, the home and community care funder, a major aged and community care provider, a home care technology supplier, a smart home environment supplier, an association of owners and operators of aged and community care facilities, an aged care consumer organisation, a multi-national manufacturer of ICT componentary, a telecommunications company and universities with researcher expertise in this or related fields.

The QSHI established its first Smart Home in an aged care campus in Brisbane, Australia in 2007. The objective was to demonstrate working technologies in a live environment. It also aimed to increase awareness, provide an educational resource and gather feedback from stakeholders. The site had around 250 visitors over 12 months and people visiting the Smart Home were invited to share their impressions. Each visit was hosted and the technology presented and explained (Soar, Livingstone & Wang, 2009).

Subsequently a study was undertaken to distil the vision, research needs, priorities and expectations of the participant organisation representatives. The aim was to arrive at a collective vision on the potential of the Smart Home project and the development of prioritised research programs. The methodology involved individual consultations and focus groups with managers and senior executives of each of the participating organisations. Semi-structured interviews covered vision, expectations, desired outputs, desired projects, anticipated benefits and other impacts. This was followed by a facilitated focus group workshop. Thematic analysis of the data assisted with analysis and further interpretation. The results highlighted the different perspectives and expectations of participants (Soar & Croll, 2007). Government agencies were concerned with managing demand for services, improving access, and enhancing independence of consumers. Care provider organisations were particularly interested in technology to assist in workforce issues. These include making aged-care a more desirable place of work, providing staff with efficiency and productivity tools, and improved work-force satisfaction and retention. Some functions that are labour-intensive could be aided or eliminated by technology. These include monitoring or taking vital signs. There was an expectation that technology offered particular potential for consumers in rural and remote locations where access was restricted by the vast distances in Australia. Technology providers were interested in knowing more about the barriers to adoption and in seeing quality research evidence that would inform policy development and resource deployment.

Privacy, security and trust in systems were consistent themes. As the consumers included vulnerable groups it was seen as important that systems could be trusted, were aged appropriate and as transparent as possible to the users.

The QSHI has now completed its first phase involving a smart home demonstrator unit. It has recently commenced a "connected-community for care" project that is supported by the Australian Research Council and industry partners. The project will examine the effect on hospital attendances, admissions and length of stay following better sharing of information in community settings. The QSHI second phase will involve a large-scale roll-out of assistive technologies into the homes of people needing support. These people will be supported by software intelligent agents to assist with reminders, access to information and decision-making. Links to a Call Centre will ensure an operator is always available when needed. The project is informed by the small but increasing number of roll-outs of assistive technologies around the world. Also as part of the QSHI second stage, a modern facsimile demonstrator home has been set up close to the city centre to allow easy drop-in access by the general public, six days a week. It is expected that the demonstrator will result in considerably greater understanding and acceptance of some of the relatively inexpensive, assistive technologies that can effectively increase the independence of frail elderly people.

CONCLUSION

This paper has covered a wide range of issues including demographic trends, the increasing prevalence of chronic disease and associated changes in demands for health care and support services. Technology has been reviewed for its capacity to improve support for frail elderly, chronic illness sufferers and people with disabilities. This includes the potential benefits for consumers, carers and the professional workforce. Further research will be required to provide models for adoption and to provide research evidence to support a shift in resourcing more towards prevention and community care supported by innovative technology. Assistive technology will play a major role in promoting new health and wellness models; it can accelerate the international healthcare reform agenda.

Finally the Queensland Smart Home Initiative was reported on as one of several consortia around the world aiming to contribute to the national and international agendas for quality care and independent living through assistive technologies.

REFERENCES

ABS. 2005). Use of information technology by older people. In *1301.0 - Year Book Australia*, 2005. Canberra: Australian Bureau of Statistics.

ABS. (2008). *3222.0 - Population projections, Australia, 2006 to 2101*. Canberra: Australian Bureau of Statistics.

ACMA. (2009). *Australia in the digital economy: Report 2 Online participation*. Australia Communications and Media Authority Retrieved October, 3, 2009, from http://www.acma.gov.au/WEB/STANDARD/pc=PC_311655

ADI. (2009). World Alzheimers report 2009. *Alzheimers Disease International*. Retrieved September 2009 from www.alz.co.uk

AHMC. (2005). *National chronic disease strategy*. Conference communiqué. Australian Health Ministers Council, 18 November 2005.

AIHW. (2006a). *Chronic disease and associated risk factors in Australia*. Canberra: Australian Institute of Health and Welfare.

AIHW. (2006b). *Australia's health 2006*. Canberra: Australian Institute of Health and Welfare.

AIHW. (2008a). *Australia's health 2008*. Canberra: Australian Institute of Health and Welfare.

AIHW. (2008b). *Disability in Australia: Trends in prevalence, education, employment and community living*. Canberra: Australian Institute of Health and Welfare.

Alcatel-Lucent. (2008). *Corporate social responsibility report 2008*. Paris: Alcatel-Lucent.

Australian Government Treasury. (2007). *Intergenerational Report 2007*. Canberra: Commonwealth of Australia.

Barlow, J., Singh, D., Bayer, S., & Curry, R. (2007). A systematic review of the benefits of home telecare for frail elderly people and those with long-term conditions. *Journal of Telemedicine and Telecare*, *13*, 172–179. doi:10.1258/135763307780908058

Bowes, A. M., & McColgan, G. M. (2003). *Evaluation of home comforts: Smart home technologies initiative*. Final report to South Ayrshire Council. Cited in Tribal - Francesca Richards, Gill Walker, Lorelei Jarvis (2006). Time to Move? A Literature Review of Housing for Older People. Scottish Executive Social Research 2006.

Bowes, A. M., & McColgan, G. M. (2005). *West Lothian interim report*. West Lothian Council and the Department of Applied Social Science, University of Stirling.

CDC. (2009). *Healthy aging: Improving and extending quality of life among older Americans*. Atlanta, GA, USA: Centers for Disease Control.

Cohen, J. E. (2003). Human population: The next half century. *Science, 302*(5648), 1172–1175. doi:10.1126/science.1088665

Cox, W. (2005). *Robot jacket to help stroke victims*. Retrieved October, 10, 2009 from http://www.gorobotics.net/the-news/latest-news/robot-jacket-to-help-stroke-victims/

Coye, M. J., Haselkorn, A., & DeMello, S. (2009). Remote patient management: technology-enabled innovation and evolving business models for chronic disease care. *Health Affairs, 28*(1), 126–135. doi:10.1377/hlthaff.28.1.126

CSCI. (2006). *Time to care? An overview of home care services for older people in England.* Report published by Commission for Social Care Inspection, London, www.csci.org.uk, October 2006.

Darkins, A., Ryan, P., Kobb, R., Foster, L., Edmonson, E., Wakefield, B., & Lancaster, A. E. (2008). Care coordination / Home telehealth: The systematic implementation of health informatics, home telehealth, and disease management to support the care of veteran patients with chronic conditions. *Telemedicine and e-Health* (10), 1118-1126.

Duras, T. (2007). Raging against the machine: Unions and technological change in Australia 1978-1996. In *Proceedings - Labour Traditions: The 10th National Labour History Conference*, 4-6, July 2007, University of Melbourne.

Dwyer, J., & Eager, K. (2008). *Options for reform of Commonwealth and State governance responsibilities for the Australian health system.* A paper commissioned by the National Health and Hospitals Reform Commission.

Essen, A., & Conrick, M. (2007). Visions and realities: Developing 'smart' homes for seniors in Sweden, *eJHI - electronic Journal of Health Informatics, 2*(1), e2.

Eysenbach, G., & Jadad, J. R. (2001). Evidence-based patient choice and consumer health informatics in the Internet age. *Journal of Medical Internet Research, 3*(2), e19. doi:10.2196/jmir.3.2.e19

Ferri, C. P., Prince, M., Brayne, C., Brodaty, H., Fratiglioni, L., & Ganguli, M. (2005). Global. prevalence of dementia: a Delphi consensus study. *Lancet, 366*(9503), 2112–2117. doi:10.1016/S0140-6736(05)67889-0

Filan, S. I., & Llewellyn-Jones, R. H. (2006). Animal-assisted therapy for dementia: a review of the literature. *International Psychogeriatrics, 18*(4), 597–611. doi:10.1017/S1041610206003322

Forlizzi, J., DiSalvo, C., & Gemperle, F. (2004). Assistive robotics and an ecology of elders living independently in their homes. *Human-Computer Interaction, 19*, 25–59. doi:10.1207/s15327051hci1901&2_3

Friedman, T. L. (2008). *The world is flat: A brief history of the twenty-first century.* New York: Farrar, Strauss and Giroux.

Giaimo, S. (2002). *Markets and medicine: The politics of health care reform in Britain, Germany, and the United States.* Michigan: University of Michigan Press.

Horner, B., Soar, J., & Koch, B. (2009). Assistive technology: Opportunities and implications, srontic nursing body of knowledge. In Nay, R., & Garratt, S. (Eds.), *Older People: Issues and Innovations in Care* (3rd ed.). Sydney: Elsevier.

Jordan, J., & Osbourne, R. (2007). Chronic disease self-management education programs: challenges ahead. *MJA, 186*(2), 84–87.

Kinsella, K., & Velkoff, V. A. (2001). *An aging world: 2001 - International population reports. U.S. Department of Health and Human Services, National Institutes of Health, National Institute On Aging and U.S. Department of Commerce, Economics and Statistics Administration, U.* S. Census Bureau.

Kralik, D., Koch, T., Price, K., & Howard, N. (2004). Chronic illness self-management: taking action to create order. *Journal of Clinical Nursing, 13*(2), 259–267. doi:10.1046/j.1365-2702.2003.00826.x

Madden, G., & Savage, S. (2000). Some economic and social aspects of residential Internet use in Australia. *Journal of Media Economics, 13*(3), 171–185. doi:10.1207/S15327736ME1303_2

Marin, B., Leichsenring, K., Rodrigues, R., & Huber, M. (2009). *Who cares? Care coordination and cooperation to enhance quality in elderly care in the European Union.* European Centre for Social Welfare Policy and Research, Affiliated to the United Nations, Vienna, 24 August 2009.

Miller, S. (2003). *Unnecessary and avoidable hospital admissions for older people - A report to the Department of Health and Ageing.* Canberra: COAWG.

National Health Priority Action Council. (2006). *National chronic disease strategy.* Canberra: Australian Government Department of Health and Ageing.

Newman, S., Steed, L., & Mulligan, K. (2004). Self-management interventions for chronic illness. *Lancet, 364*(9444), 1523–1537. doi:10.1016/S0140-6736(04)17277-2

NHHRC. (2009). *A healthier future for all Australians: Final report June 2009.* Australia: National Health and Hospitals Reform Commission.

NHS. (2007). *The expert patients programme.* UK: Department of Health, Chief Medical Officer, National Health Service.

NIH. (2000). *Self- management strategies across chronic* diseases. Bethesda, Maryland, USQ: National Institute of Health.

Rice, D., & Fineman, N. (2004). Economic implications of increased longevity in the United States. *Annual Review of Public Health, 25*, 457–473. doi:10.1146/annurev.publhealth.25.101802.123054

Richards, T.F., Walker, G., & Jarvis. L. (2006). Time to move? A literature review of housing for older people. *Scottish Executive Social Research.* UK Audit Commission (2004). Older people: Assistive technology: Independence and well-being No. 4.

Soar, J. (2008). *Information management in modern healthcare organisations.* Proceedings IBIMA, 4-6 January 2008, Marrakesh, Morocco

Soar, J., & Croll, P. (2007). Assistive technologies for the frail elderly, chronic illness sufferers and people with disabilities: A case study of the development of a Smart Home. In Toleman, Cater-Steel & Roberts (Eds.), *ACIS 2007: Proceedings of the 18th Australasian Conference on Information Systems*, University of Southern Queensland, Queensland

Soar, J., Livingstone, A., & Wang, S. Y. (2009). A case study of an ambient living and wellness management health care model in Australia. In M. Mokhtari, I. Khalil, J. Bauchet, D. Zhang & C. Nuget (Eds.) *Ambient Assistive Health and Wellness Management in the Heart of the City*, Refereed Proceedings of the 7th International Conference On Smart Homes and Health Telematics (ICOST2009) 1-3 July, 2009–Tours, France, Springer.

Soar, J., & Wang, S. Y. (2009). Information for guided chronic disease self-management in community settings. In Sintchenko, V., & Croll, P. (Eds.), *Frontiers of Health Informatics – Redefining Healthcare, HIC 2009 Proceedings.* Health Informatics Society of Australia.

Taskforce, A. C. T. G. P. (2009). *Issues and challenges for general practice and primary health care*. A Discussion Paper, Canberra, June 2009.

Weinert, C., Cudney, S., & Hill, W. G. (2008). Rural women, technology, and self-management of chronic illness. *Canadian Journal of Nursing Research*, *40*(3), 114–134.

Wessels, R., Dijcks, B., Soede, M., Gelderblom, G. J., & De Witte, L. (2003)... *Technology and Disability*, *15*(4), 231–238.

WHO. (2002). *Innovative care for chronic conditions: building blocks for action: Global report*. Geneva: World Health Organisation.

Wilson, J. (1999). Acknowledging the expertise of patients and their organisations. *BMJ (Clinical Research Ed.)*, *319*(7212), 771–774.

Zhang, D., & Nunamaker, J. (2004). Powering e-learning in the new millennium: An overview of e-learning and enabling technology. *Information Systems Frontiers*, *5*(2), 207–218. doi:10.1023/A:1022609809036

Chapter 3
A User-Driven Approach to Developing Ambient Assisted Living Systems for Older People:
The SOPRANO Project

Andrew Sixsmith
Simon Fraser University, Canada

Sonja Mueller
empirica Gesellschaft fur Kommunikations und Technologieforschung, Germany

Felicitas Lull
empirica Gesellschaft fur Kommunikations und Technologieforschung, Germany

Michael Klein
CAS Software AG, Germany

Ilse Bierhoff
Smart Homes, The Netherlands

Sarah Delaney
Work Research Centre, Ireland

Paula Byrne
University of Liverpool, UK

Sandra Sproll
University Stuttgart, Germany

Robert Savage
Simon Fraser University, Canada

Elena Avatangelou
Exodus, SA, Greece

ABSTRACT

This chapter describes some of the results of the EU-funded SOPRANO project to develop an Ambient Assisted Living system to promote active ageing and ageing-in-place. The chapter outlines SOPRANO's experience and application research approach to ensure that end-users are involved in all stages of the research and development. A number of key areas for application development were identified and developed as a set of use cases (or descriptive models), for example for medication reminding, and to support exercise. These use cases were further refined through visualization and iterative prototyping techniques with end-users to ensure usability, usefulness and acceptability for users. The SOPRANO prototype system is described together with future plans for deployment in demonstration sites and field trials.

DOI: 10.4018/978-1-61520-825-8.ch003

INTRODUCTION

The challenge of an ageing population requires innovative approaches to meet the needs of increasing numbers of older people within society (Sixsmith & Sixsmith, 2008). In particular there is a need to move from a health and social agenda that emphasizes dependency to one that promotes active ageing and creates supportive environments to enable healthy ageing in the settings where older people live. Emerging information and communication technologies (ICTs) such as "pervasive computing" and "ubiquitous computing" have considerable potential for enhancing the lives of many older people throughout the world and helping them to "age-in-place" (Sixsmith & Sixsmith, 2008). Ambient Assistive Living (AAL) refers to information and communication technology (ICT) systems, products and services that integrate sensors, actuators, smart interfaces, artificial intelligence and communications networks to provide supportive environments for frail and disabled older people (AALIANCE, 2009). AAL has been an important emerging area of research over recent years involving collaboration between domain experts (health sciences, rehabilitation, gerontology and social sciences etc.) and technical experts (engineering, computing science, robotics, etc). Research and development (R&D) within AAL has aimed to develop applications and systems to facilitate independence (AALIANCE, 2009) such as activity monitoring to detect potential emergencies; reminder devices for supporting and encouraging mobility and activities of daily living; monitoring activity patterns as indicators of change in cognitive and physical status; and smart interfaces to help people control their everyday environment. This chapter will review some of the initiatives in the area of AAL and will describe the user-driven approach adopted in the European Union (EU) funded SOPRANO project to ensure that technological development is usable, useful and acceptable in the everyday life context of older users. The chapter presents the results from initial requirements capture and prototype development and testing. The paper concludes by discussing the benefits of the user-driven approach and plans for system demonstration and large-scale field trials.

BACKGROUND

Initiatives and Challenges in AAL

The Ambient Assisted Living Joint Programme of the European Union (AAL Joint Programme, 2009), set up in June 2008 with support of 23 member states of the EU, has an overall objective to use ICTs to improve the quality of life of older people. The budget of AALJP is in the order of 55-60 million Euro per year (2008-2013) to fund the development of innovative ICT based solutions to extend the time older people can live independently at home, and at the same time to support European industries to develop competitive products and services.

Specific objectives are to:

- Allow people to "age-in-place" by increasing their autonomy, self-confidence and mobility.
- Support health and functional capability.
- Promote active and healthy lifestyles.
- Enhance security, prevent social isolation and maintain the support network of the individual.
- Increase the resource efficiency and effectiveness of health and social services.

AALJP is perhaps the most extensive systematic initiative worldwide in the area of AAL and represents a major commitment to, and belief in, the potential of using technology to support older people at home. There are also other major initiatives around the world (see, for example, Sixsmith, 2008) making AAL a significant emerging focus for research within engineering and computing science. However, despite its potential, the impact of the R&D has so far been limited in terms of bringing new products and services to the market, with a number of factors limiting exploitation. Indeed, there is still little hard evidence to suggest that AAL-based products and services have significant benefits for end-users or service providers (Sixsmith & Sixsmith, 2008; Martin 2008). A key problem is that much of the R&D effort has been technology-driven, focusing primarily on technical development and issues of usability, where applications are developed to address the so-called "problems" facing frail and disabled older people living at home. This technology-driven approach can miss the point of how technology may be, or may not be, impacting on the everyday lives of older people and how it could positively enhance their quality of life. Without a user-driven research approach that takes these issues seriously, there is a danger that ill-conceived technologies will at best be irrelevant or inappropriate, and at worst will reinforce some of the negative ageist assumptions that frame much of society's response to ageing.

SOPRANO (http://www.soprano-ip.org/) is a EU-funded project to develop an AAL system. SOPRANO (Service-oriented Programmable Smart Environments for Older Europeans) is a consortium of commercial companies, service providers and research institutes with over 20 partners from Greece, Germany, UK, Netherlands, Spain, Slovenia, Ireland and Canada. As well as technical issues, research and development within SOPRANO has dealt with a number of challenges, not least being how we should explore, visualize and map out this uncharted area in order to exploit this potential. Sixsmith (2008) outlined a number of key questions: What are the important directions for research and development? How can we ensure that older people benefit from these technologies? How can we ensure that some people are not excluded from accessing these technologies? What are the potential disadvantages and how can these be avoided? How can we improve the design and development process to ensure that new technologies are "user-driven"? A key question is therefore how the technical systems being designed in the SOPRANO project are embedded in the process of delivering new ICT-based services. Thus the SOPRANO system and its technical components should be explicitly conceived and designed as part of a "socio-technical" system that models both the human and machine domains within a single conceptual framework.

APPROACH AND METHODS

Against this background, SOPRANO has been highly innovative both in terms of its approach to the research and development process and in terms of the social and technical work being carried out. A major aim within the project has been to move away from technology-push and problem-focused approaches to user-driven approaches and efforts to explore, visualize and map out an AAL system that will have practical benefits for users in their everyday lives.

The Experience and Application Research (E&AR) design methodology adopted in SOPRANO involves research, development and design by, with and for users, involving users in all stages of a product development lifecycle, not just at the end phases. The methodology of SOPRANO is based upon the Human-Centered Design process (ISO 9241-210) and has taken the approach further. Human-Centered Design typically involves users for the specification of the context of use, the collection and analysis of user needs and requirements, and the assessment of prototypes. However, "experts" define functions, services and interactions with the device or system. In SOPRANO the idea of a user-driven approach involves older people and their carers directly in developing the conceptual design, and later, the prototypes. It is not the user who responds to the ideas of experts, rather the experts listen to the suggestions of older people and their carers and respond to their input (Figure 1.).

Figure 1. SOPRANO iterative approach to research and development

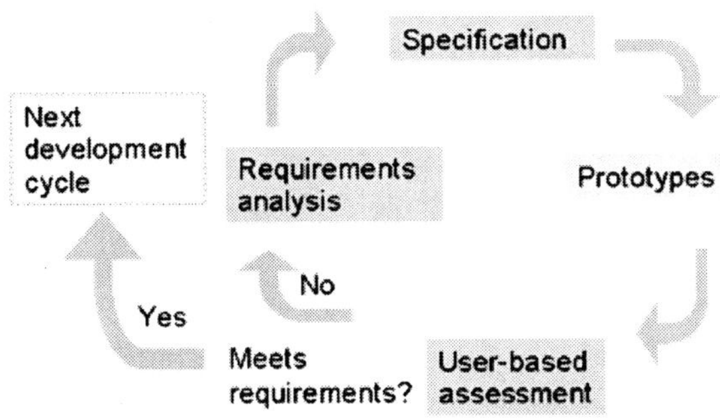

The SOPRANO R&D process can be subdivided in four stages of user involvement. The aim of the first phase was to understand and specify the context of use and to also specify user and organizational requirements. The gathered information was transformed into use cases, or descriptive models, of how an AAL-based service can interact with a user in relation to a particular problem scenario such as reminding a person about medication. In a second phase, use cases were transformed into multimedia demonstrators and dramatized scenarios to allow users to visualize, validate and develop the use cases to provide the basic high-level requirements for system development. In a third stage, system and component prototypes were tested with users in a laboratory context, focusing on user feedback to optimize usability. Finally a close-to-final prototype will be tested both in demonstration homes and in large-scale field trials in order to evaluate the system's impact in real-life situations.

The approach adopted throughout this cycle was primarily qualitative and ethnographic. The aim was to allow potential users to express their needs, concerns and goals in their own words and define their own agendas and ideas about SOPRANO and its potential benefits, problems, and improvements. Participant recruitment and the research sessions were facilitated by the user organizations within the SOPRANO consortium in Spain, UK, Germany and the Netherlands. Research sessions were carried out in informal and non-threatening settings and were subject to the ethical guidelines and procedures for each country. Sessions were audio or video recorded for subsequent analysis. User feedback has been analyzed and evaluated according to key criteria of acceptability, usefulness and usability.

Results

The methods and results of the user research in stages 1-3 are presented in this chapter: exploration of user requirements; use case development and refinement; and prototype development. Conclusions about key results, and the future direction of the project are presented in the concluding section of the chapter.

Exploration of User Requirements

Potential users provided input into SOPRANO in terms of the key challenges to their independence/ quality of life without specific reference to how technology could be used to cope with these challenges. The aim was to identify "opportunities" for introducing technological support, without being driven by a predefined technical agenda. A qualitative approach involved focus groups and individual interviews. Fourteen focus groups (with more than 90 users) were conducted with older people, informal carers and care professionals in the UK, The Netherlands, Spain and Germany. Individual interviews with older people took place in Germany, Spain and The Netherlands. Methods for sampling and recruitment were pool-based in Spain. In Germany, the UK and The Netherlands, snowball sampling was used, in which members of existing groups were asked whether they would like to participate. Semi-structured interview schedules were used in both the focus groups and the individual interviews. The interview schedule comprised an agenda to explore the key challenges that faced older people in living independently and the required supports that SOPRANO should offer to help them overcome these challenges. The metaphor of the 'Guardian Angel' was used during the interviews to allow researchers to discuss possible supports and solutions to challenges faced by older people without referring to technological concepts straightaway, and to allow for freedom in coming up with ideas. However, many of the participants were already familiar with assistive technology and able to imagine solutions based on existing technologies. This had benefits in that potential users could think of improvements or additions to existing technological solutions. However, this familiarity with existing solutions was a significant constraint in terms of generating new ideas. All interviews were transcribed in full and analyzed internally, across interviews and across countries. A thematic analysis approach was used, where recurring themes were identified and analyzed. However, exceptions and unexpected findings were also identified and discussed. A number of themes emerged from the user research (Mueller & Sixsmith, 2008):

- **Social isolation** can lead to loneliness, depression, boredom, social exclusion and disruption of patterns of daily living.
- **Safety and Security** includes falls, disorientation and getting lost, and control of potentially dangerous household equipment.
- **Forgetfulness** undermines independence, for example, taking medication, finding objects in the house and carrying out activities of daily living, especially for people with cognitive impairments.
- **Keeping healthy and active** involves physical and mental activity, exercise, good nutrition, daily routines and adherence to medications.
- **Community participation and contribution to local community** is an important component of the quality of life of some people.
- **Accessing information/keeping up to date** is an important issue, as well as finding help and tradesmen to do little jobs around the home.
- **Getting access to shops and services** can be a problem for people who have difficulty getting out of the house.
- **Quality of care provision** is important to ensure that the right amount and right quality of care is delivered to help people remain living at home.
- **Mobility** includes getting around inside the house and mobility in terms of walking in the neighborhood and use of public transport.

Ambient Assisted Living has a potential role in all these areas, and the results were used to drive the technological development in the next phase of the SOPRANO project.

Use Case Development and Refinement

Based on the results of the user research above, the next stage was to develop ideas for services to enable older people to stay in their own home as long as they wish, and to increase quality of life. This was done by considering features of technology seen as desirable by focus group participants and also by identifying aspects that were seen as less desirable, intrusive or unnecessary. SOPRANO use cases do not merely reflect the development of a technical system and components, but include a strong reference to the social world within which the person lives. The key to creating useful and acceptable technology-based services is to understand how they are embedded in a person's everyday life. The initial user research provided input into top-level system ideas in terms of a set of use cases (descriptive models) that describe in a straightforward way the interactions between users and the system itself. These use cases not only reflected functionalities of the prospective technical system, but also the processes, actions and interaction of components of the overall socio-technical system, i.e. the assisted person, informal and formal careers, and service providers within which SOPRANO is embedded. The following use cases were developed:

- **Medication Reminding** addressed how SOPRANO could help a person who keeps forgetting to take medicine. Medication reminding is one of the key challenges people face with old age, and medication reminders are one of the top concerns of care professionals.
- **Safety and Security.** Security issues were mentioned as crucial issues in all discussion settings. Different aspects and different sources of risk within the home environment are important here and support in this area is seen as very convenient and desirable. Use cases that were developed in this area:
  - **Open Door** addressed safety and security aspects of access into and out of the home.
  - **Safe** involved activity monitoring for signs of problems.
  - **Fall** focused on detection and response to falls at home.
  - **Easy-to-use Home Automation** demonstrated smart home components supporting independent living.
- **Exercise** focused on helping older people to follow rehabilitation programs after discharge from hospital. Exercise support has enormous potential in rehabilitation.
- **Active** aimed at monitoring and supporting healthy and active routines. Supporting good routines has enormous potential in alleviating associated problems such as insomnia at night or malnutrition.
- **Remembering** provided support for people with cognitive impairments. Forgetfulness is a key challenge to independence. Forgetfulness concerns finding objects in the house as well as forgetting appointments. Technological support in this area is very promising in relation to maintaining independence of older people.
- **In Touch** is aimed at combating social isolation. Social isolation and increasing loss of social contacts is a huge problem in relation to living independently and is often associated with physical limitations.
- **Entertained** focused on leisure and counteracting boredom. Boredom is related to social inclusion/exclusion since the potential for boredom generally correlates with social isolation.

A detailed description of each of these is not possible within this chapter, but to illustrate, a simplified "Remembering" use case is presented:

"Remembering" *focuses on people who experience increasing forgetfulness in daily life. The user research uncovered some specific challenges that occur commonly in particular situations during the daily routine, including leaving the house without closing the windows or terrace door, forgetting the house key or leaving applications (TV, lights etc.) running, and also forgetting important appointments. Depending on the scenario, a family member may live in the same household as the assisted person (AP).*

A SOPRANO in-home system along with the necessary peripherals (including a touch screen panel beside the front door and window sensors, power consumption sensors, RFID tags for keys etc., depending on the situation) is installed and operated by a care provider organization (CPO).

When the AP opens the front door to leave the house, SOPRANO checks the installed peripherals to determine if anything was forgotten (e.g. a window was left open). In that case, an alert message will be displayed on the touch screen informing the AP of the things that are not in order. The AP can either react to this alert by rectifying the situation (e.g. turning off the TV) or by defining certain conditions as "normal" (e.g. the open window). In both cases the alert will be cancelled for the present time. Using a doorbell sensor the system is also capable of distinguishing between the door being opened to let in a visitor (no alert will be raised) and the door being opened to leave the house.

Further to this, the AP or a family member living in the household can enter important appointments into the system via the user interface and the AP will be reminded of these appointments by SOPRANO.

Following this, user research was conducted to validate and refine the use cases. The idea in SOPRANO was that the technology developers should listen to and act on the input from end users. A challenge was to help potential users to provide design ideas and evaluate a system that did not yet exist. Considerable effort was put into creative methods that would ensure the effective involvement of users at the very early stages of prototype development, both in terms of design idea generation (eliciting ideas from end users) and design idea evaluation (refining design decisions from previous activity sessions). SOPRANO used two approaches for use case validation and refinement. Both were adaptations from a methodology known as Scenario Based Design for prototype testing (Rosson, Carroll, Seals, & Lewis 2002; Machate & Burmester, 2003). Here, two specific methods of user involvement were employed for both design idea generation and design idea evaluation, namely, multimedia demonstrators, and live dramatizations. The goal was to present the SOPRANO use cases to the potential end-users in order to help them 'visualize' the SOPRANO services and stimulate discussions for both idea evaluation and idea generation. The various use cases were transformed into a drama workshop or animated within a multimedia demonstrator, which were viewed interactively and discussed within small groups of users.

All use cases presented in the multimedia demonstrator were divided into two categories, those for idea evaluation purposes (Open Door, Remembering, Medication 1, Holiday, Entertained) and those for idea generation purposes (Medication 2, Fall, Exercise, Active, In Touch, Safe). In order to support the idea generation sessions, alternative solutions were developed for the respective use cases. The multimedia demonstrator was developed in the four languages (English, German, Dutch, Spanish) of the user session participants.

The demonstrator starts with a side-view presentation of a prototype SOPRANO house.

Figure 2 shows a screen shot of the multimedia demonstrator.

The multimedia demonstrator enabled the session moderator to use it in two modes: (a) in a scene-by-scene mode where there is a pause after each scene and the moderator needs to explicitly move on the next scene, thus enabling discussion among the session participants; and (b) in a video mode, where the specific scenario plays continuously until its end, thus being suitable for use during a demonstration, or an exhibition. A total of 72 potential users participated in

Figure 2. Screenshot of a multimedia demonstrator scene of use case: "Remembering", displaying messages when the user is leaving the house

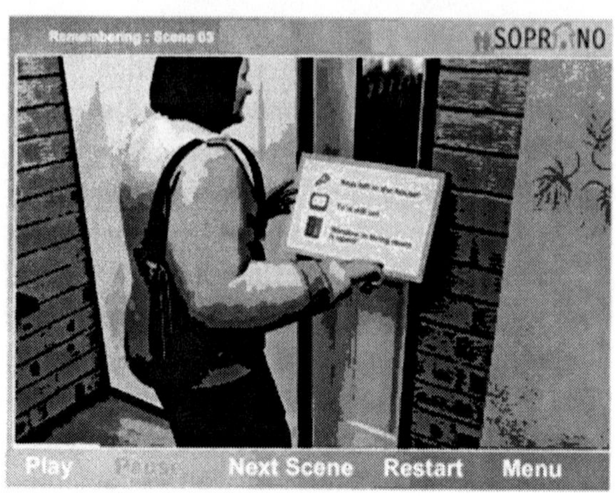

27 sessions conducted in the 4 different countries. Figure 3 shows how a multimedia demonstrator focus group in The Netherlands took place.

Theatre methods were applied with use cases 'Exercise' and 'In Touch' in Newham, London. Theatre methods are an innovative approach to supporting the process of design idea generation. These two use cases were selected because they provide the best examples of complexity, human interaction and human-technology interaction.

As a first step, both use cases were transformed into a script by a professional scriptwriter. This was necessary to help the theatre group prepare the session. During the session itself, the problem area was enacted by the theatre group, and a focused design discussion was conducted. Initial ideas generated by participants were noted on a flip chart as well as in audio and video recorded. The actors then played the design solution of the use case, and participants were invited to give feedback and compare the presented solution to the ideas they had come up with themselves. Ultimately, one specific design solution was agreed on for each use case.

The overall aim of the analysis of the sessions with users was twofold: On the one hand the objective was to elicit design ideas from end users and incorporate these ideas into the existing use cases. On the other hand, results from design idea evaluation sessions were analyzed in order to refine/detail user requirements in relation to functionality, modality, interaction sequences and input/output elements. All this has been accomplished by applying qualitative analysis methods supported by quantitative analysis of the questionnaire results (Mayring 2000; Padgett 2004; Barbour 1998).

Figure 3. Lively discussion with users on the presented scenario via the multimedia demonstrator

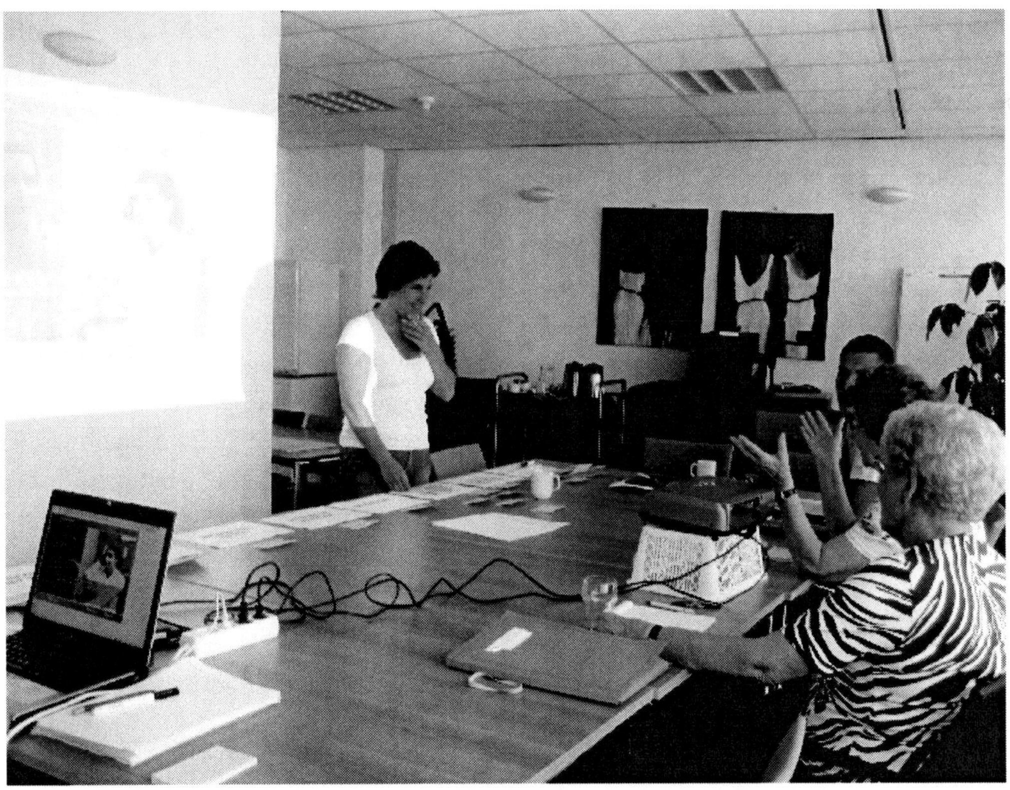

The multimedia demonstrators and theatre groups successfully revealed specific refinements to all the use cases in relation to functionality, interaction sequence and modality. Some general requirements also emerged, notably that the system must be easy to operate; the modality for reminding, informing and alerting must be configurable; user control over the system is essential; reminders/notifications should not interrupt activities such as TV watching; the system must take into account that users do not want to leave appliances on stand-by; information about what has been done (help is underway, appliances switched-off, a third person has been informed etc.) should be provided; and device location, such as touch screen, camera etc. is important. An example of how user input was incorporated into design was that feedback suggested that the TV should not automatically be used as an information device to communicate with the user. Although the TV had been planned to be the primary interaction device of SOPRANO, other input and output modalities (such as touch screen, speaker, flashing light) were selected for use in a context-aware manner. Additionally, the user should have the possibility to define a preferred output device.

An example of how input from a focus group further developed the original SOPRANO use cases is provided by medication reminding: The SOPRANO medication use case addresses APs who experience light to moderate forgetfulness and who also have to take medication prescribed by a doctor at regular intervals (e.g. twice a day). Depending on the scenario, a family member or other informal carer may be involved.

A SOPRANO system along with the necessary peripherals (including a pill dispenser) is installed and operated by a CPO. The system is configured by the CPO to the medication regime of the AP, including information on the time of day medication needs to be taken, the size of dose at each time and the name of the medication. The configuration also includes time spans for repeated reminders in case the pill dispenser is not opened after the first alert, and time spans for an escalation to the CPO or an informal carer when the dispenser is not opened after repeated reminders.

At the pre-set times, a reminder buzzer will sound to alert the AP to open the dispenser and take the medication. The AP will also get a reminder message on the TV. If the dispenser is not opened, repeated alerts will sound and after a certain period of time a message will be sent either to the CPO or the informal carer. Depending on the scenario, the dispenser will be refilled either by the CPO or by the informal carer.

Mobile reminding for medication was not foreseen in this original use case developed during the early phases of SOPRANO. In the first cycle of user involvement, users suggested that mobile medication reminding is crucial since people will not stay in the house the whole day and expressed the idea that receiving a reminder when being outside the home would be very valuable. Experts also rated this idea as very valuable. SOPRANO thus will send a reminder message when the AP is outside the home.

Both the Theatre Method and the "Multilevel Prototyping" turned out to be valuable methods for replacing experts input in the development of conceptual design ideas and solutions with input driven by users. These methods enable the user to identify with the problem area and generate ideas according to the respective mental models and perception. This methodology represents an important advance in AAL research, because experts are not able to completely identify with the older adult users and to take over their mental models in order to generate the ideal appropriate design solution. Moreover, the "Multilevel Prototyping" was not only an innovative approach for involving the user in the generation of the conceptual ideas, but also for the user based assessment of the created design solutions.

SOPRANO Prototype System

User feedback was crucial in finalizing an architecture for the SOPRANO system. A common hardware setup is envisaged to support all use cases. A detailed description of the software and hardware architecture is not possible in this paper (more details can be found at the SOPRANO website). However, the principal device setup (see Figure 4) for a large-scale roll-out in the demonstration phase of the project (see Conclusion) will concentrate on two rooms: hallways and living rooms with some additional sensors in the kitchen. The main components are:

- Home hub (Tunstall Connect+ box which will be connected to the SOPRANO PC).
- Passive user activity sensors (door/window sensors, Tunstall motion detectors) to detect occupancy and movement.
- Device sensors (door bell sensor, TV usage, sensors connected to possibly dangerous devices in the kitchen).
- Emergency sensors (Tunstall fall detector and Tunstall security red button to be worn by the assisted person, if needed).
- Medication dispenser connected wirelessly to the SOPRANO system.
- Interface devices (Dialoc Touch Screen Terminal to display messages when leaving the house, TV tuner and remote control to show the SOPRANO GUI and Avatars, PC loudspeaker to play sound messages, Flashing light connected by wire to the Connect+ box to be used in all cases that the SOPRANO system wants to output a message).
- Connection devices (DSL internet router connected to the SOPRANO PC to obtain broadband internet access, Short Message Service (SMS) gateway to be able to send text messages from the SOPRANO PC).

Additionally, a full-function system is envisaged for the demonstration phase, where more sensors and actuators will be deployed to support all the use cases.

Lab-Based Testing of Prototypes

While the previous user interaction cycles aimed at eliciting user requirements, and generating and evaluating design ideas with potential end users of the system, this interaction cycle aimed at testing real component prototypes of the SOPRANO system with end users for the very first time and to help technical designers to improve the prototype components and overall system.

Guided by the results derived from previous user research within SOPRANO, components were improved and further developed taking ideas and requirements from SOPRANO end users into account. This focused on testing and evaluating those components that were: (a) developed within the SOPRANO project; and (b) used as interaction devices/components by older end users. Components were tested in single interviews and the tests were embedded in a use case scenario in order to stimulate user feedback, to support the user to imagine the situation with the components coming into play, and to make the tests more lively and interactive, thus facilitating evaluation of the components to be tested. This made the development of test sets necessary that, apart from the component to be tested, also included other SOPRANO equipment and devices. Thus, four test packages have been developed:

- Package I: Graphical User Interface (GUI) + digital TV + remote control: embedded in medication use case.
- Package II: GUI + touch screen: embedded in remembering use case.
- Package III: Avatar, digital TV, remote control, speech generation and speech recognition: embedded in exercise use case.

Figure 4. Principal setup of SOPRANO system for the large-scale field trials

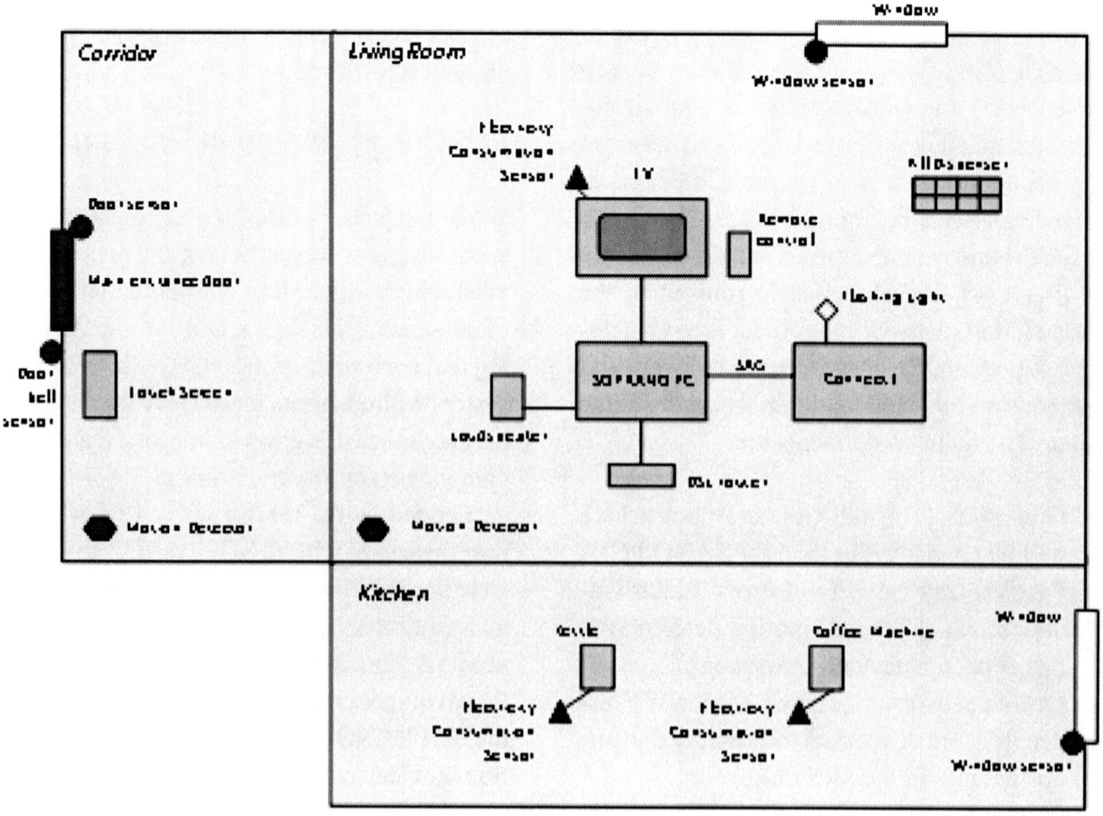

- Package IV: Digital TV, remote control, speech generation and speech recognition: embedded in open door use case.

Each test applied a mixture of scenario-based task execution, observation, user walk-through and questionnaires. The system response was provided by the prototype component. In order to ensure comparability of the tests across the different sites, detailed implementation schemes and test protocols were developed. The first section of the test protocols consisted of a list of research questions (for instance, testing of graphical design, look and feel in general icon comprehensibility, and acceptability of the avatar) that could be used as a checklist by the researchers to make sure that every issue was discussed with the participant.

Results from this cycle of user involvement aimed to help technical designers to improve the prototype components and overall system. Prototypes were lab-tested in four countries with more than 50 users between November 2008 and February 2009. Figure 5 shows component testing in Eindhoven.

The lab-testing of prototypes focused on testing and refining usability of the different SOPRANO components, for example revising the menu structure for the user interface or facilitating the understanding of assignment of functionalities to remote control buttons. The components tested were digital TV, speech generation, speech recognition, remote control, avatar, touch screen and web-based GUI. The data from this phase of the user research was still being analyzed at the

Figure 5. Woman using the touch screen (left) as part of the Remembering use case and a man copying the movements of the avatar (right) as part of the Exercise use case

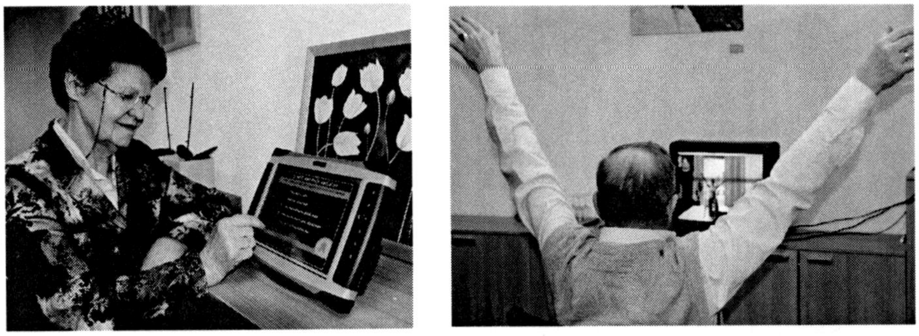

time of writing however, some examples of refinements are:

SOPRANO menu structure: Various alternative designs of the SOPRANO menu have been tested. Results revealed that navigation using numbers rather than icons seems to be easy to understand and use. Navigating "back" and "forward" in the menu is still possible with the arrows on the remote control (Figure 6).

Menu colors: Tests with users revealed that preferences for background and font colors differ between users. Thus, user-defined combinations of background/font colors will be implemented.

Remote control: User tests indicated that the remote control was easy to use, but highlighted improvements in assigning functions to remote control buttons and the intuitiveness of the remote control itself. The tests highlighted the advantages of using arrow navigation in conjunction with the numbers menu.

Reminder sound: As demonstrated in the previous user iteration, addressing more than one sense is important in order to maker sure that the user attends to reminders/information. This also enables acknowledgement of differing abilities of potential users. A reminder is thus visually displayed on the TV in combination with a sound. User tests showed that for many people the sound was not loud enough.

Reminder design: Results from the first phase of prototype tests revealed that the users preferred to continue watching TV programs when SOPRANO reminders or displays appeared on the TV screen. This was also expressed during the second cycle of user interaction. This requirement from the users was considered in two ways: (a) A small TV screen was displayed at the upper left corner of the TV screen when the SOPRANO menuwas displayed (Figure 7); and (b) a subtitle reminder was implemented that does not cover the whole TV screen, and does not immediately interrupt the TV program. Results from prototype testing revealed that preferences followed individual needs and circumstances, and no definite decision for implementing subtitle reminder or full screen reminder could be drawn. Observation by the researcher, however, often showed that the subtitle reminder was not recognized immediately by some participants. The resulting design solution suggested that the reminder should be displayed as a subtitle and then, if not recognized by the user, as a full screen reminder.

Accept button in touch screen menu: Many test persons did not recognize the accept button at all and those who recognized it did not always identify it as being touchable. Since the accept button was one of the most important functionalities in the "house status" menu, certain design improvements were needed. Some of the test persons mentioned that a renaming would be helpful and suggested ""I have done it", "done" or "approved" as examples. These suggestions

Figure 6. SOPRANO GUI and remote control

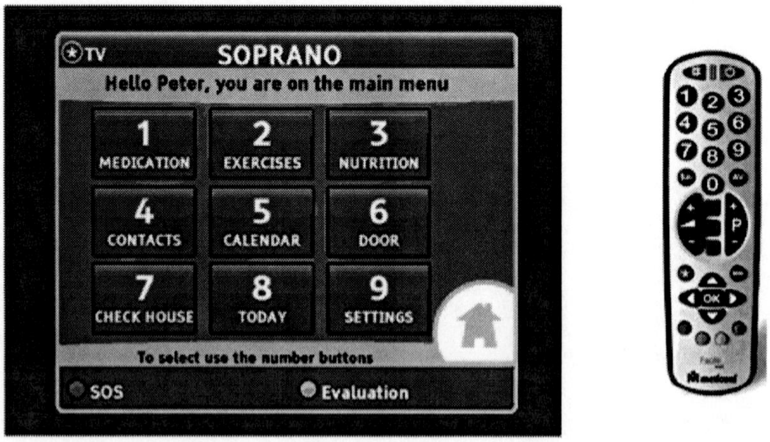
TV
SOPRANO
Hello Peter, you are on the main menu
1 MEDICATION
2 EXERCISES
3 NUTRITION
4 CONTACTS
5 CALENDAR
6 DOOR
7 CHECK HOUSE
8 TODAY
9 SETTINGS
To select use the number buttons
SOS
Evaluation

Figure 7. Small TV screen

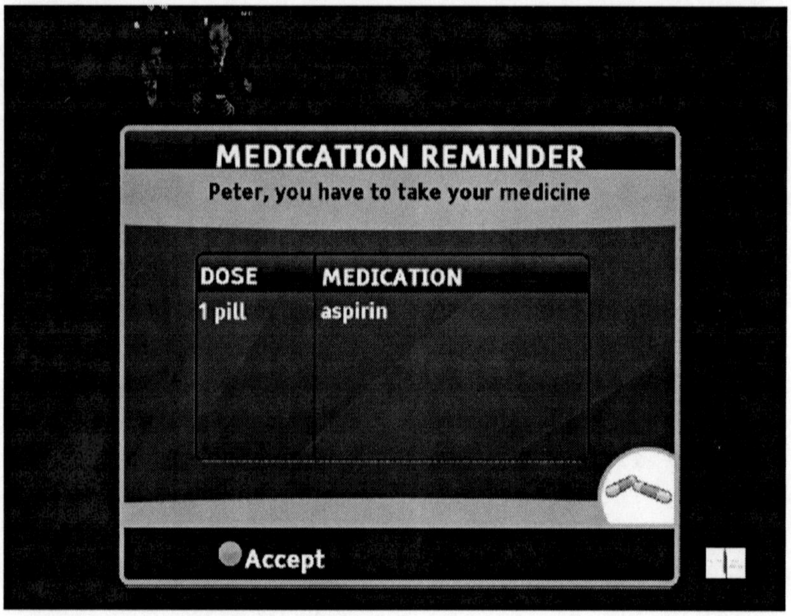

have been taken into account, and the "accept button" has been renamed in "I have done it" (Figure 8). This now also considers concerns users previously had when they were asked to "accept" that the oven is switched on.

Avatar: In general, users liked the system and design. They thought that the system was useful, and the avatar in the exercise use case motivated them to exercise at home. In most cases, users did not have a problem recognizing the avatar as a tutor, and they followed its movements. Even in some cases where the instructions and the movements of the avatar were not in concordance, people followed the movements, which showed the power of visual guides to explain activities. The research shows that using an avatar as an interface to guide exercise seems to work very well. All test persons were able to follow the

Figure 8. Original and improved design of a touch screen menu

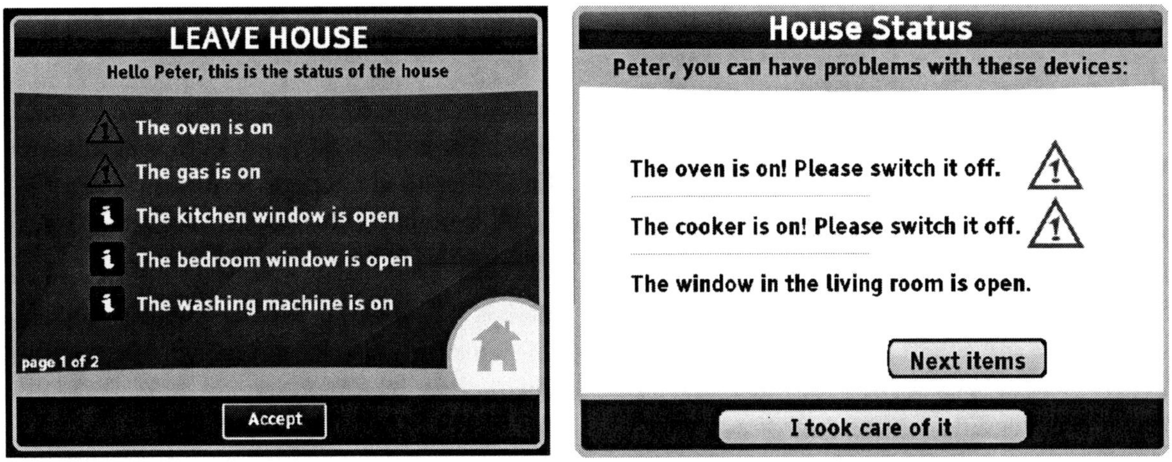

movements of the avatar without explanation or guidance from the researchers. The avatar also reduced the complexity of the exercise movements to the important things people have to focus on without distracting them with irrelevant details. However, one suggestion was that the avatar should count out the exercises. This was assessed as being of high importance for the further development of the system and the avatar itself. However, since the avatar already explains the exercises, it could be difficult to also have it count so the researchers looked for an alternative to address the underlying user need. As a consequence, the counting out of the exercises will be displayed on the screen.

CONCLUSION AND FUTURE DIRECTION

This paper has outlined the methods and results of an iterative, user-driven approach to developing the SOPRANO AAL system. The paper demonstrates the usefulness of the approach for involving users in all stages of R&D and in generating and evaluating ideas for prototype development. User involvement has been facilitated through continuous dialogue using methods that have been tailored to meet the specific information needs at each stage of the research process. This involvement should maximize three key outcomes: usability, usefulness, and acceptability. User involvement was beneficial not only in a technical sense (system and component usability), but also in terms of the practical benefits conferred to the user (usefulness) and its appropriateness to their everyday living context (acceptability).

In the final phase of the project, the SOPRANO system will be deployed in two ways. First, full-function demonstration facilities will be set up in demonstration homes in the UK, The Netherlands and Spain. As the technology and services developed within SOPRANO are innovative, some parts will still be at the design stage and will not have been tested and proven to be reliable. However, it is still important to get feedback from users at this stage either as input to the design process and/or as evaluation on the functionality of the total SOPRANO system. The full function trials will support all the use cases described above. However, some of the use cases may be deployed in a slightly limited manner. Large-scale field trials of a more limited version of the SOPRANO system are also planned to evaluate its impact in real-life situations with 600 users across Europe. The large-scale trials will fully support the "medication", "remembering" and "fall" use cases and partially support the "active" and "entertained" use cases.

The information from the demonstration phase will provide critical information on the practical and commercial deployment of the SOPRANO AAL system. As discussed earlier, the recent European financing of over €1 billion certainly represents a major commitment to and belief in the political and commercial potential of AAL. This is interesting given that the actual and potential benefits of ICT-based solutions, clinical, social, commercial, or otherwise have yet to be demonstrated (Martin et al., 2008). Sixsmith (2008) points to the very limited nature of any evidence to support large-scaleimplementation. The planned SOPRANO field trials should contribute to providing such evidence.

ACKNOWLEDGMENT

SOPRANO (http://www.soprano-ip.org/) is an Integrated Project funded under the EU's FP6 IST programme Thematic Priority: 6.2.2: Ambient Assisted Living for the Ageing Society (IST – 2006 – 045212). The authors acknowledge the input and role of the SOPRANO consortium and would also like to thank the many people who volunteered in the various stages of user research described in this paper.

REFERENCES

AALIANCE. (2009). *The European Ambient Assisted Living Innovation Alliance Website.* Retrieved December 11, 2009, from http://www.aaliance.eu/public/

Ambient Assisted Living Joint Programme. (n.d.). "What is AAL?" Retrieved January 20, 2009, from http://www.aal-europe.eu/about-aal

Ambient Assisted Living Joint Programme. (n.d.). AAL: Preparation of a new European Initiative for IT supported solutions. Retrieved January 20, 2009, from http://www.aal169.org/intern/Work-packages/wp0/networking/AALflv2.pdf

Barbour, R. (1998). Mixing qualitative methods: Quality assurance or qualitative quagmire? *Qualitative Health Research*, *8*(3), 352–361. doi:10.1177/104973239800800306

Machate, J., & Burmester, M. (2003). *User interface tuning*. Germany: Software and Support.

Martin, S., Kelly, S., Kernohan, G., McCreight, B., & Nugent, C. (2008). Smart home technologies for health and social care support. *Cochrane Database of System Reviews.* Retrieved January 22, 2009, from http://mrw.interscience.wiley.com/cochrane/clsysrev/articles/CD006412/frame.html.

Mayring, P. (2000). Qualitative content analysis [Electronic version]. *Forum Qualitative Sozial Forschung, 1*(2).

Mueller, S., & Sixsmith, A. (2008). *User requirements for Ambient Assisted Living: Some evidence from the SOPRANO project.* Paper presented at the 6th International Conference of the International Society for Gerontechnology/, Pisa, Tuscany, Italy, June 4-7.

Padgett, D. (2004). *The qualitative research experience*. USA: Wadsworth.

Rosson, M. B., Carroll, J. M., Seals, C., & Lewis, T. (2002). Community design of community simulations. [New York: ACM.]. *Proceedings of Designing Interactive Systems: DIS, 2002*, 74–83.

Sixsmith, A., & Sixsmith, J. (2008). Ageing in place in the United Kingdom. *Ageing International*, *32*(3), 219–235. doi:10.1007/s12126-008-9019-y

Sixsmith, A. (2008). *Ambient technologies: Developing user-driven approaches to research and development.* Paper presented at the Gerontological Society of America 61st Annual Scientific Meeting, Gaylord National Resort and Convention Center. *MD Medical Newsmagazine*, (Nov): 21–25.

Chapter 4
Falls Prevention in the Home: Challenges for New Technologies

Rose A. Kenny
Trinity College, Ireland

Cliodhna Ni Scanaill
Intel, Ireland

Michael McGrath
Intel, Ireland

ABSTRACT

Approximately 1 in 3 people over the age of 65 fall each year; therefore it is of little surprise that falling is often accepted as a natural part of the aging process. Many falls are simply managed using alarm pendants to notify others when a falls event occurs. However, falls technology extends beyond simple notification; technology can be used to screen for falls risk, or to prevent a fall from occurring. In this chapter, we review the latest best practices for the identification of falls risk. We review the technology, if any, developed to support these practices, and discuss the challenges of using technology for in-home falls prevention, risk assessment and falls detection. Recommendations and suggestions for future research directions are discussed.

INTRODUCTION

Falls are of significant social and economic concern, due to the high incidence of falls among the rapidly growing "old" and "old old" populations and the direct and indirect cost of each fall. Approximately 28-35% of people aged 65 and over fall each year, increasing to 32-42% for those over 70 years of age (World Health Organization, 2008). However, it is the impact rather than the occurrence of falls in older adults which is of most concern. Older adults are typically frailer, more unsteady, have slower reactions and thus are more likely to be injured than toddlers and athletes, who also fall regularly. Approximately 40-60% of all reported falls in older adults lead to injuries, of which 30-50% are minor injuries, and 5-6% result in fractures. Most older adults who sustain a fracture following a fall report never regaining previous levels of mobility, and 20% of falls-related hip fractures result in death within 1 year. An injurious fall in a person over 65 can cost the healthcare system US$1049 in Australia (Hendrie et al., 2003) or US$3611 in Finland

DOI: 10.4018/978-1-61520-825-8.ch004

(Nurmi I. & Lüthje P., 2002). If falls rates are not reduced in the immediate future, the number of injuries caused by falls is projected to double by 2030 (Kannus et al., 2007).

Falling also incurs social and psychological consequences. Socially, a fall can lead to loss of independence and loss of social engagement, as well as broader societal costs and consequences. Psychologically, 54% of people aged over 70 express a fear of falling (G. A. R. Zijlstra et al., 2007), resulting in reduction in their physical and social activities. The main consequences of fear of falling are a decline in physical performance, a decline in mental performance, an increased risk of falling, and progressive loss of health-related quality of life. A fall event can also affect the spouse, family and friends of the person who falls, in particular generating concern for the safety of their loved one. This can result in an increased focus on caring for the older person including considering hiring a carer. It is unsurprising, given the incidence of injury and development of fear of falling, that a recent fall is one of the primary reasons given for moving into nursing homes.

The majority of falls do not result in injury, and many minor trips and stumbles are not reported and are quickly forgotten. However, multi-factorial fall risk assessment is recommended if a fall results in a soft tissue or fracture injury, two or more falls events within a year (recurrent falls), difficulties in walking and balance, or fear of falling are reported. A multi-factorial fall risk assessment can reveal factors that put an individual at risk of falling and can help identify the most appropriate interventions. The risk of falling increases dramatically as the number of risk factors increase. Technologies associated with the falls arena can generally be classified as assisting with detection, assessment, or prevention, and further sorted by the setting to which they belong – acute hospital, nursing home or domiciliary. A variety of falls technologies exist for non-fallers, recent fallers, and recurrent fallers, although the technology requirements vary for each group. An alarm pendant to summon help which may be very useful for a recurrent faller is unnecessary for a non-faller or someone who experiences an occasional accidental fall. Similarly, a challenging balance training game which reduces the risk of falling in non-fallers would be dangerous for a recurrent faller with balance issues.

In the background section of this chapter, we review the strategies developed to identify and treat falls risk factors. We then discuss the role of technology in quantifying and treating these risk factors. In some situations, falls cannot be prevented but the impact of the fall can be reduced through an appropriate application of technology. We then discuss the challenges of developing falls technology for the home and suggest some future research directions. Although older persons in long-term care or older persons with cognitive impairment are at high risk of falling, technology developed specifically for these populations is outside of the scope of this chapter.

BACKGROUND

There is no standard definition for a fall, but the most commonly adopted definition is "an event whereby an individual comes to rest on the ground or another lower level with or without the loss of consciousness". Each fall event can be further classified (Kenny et al., 2009) according to their self-reported mechanism (explained/unexplained), objective mechanism (extrinsic/intrinsic), severity (non-injurious/injurious) and frequency (single/recurrent). The definition of a faller also varies in the literature but a faller is usually described as someone who has fallen at least once within a set period of time. The latest AGS guidelines (American Geriatrics Society, in press) recommend screening older persons for falls every 12 months.

There are several reasons why older adults fall. Some reasons such as age and gender cannot be modified, and others such as medications,

Table 1. Common falls risk factors

	Intrinsic	Extrinsic
Non-modifiable	Age, Gender History of previous falls Acute or chronic medical problems (e.g. Parkinson's, osteoporosis, cardiovascular disease) Neurological function	Environment outside of home (e.g. uneven paving, ice)
Modifiable	Gait, Balance, Mobility levels, Lower extremity joint function Lower extremity muscle strength Cardiovascular status (e.g. blood pressure, heart rate and rhythm) Visual Acuity Self-efficacy, and Fear of Falling	Poly-pharmacy Footwear Home environment (e.g. loose rugs, steps)

muscle weakness and vision can be modified. Table 1 categorizes the most common falls risk factors according to their objective mechanism, and whether or not they can be modified. The presence of more than one risk factor is common, and several studies have shown that the risk of falling increases dramatically as the number of risk factors increases. A recent Cochrane review on falls interventions (Gillespie et al., 2009) found that multi-factorial interventions were the most beneficial in reducing falls; however, the most successful interventions only reduced falls by 35%.

There are several evidence-based clinical guidelines that prescribe clinical pathways for fall assessment and interventions. The NICE (National Institute for Clinical Excellence (NICE), 2004), ProFaNE Clinical Assessment Tool (Profane), and AGS Guidelines (American Geriatrics Society, in press) prescribe screening all older adults (aged over 65) for recent falls and/or poor gait/balance (Figure 1). If these preliminary risk factors are identified, a multi-factorial risk assessment and intervention are prescribed. A health professional or team should conduct this fall risk assessment, and directly implement the interventions or ensure that the interventions are carried out by qualified healthcare professionals. Technologies that can be used to quantify many of these risks and support falls interventions are described in the next section.

FALLS TECHNOLOGY

Alarms and Falls Detection

There has been significant interest in falls both from a research and commercial perspective for many years. A variety of approaches have been taken technologically towards falls detection with varying degrees of success. Falls detection devices can be categorized as Wearable Alarms and Passive Sensing Alarms.

Wearable Alarms

The most commonly known falls technologies are devices that a faller can manually use to summon help following a fall event. These alarms typically consist of an alarm button and a wireless transmitter or transceiver, which are worn by the faller as a pendent or a bracelet. When a falls event occurs, the user presses the alarm button, which wirelessly connects to an alert unit installed in the faller's house, which in turn notifies a remote monitoring center (such as the Philips Life Line (Philips) or MedicalAlarm.com (Connect America) monitoring centres) via a telephone or broadband connection. However this approach does have a significant drawback, as it is unsuitable for individuals who are unable to activate the alarm due to physical impairment

Figure 1. AGS Algorithm summarizing the assessment and management of falls. (reproduced from (American Geriatrics Society, in press))

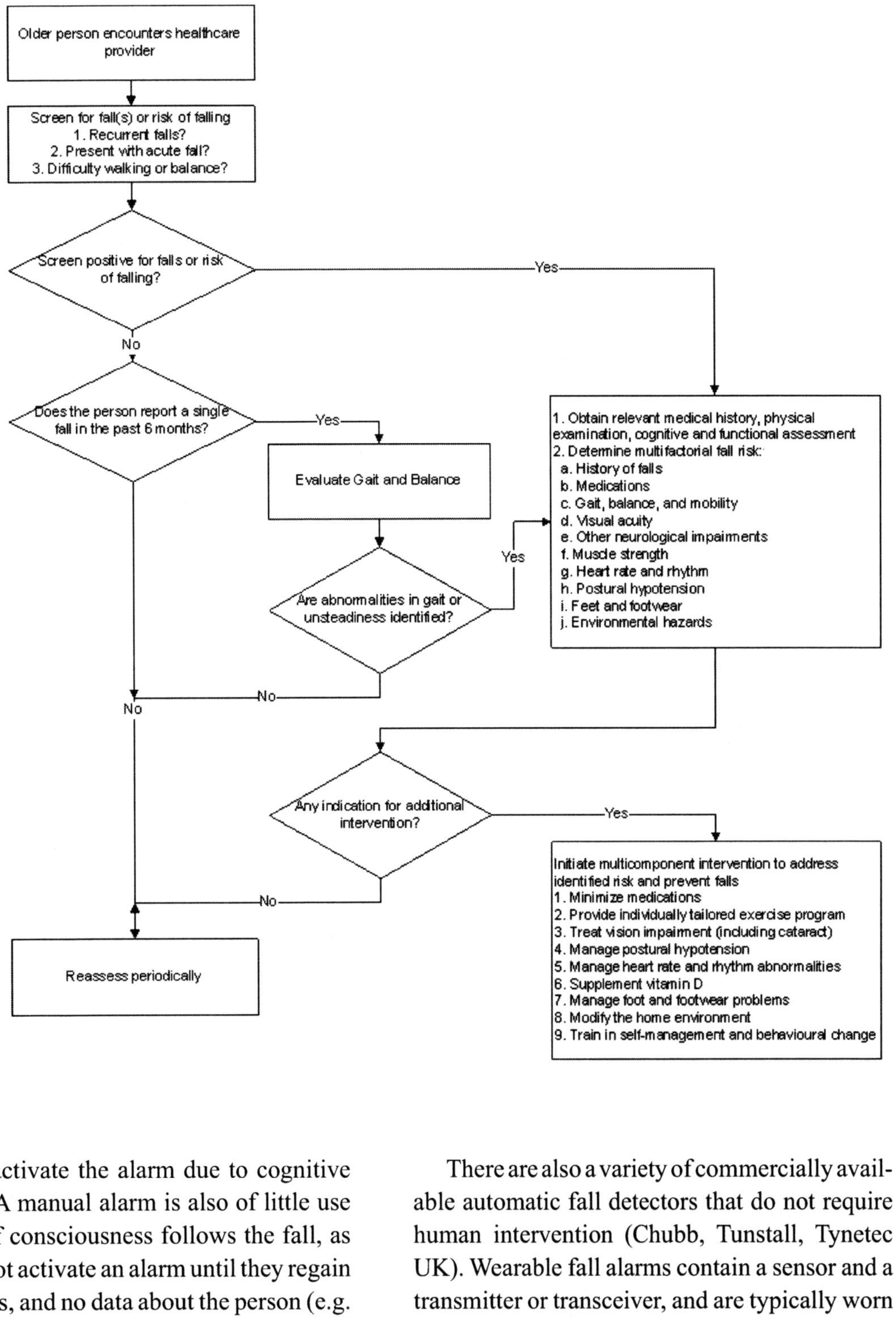

or forget to activate the alarm due to cognitive impairment. A manual alarm is also of little use where loss of consciousness follows the fall, as the user cannot activate an alarm until they regain consciousness, and no data about the person (e.g. changes in blood pressure) or circumstances (e.g. duration of the event) are recorded.

There are also a variety of commercially available automatic fall detectors that do not require human intervention (Chubb, Tunstall, Tynetec UK). Wearable fall alarms contain a sensor and a transmitter or transceiver, and are typically worn on the chest, hips or waist, wrist or forearm, knee or thigh (Rajendran et al., 2008). Most automatic wearable fall detectors are designed to detect sudden impact on the floor usually indicated by a significant downward acceleration towards the floor followed by a person remaining in a horizontal orientation (determined by a gyroscope or tilt sensor) for a specified period of time. The use of multiple sensors helps to reduce the number of false positives (e.g. distinguishing a fall from someone sitting down quickly). Researchers at the University of Singapore have demonstrated pre-impact detection with body worn sensing with an average lead time of 700 ms, 100% specificity and a sensitivity of 95.2% using a combination of a tri axial accelerometer and 2D gyroscope (Nyan et al., 2008).

Wearable falls alarms rely on seamless integration between the body worn sensor and the call centre. The typical approach requires an intermediate device which receives the alarm from the sensor wirelessly and forwards the alert to a call centre over a telephone line or some form of broadband connection. The intermediate steps are obvious points of failure due to various forms of communication failures (e.g. radio interference). Such systems can only work when the person is located in their home or in close proximity (limited by the range of the sensor's radio). Research has focused on integrating 3G communications into the sensor platform to provide reliable and flexible communications not restricted by time or location. The EU 6th Frame project HEBE (Azkoitia, 2004) focused on the detection of falls and monitoring of older people using a GPS locating device with a bi-axial accelerometer, all connected to a call centre using GSM/GPRS technology. For body worn devices to be effective, user compliance is of critical importance especially when the person is moving during their normal daily activities. Conspicuous fall alarms that are worn on the body can often be perceived by the users as stigmatizing them as fallers among their peers. Significant opportunity remains to improve their aesthetic design such as their inclusion into everyday objects e.g. Philips Lifeline Tempo Watch (Philips) and Emporia Life Plus mobile phone.

Passive Sensing Alarms

Video monitoring systems use cameras that attempt to detect a fall event using image-processing algorithms and that are programmed to identify unusual inactivity, which may occur following a fall. The fall detectors under this category are passive as the older person does not have to wear any device. This form of approach remains an active area of research within the academic community focusing design variations in image-processing algorithms and monitoring/transmission systems. The UbiSense project (Lo, 2005a, 2005b) at the Imperial College London is focused on developing a non contact, unobtrusive health-monitoring system for the older person by using embedded vision techniques to detect changes in posture, gait, and activities. Privacy issues are addressed in UbiSense by filtering the images at the device level into blobs. These blobs only contain the person's silhouetted outline and motion information. As images are not stored or transmitted, the original image cannot be recreated, therefore ensuring privacy. Pham et al. (2008) have demonstrated a multifunctional video monitoring system which supports real-time posture discrimination to determine emergency situations such as a fall event. Alternatively an alarm can also be triggered by suspected immobility in an unusual location. Privacy is supported by the utilization of a silhouetting technique. An alternative approach to standard video cameras which addresses many of the privacy issues is the SIMBAD system reported by the University of Liverpool. The Smart Inactivity Monitor Using Array-Based Detectors (SIMBAD) fall detector is based on a low-cost array of infrared detectors to capture low-level images of the resident and analyze the subject's motion to detect a fall event (Sixsmith & Johnson, 2004). Falls are detected using a neural model based on the velocity and acceleration of the tracked object. The findings indicated good specificity in terms of low false-alarm rates; however the model could only detect 30% of emulated falls. Despite the ability of video-based fall-monitoring systems to automatically detect falls with no user intervention, the fear of intrusion of privacy is extremely prominent in this approach. Although a variety of solutions have been developed to ensure privacy, people in homes still experience the feeling of "being-watched", making the technology unacceptable in many cases.

Floor vibration solutions fall into two categories: Acoustic Sensing Solutions and Vibration Sensing Solutions. Acoustic detection of falls events has generated recent interest. This approach uses an accelerometer in combination with a microphone to detect the sounds made when a person falls and contacts a solid object or surface, such as the floor. There are limitations to the technique associated with surfaces such as concrete with carpet overlay, for example. Doukas and Maglogiannis (2008) reported a system which wirelessly transmits acoustic data from a microphone to a monitoring unit, where Short Time Fourier Transform (STFT) and spectrogram analyses are applied. Support Vector Machines were utilized for event classification. They report 100% success in the detection of falls events. Litvak et al. (2008) report similar results with a system of a microphone and an accelerometer attached to the floor. The sensors are connected to a data acquisition unit which then transmits the signals at 16 KHz to a PC. They report detection of falls events with a sensitivity of 97.5% and specificity of 98.5%. The second type of floor vibration solution uses conversion of the mechanical energy that is generated when a person impacts an object/surface such as a floor; the energy is converted into electrical energy using piezoelectric sensors. The selectivity of the sensors is based on the hypothesis that the vibration signature of the floor generated by a fall is significantly different from those generated by normal daily activities such as walking, and that the vibration signature of a human fall is significantly different from those of falling objects. The Medical Automation Research Centre (MARC) at the University of Virginia has demonstrated a sensor based on this approach. In controlled experiments using a dummy, this fall detector attained 100% true positives and 0% false alarms with a detection range of 20 feet (Alwan et al., 2006). The significant disadvantage of both video and floor vibration approaches is that they only detect falls that occur within the home environment and only in rooms within the home that have the cameras or sensors installed in them. Controlled environments and small participant numbers curtail generalizability of results.

Assessing Falls Risk Factors

Balance Assessment

Balance can be defined as the ability of an individual to maintain the position of the body or more specifically, its centre of mass, within specific boundaries of space. Maintaining balance requires the integration of sensory information of the body relative to the surroundings, and the ability to generate forces to control body movement. As we age, the sensory inputs required for balance deteriorate; the processing system, which informs anticipatory and reactionary movements, is slower and sometimes incorrect; and the musculo-skeletal systems, which are required to maintain balance, can be weaker and painful. These age-related deteriorations can be further exacerbated by illness and disease. Static balance, also known as postural sway, describes the small movements and corrective actions required to keep the body standing upright. Balance is typically assessed in a clinical setting using functional performance scales (Tyson & Connell, 2009), such as the Berg Balance Scale, or the Performance-Orientated balance and Mobility Assessment (POMA). These assessments require the older person to perform a series of tasks which require steady state or anticipatory postural control. Their ability to complete these tasks is subjectively scored by a clinician.

Technological methods to assess and quantify balance are rare in falls clinics, but force plate, pressure measuring, and posturography equipment can be found in specialist rehabilitation and motion analysis laboratories. Force plates are measuring instruments that measure the ground reaction forces generated by a body standing on or moving across them, to quantify balance, gait and other parameters of biomechanics. Force plates measure three-dimensional components of the force applied to the surface of the force plate, the centre of pressure, and the vertical moment of the force. Pressure measuring systems also quantify centre of pressure, but do not directly measure the applied force vector. These systems are useful for quantifying the pressure patterns under a foot over time but cannot quantify horizontal or shear components of the applied forces. Posturography is used to objectively identify abnormalities in the three sensory systems (visual, vestibular, somasensory) and balance processing system by measuring anterior-posterior sway and response time when the individual sensory inputs required for balance are challenged.

NeuroCom developed a range of products (Equitest®, BalanceMaster®, VSR™), which use dual force plates with rotation capabilities to challenge the balance and measure the vertical forces exerted by the patient's feet. These products provide a number of methods to assess and rehabilitate patients with balance and mobility disorders. The Metitur Good Balance System is a triangular force platform made of fiber glass composite material, which is used to measure postural control in different static and dynamic testing conditions. This system then uses visual and auditory biofeedback to aid rehabilitation of balance and asymmetric posture. TechScan develops pressure measurement systems that measure the underfoot pressure using insoles, sensor mats and sensor walkway. They have developed a Sway Analysis Module (SAM) add-on and a centre of mass module (CoM'nalysis®) add-on to supplement their gait analysis products. Accelerometry has been shown to be a reliable method for the assessment of balance and gait in the clinic (Moe-Nilssen, 1998). In a recent study, O'Sullivan et al. (2009) demonstrated that a commercial tri-axial accelerometer (ActivPAL Trio) can distinguish between sway responses between fallers and non-fallers, and demonstrated a high correlation between accelerometry and standard clinical assessments (Berg Balance Scale and Timed Up and Go). The Nintendo Wii has brought fitness gaming to the mass market. The Wii Balance board accessory uses 4 pressure sensors to measure the user's center of balance and weight. The associated WiiFit games challenge the user to maintain or move their centre of balance in a controlled manner. The WiiFit software has features to allow the users to track improvements/decline in their balance, thus encouraging continued use of the system. Ross (2009) recently compared the Wii Balance Board to the Force Plate and found that the Wii Balance Board is a valid tool for assessing standing balance.

Force-plate based systems require careful installation, and are typically only found in specialized motion analysis laboratories. The TechScan and Metitur products are less specialized and are targeted towards physiotherapists, chiropractors, and falls clinics. Kinematic sensing (accelerometers and gyroscopes) offer a low-cost, reliable, and portable method to objectively measure balance in any setting. However, to date there is no commercial clinical product which uses accelerometry to assess balance. The WiiFit system has focused attention on the topic of balance training in the home. It has been readily adopted by all generations, including older adults, who wish to improve their balance. The games were not developed for the rehabilitation of fallers and the Wii does not claim to be a rehabilitation device; in fact, it is possible that the challenging games may be unsafe for those who have serious balance issues. Researchers at the University of Aberdeen and

NHS Grampian in Scotland began a study in early 2009 to investigate if people aged 70 years and older can improve their balance through regular use of the WiiFit.

Gait Assessment

Human gait is a complex balance challenge, in which a person must initiate a fall forward and recapture their momentum through the appropriate placement of their leading foot. Deficits in balance and gait are the most predictive risk factors for falls. The potential for loss of balance during walking is significant, and it is not surprising that over 50% of falls in older adults occur during walking (Lord et al., 2007). Stumbles are increasingly common among older adults, as foot clearance is lower and slower during the swing phase of gait. Slower reaction times, due to impaired processing of sensory inputs, painful joints, and increased muscle risks, further increase the risk of falling. The risk of falling is higher in people with Parkinson's, due to the increased incidence of orthostatic hypotension, freezing mid-motion, and "hurrying gait", and following a stroke, due to muscle weakness and difficulties in coordination. Gait impairments can be assessed using a number of methods, ranging from optical motion systems in motion analysis labs, to subjective observation of a person walking over a short distance.

A popular approach to gait analysis is stereophotogrammetry, based on either conventional photography/video (Wang et al., 2003) or optoelectronic sensors image processing systems (Cappozzo et al., 2005). Systems such as CODA from Codamotion (Charnwood Dynamics Ltd.), and Vicon have gained popularity for Gait Analysis (Lee & Hidler, 2008; Monaghan et al., 2006). The Codamotion optical systems consist of body worn markers that have in-built infra-red LEDs. These markers are attached to the body in different positions depending on the clinical protocol. As the person moves, the position of the markers is tracked at 42 μsec intervals using tripod-mounted motion capture units (CX1). The resulting data are connected to a data acquisition unit and then finally to a PC where the measurement information can be displayed in real-time and derived variables, such as joint angles, moments and powers, are calculated. Optical motion analysis systems can be further enhanced by integrating then with other devices such as force plates and EMG systems. The GAITRite system from CIR System Inc is one of the most popular methods for the objective measurement of Gait parameters in a clinical setting (Besser et al., 2001; Bilney et al., 2003). The GAITRite system automates the measurement of the temporal (timing) and spatial (distance) parameters of Gait via an electronic walkway connected to a PC. The standard GAITRite system is approximately 366cm long and contains 13824 sensors spaced at 1.27 cm apart. As the patient walks across the walkway the system dynamically captures pressure data with respect to each footstep and calculates both temporal and spatial parameters for the walk.

The major advantage of these laboratory based assessments is their ability to provide objective and quantitative measurement of gait. However a major drawback is the need for a permanent laboratory setting with skilled personnel to run them. A second major disadvantage is that gait sample, captured in the lab, is often not truly representative of the environment leading to a fall in the home (W. Zijlstra & Aminian, 2007), which contains many physical and cognitive obstacles. 'White coat' syndrome is often evident in the laboratory, and people significantly improve posture and gait during the period of the test. In an effort to address some of these limitations, there has been growing interest in the use of kinematic sensors as a low cost alternative for Gait analysis (Aminian & Najafi, 2004; Daniele, 2006; Giansanti et al., 2005; Mayagoitia et al., 2002; Narayanan et al., 2007). Accelerometers are commonly used to measure acceleration of body segments in 3-D. Miniature gyroscopes, which use a vibrating mechanical element to sense angular velocity,

Figure 2. Overview of the TRIL gait analysis platform

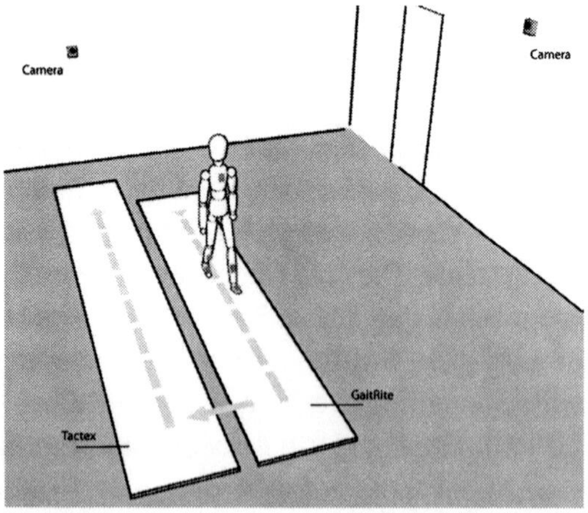

are also commonly employed. A third approach is pressure sensors or foot switches attached to the shoe or foot sole; these can be used to detect contact of the foot with the ground. Goniometers have also been utilized to measure a person's range of motion (Carnaz et al., 2008; Piriyaprasarth et al., 2008). The goniometer is attached to the joint segments, and produces a voltage output that is proportional to the angle between these two axes. The key advantage of the body worn sensing approach is the ability to record objective data in non tethered conditions. Thus, the distance or location of a clinical gait assessment can be altered without moving or purchasing additional equipment. Wearable sensors can also be worn at home for an extended period of time to provide a true measurement of the person's normal gait pattern. The body worn sensing approach to gait analysis is clearly advantageous; however, further development of such systems is required to provide reliable temporal and spatial parameters of gait with turnkey ease of use. Nonetheless, extended use in a home environment has many of the limitations associated with body worn falls detection devices.

The TRIL Centre developed a gait analysis system (Figure 2) which uniquely combines a floor mat sensor, body worn sensors, video capture, and a software user interface for clinicians. The SHIMMER wireless sensor platform (McGrath D et al., 2009) was used to record gait and heart rate. O'Donovan et al. (2009) reported favorable comparison between gait analysis measured using SHIMMER kinematic sensors and gold standard optical (Codamotion) measurement. The SHIMMER (Barton & Jung, 2009; Lorincz et al., 2007; Patel et al., 2007) sensors are controlled by and communicate data to a master PC via a Bluetooth radio stack. The application software was developed using the BioMOBIUS (2009) software environment that supports data capture at rates up to 100Hz for kinematic SHIMMERs and up to 500Hz for ECG SHIMMERs. During clinical trials three SHIMMERs are worn by the subject: two kinematic SHIMMERs, one attached to each leg, are used to determine the temporal parameters of gait; and a third ECG SHIMMER unit attached to the chest is used to determine heart rate. A floor-mat sensor, developed by Tactex Technologies, was used to measure underfoot pressure as the older adults walked along the floor mat. The 457cm floor mat consists of 1296 pressure points spaced 2.5cm apart. The floor sensor measures pressure under the foot as the person walks along the walkway. The sensor can therefore be used to detect the location and timing of each footfall, as well as dynamic pressure changes under the foot during gait. The system's user interface allows clinicians to select and adjust what data are being collected and how the data is processed. The software encapsulates data acquisition and signal processing modules, and allows customization of the sensors (K. O'Donovan et al., 2008).

Neurocardiovascular Assessment

Postural hypotension can result in a loss of balance due to low blood pressure and associated cerebral hypoperfusion. It can occur due to dehydration as well as medication, and is common in people with Parkinson's disease. Postural hypotension is a transient event that is diagnosed by measuring beat-to-beat blood pressure when lying, moving from sitting to standing, and standing. It is difficult to detect this condition, as the drop and subsequent recovery in blood pressure following a postural transition may occur too quickly for traditional arm-cuffs to detect. The bedside Finometer and portable Portapres (Finapres Medical Systems) measure beat-to-beat blood pressure using a small finger cuff inflated to a pressure equal to the pressure in the artery. The cuff incorporates an infra-red transmitter on one side of the finger and a receiver on the opposite side. The transmission of the infra-red light through the finger is measured and found to oscillate with the cardiac cycle. The cuff pressure that produces the largest amplitude oscillations corresponds to the mean finger arterial pressure. This equipment is specialized and requires clinical expertise to interpret the results. There is currently no equipment capable of measuring beat-to-beat blood pressure in the community or the home.

Abnormal heart rhythms are common among older adults. Some people may experience these abnormalities continually, thus the abnormality is still present during a post-fall assessment. However in some people these abnormalities occur intermittently. In these cases, it is difficult to establish if an intermittent abnormality is the cause of a fall, as the clinician does not have access to a recording of the faller's heart rhythm at the time of the fall and the abnormality may not occur during the post-fall assessment. Portable heart rate monitors (Holter monitors), which can record a person's heart rate and heart rate variability for extended periods (24 hours to 2 weeks), are given to fallers when a clinical ECG appears to be normal and an intermittent heart rhythm is suspected. If an abnormality is not captured in this time period, an implantable device, such as Reveal (Medtronic), is inserted under the skin above the breast. These devices can record heart rhythms for up to 18 months, but require a minor operation to insert and remove. Wearable wireless sensors, such as the Intelesens Vitalsens platform (Intelesens), can integrate into existing home monitoring stations, and can warn if changes in vital signs are detected.

Falls Prevention

Education & Peer-Support

All falls prevention programmes include education components, intended to raise awareness about risk factors and interventions that reduce risk, for the purpose of preventing future falls. There is no evidence that education alone reduces falls, but it is a vital part of any multi-factorial intervention. The internet has become an expedient tool for dissemination of knowledge among falls experts and their peers, from falls experts to fallers, and among fallers. Resources, such as the Profane discussion board (www.profane.eu.org), allow falls researchers to share their expertise and latest findings among their peers, thus reducing unnecessary duplication, and ensuring that falls knowledge is collectively progressed. The internet is also a useful resource for fallers and their carers to learn more about falls, falls risk factors, and coping strategies. Although the current generation of older adults typically relies on a healthcare professionals for advice and support; future generations, beginning with the baby boomer generation, will question medical advice, and actively seek more information and methods to empower themselves. It is important, therefore, that information published online regarding falls interventions is safe and targeted to the person reading it. The Balance Training website (http://www.balancetraining.org.uk/fallsAdvice/findPath.do) tailors their advice by requiring the user to fill in a questionnaire before accessing advice. Social networking tools, such as Skype, Facebook, Twitter, and the TRIL Building Bridges project (Wherton & Prendergast, 2009), may all play a role in destigmatizing falls and reducing the onset of fear of falling through peer support. However, it is important that these forums are carefully moderated, to ensure that incorrect (and potentially dangerous) advice is not shared among members.

Exercise

Exercise programs are a recommended falls prevention strategy, both on their own and as part of a multi-factorial intervention (Gillespie et al., 2009). The style of exercise (tai-chi/yoga, group balance and strength training, OTAGO) and delivery method (group training or one-on-one training) is dependent on the balance status of the older person. To be successful, a falls prevention exercise program must include a combination of strength, gait and highly challenging balance training (Sherrington et al., 2008). Exercise should take place at least twice a week for a minimum of 6 months, and should be progressed as the individual improves. Walking is contra-indicated, and a walking program may actually increase the risk of falling for an individual with poor balance. Wellness training, such as yoga and tai-chi, are useful for maintaining and improving balance in older adults who do not have balance issues. In a systematic review of exercise interventions, Sherrington et al. (2008) concluded that Tai Chi was an "effective program" for the reduction of falls and falls risk for those with mild deficits of strength and balance. Tai-chi reduces fear of falling and improves self efficacy but does not reduce falls in people with a history of falls. The Otago Exercise Programme is an in-home strength and balance training program developed by a research team at the University of Otago Medical School, New Zealand and evaluated in both research and routine healthcare services in 1016 people aged 65 to 97 living at home. This program is prescribed by trained health/fitness professionals and tailored to the ability of the individual. The exercise is progressed as appropriate during the 6-month program. Overall the exercise program was effective in reducing by 35% both the number of falls and the number of injuries resulting from falls, and was most successful in training adults aged over 80.

Tai-Chi, Yoga, and balance training DVDs specifically developed for falls prevention are available to purchase on the internet and from specialist shops. DVDs are useful to guide an older adult through an exercise program, and provide correct pacing, sequence and instruction not available from a paper-based exercise program. However, DVD-based exercise programs developed for the generic market are less likely to be adapted to the abilities and disabilities of an older individual. As a passive system, a DVD has no method of tracking whether the person is doing the exercises correctly or has completed any exercises. Another method of self-prescribing exercises is to download an exercise program from the internet. The Balance Training (www.balancetraining.org.uk) website provides a tailored exercise program for older adults after they have filled in a questionnaire describing their health, balance and falls status. However, there is no method to ensure correct completion of the exercise or to progress the exercise program. In-home exercise with biofeedback was a small specialized area until Nintendo launched the Wii and WiiFit products to the mass market. These products were not developed for falls prevention and/or risk reduction, but following its widespread adoption by older adults and community care settings, the benefits of the Wii for balance training in older adults are now being investigated.

FALLS PREVENTION TECHNOLOGY: THE CHALLENGES

Issues, Controversies, Problems

Scientifically, there are still many challenges in falls prevention. Currently, there is no worldwide consensus on what a fall is, although the Profane and NICE definitions are increasingly being adopted; nor is there a standard definition for a "faller". The recently published AGS guidelines may be adopted by the research community in future studies. Previously, the definition of a faller was defined within the scope of individual studies, where a faller is labeled as a person who has experienced a fall within a fixed period of time. Profane recently published a falls prevention classification system (Lamb et al., 2007), which aims to standardize the reporting of falls, and outcome measures from fall interventions. If adopted by the falls community, this system should make the task of rating efficacy of interventions easier.

There has been little progress in falls research in recent years, with many new studies simply reiterating previous knowledge. Consequently, there has been little progress in falls technology in recent years. Despite understanding the main risk factors for falls, the most risky periods of the day for falls, and the most common location for falls, there is still no method to predict that a fall event is likely to occur and understand the cause of that particular fall. A clearer understanding of the circumstances which influence falls events in the home (time, contributing factors, and changes in behavior prior to a fall) across a large population is required before falls can be understood and subsequently predicted. Falls diaries are the most common method to record the details of a fall; however, they are ineffective if someone blacks out and does not remember their fall. What if someone is too embarrassed to admit falling and claims that they tripped? What if someone has poor memory (40% of over 80 year olds) and forgets that the event has occurred? Wearable and/or ambient technology can provide more objective descriptions of a fall event than a self reported description. However, there are also difficulties in acquiring these data due to the multi-factorial nature of falling and the difficulty in capturing a fall in the community. To capture the precise moment of a fall, the faller would have to be monitored continually; and a large number of people would have to be observed to develop a sufficiently large database. Following recent sensor technology advances, there are few technological limitations to undertaking such a study, but there are several scientific questions to be answered. For example, what risk factors should be measured? Should these be tailored to the type of faller? How frequently should these factors be measured? Should they be measured continually? What is the diurnal variation of falls risk factors? The Falls BioRythms study carried out by the TRIL Centre is designed to answer some of these questions. This study assessed 20 fallers and 20 non-fallers in their homes for one day. Each subject was assessed for five falls risk factors (gait, balance, continuous blood pressure, heart rate variability and attention) at four time points throughout the day. Preliminary results from this study indicate more pronounced blood pressure drops in fallers following lunch. This finding has implications for the timing of clinical assessment, home monitoring, timing of medications and treatment of fallers.

Older people who fall are unlikely to label themselves as "fallers" and many do not hear this word until they interface with the health system following an injurious fall. Even those who are aware of the label "faller" are unwilling to apply it to themselves. It is not uncommon to hear a 70 year old, who has previously experienced an injurious fall to say "older people fall, not me". The social stigma associated with falling affects the reporting of falls and the uptake of falls interventions, often with negative consequences. It is not uncommon for health care professionals to be dismissive of falls –'what do you expect at your age?" (The Economist Intelligence Unit, 2009). If someone who frequently trips or stumbles does not consider themselves to be a faller, they are unlikely to receive treatment until a serious event occurs. If falling is destigmatized, use of falls prevention and prediction technology should in turn be destigmatized. Lack of knowledge of technology and lack of access to technology are common issues among older adults, and compliance with known technologies, such as falls alarms, is generally poor. There are many issues that affect compliance: many older adults fear that using falls technology labels them as "old", "incapable", or "frail"; the technology may be too complicated, difficult, or "boring" for them to use; or they may simply forget to use the device. Falls prevention is a life-long process so it is imperative to properly understand the factors that motivate a faller to carry an alarm as well as the factors that dissuade him/her from doing so. Ethnographic research and a collaborative user-centered design process are required to develop a device which users are motivated to use all day, every day, for the rest of their lives.

Solutions and Recommendations

Falls are inevitable and it is unlikely that any falls prevention or prediction strategy will be able to prevent the occurrence of all falls. It is therefore imperative that falls research focuses on reducing the impact of falls as well as reducing the occurrence of falls. Mechanical solutions such as hip protectors, soft floors and wearable airbags have all been implemented to distribute the force of an impact, thus preventing hip fractures. If a fall occurs, strategies such as getting up correctly following a fall or keeping warm until help arrives can reduce the side-effects associated with a long period of lying immobile. Multi-factorial interventions, which include tailored strength and balance program, medication review, and home modifications, have been shown to be the most successful method to reduce falls risk (Gillespie et al., 2009). However, if these interventions are not part of a lifelong lifestyle change, the risk of the individual falling will return to pre-intervention levels within months of ceasing the intervention. Patient compliance is one of the greatest challenges facing in-home interventions. Once the initial novelty of the intervention has abated, and the user feels that they have been "cured" of falling they are unlikely to maintain their new lifestyle. Interactive technology, which engages the user though tailored feedback, challenging targets and interaction with others may be the solution to this issue, as the unexpected adoption of the Wii platform by older adults demonstrates.

Screening for falls risk must become as common as screening for blood pressure among at-risk populations. This screening should be more sophisticated than simply asking "Did you fall in the last year?" as awareness and early treatment of the symptoms of falls risks could prevent a serious fall event from ever occurring. The latest AGS guidelines (American Geriatrics Society, in press), recommend that all older adults are screened for falls risk every 12 months, by asking if the individual (1) reported recurrent falls in the previous 12 months or had to seek medical attention following a fall, (2) has experienced difficulties in walking or balance, or (3) has a fear of falling. If the individual screens positive for any of these risk factors they are then referred for multi-factorial risk assessment. This screening mechanism is open to individual interpretation, particularly for those who have not fallen yet; thus many "worried well" individuals may be needlessly referred for further evaluation, while some who require evaluation may not be referred. An objective, repeatable, and reproducible screening tool for assessing falls risk is clearly required. Unfortunately, "no prospective study has been published that permits selection of a specific test of balance and gait, nor is there adequate validation of cut-off score for any of the tests for identification of future falls" (American Geriatrics Society, in press). A large, longitudinal, prospective study is required to validate existing scales (e.g. Timed Up and Go, Berg Balance Scale, Performance-Orientated Mobility Assessment, or Gait Assessment) or to develop a new falls risk assessment tool. This study should periodically assess the user's falls risk, over a period of years, to track improvements\decline in their scores. Supplementing these assessments with sensors will improve objectivity, ensure repeatability and reproducibility, and perhaps extract new features from these assessments which could not be measured otherwise. An objective screening tool, which has been proven to predict increased falls risk, could prevent a serious fall by enabling early referral for specialist assessment and intervention.

The underlying mechanisms of falls are not well understood - what caused a person to fall at that particular time and at that particular place? Was it an intrinsic or extrinsic risk factor or an accumulation of risk factors? Currently, we prescribe interventions based on the retrospective, and often self-reported, identification of risk factors which the individual has in common with other fallers. Whether these risk factors contributed to a particular fall event is not always clear. Large-scale, longitudinal research, which continuously monitors the main risk factors for falling, is required to further understand the mechanism of falls. While gait and heart rate can be readily assessed through kinematic and ECG sensors worn on or embedded in clothing, continuous neurological measurement would require visible sensors, which may dissuade potential subjects from wearing them, and there is currently no method for the continuous measurement of beat-to-beat blood pressure. Availability of an unobtrusive, beat-to-beat, 24hr continuous ambulatory blood pressure monitoring device would greatly enhance our knowledge of cardiovascular falls mechanisms. Meanwhile, a comprehensive, well-defined study measuring gait and heart rate continuously over a period of one year would help us identify the mechanisms leading to falls and whether or not these mechanisms were identified as risk factors during "care as usual". In addition, such a study could help to determine which parameters are worth tracking and which are not, the time and frequency of measurements, and to identify the diurnal variation of falls risk factors. Successful completion of such a study would rely heavily on the design of the sensor technology: it must be discreet, comfortable, and easy to use to ensure 24-hour compliance for an extended period.

It is clear that many fundamental research questions regarding falls still remain. To answer these questions, it is important that a collaborative, multi-disciplinary approach is taken. The TRIL Centre is a coordinated collection of research projects addressing the physical, cognitive and social consequences of ageing, all informed by ethnographic research and supported by a shared pool of knowledge and engineering resources. Active research collaboration between engineering, ethnographic and clinical disciplines challenges preconceptions, inspires new viewpoints, and helps to ensure that the faller's best interests are central to all decisions.

Until recently, technology development for biomedical research required significant hardware and software development time before a hypothesis could be tested. Advances in reusable and interoperable sensors such as the SHIMMER platform (McGrath & Dishongh, 2009), modular software platforms, for example, the free BioMOBIUS platform (McGrath & Dishongh, 2009) and standards for interoperability of medical devices (the Continua Health Alliance) have enabled rapid development of research prototypes to test clinical hypotheses, thus maximizing the time spent answering the research question and reducing the need for new technology.

FUTURE RESEARCH DIRECTIONS

Prospective validation of a falls risk assessment scale is an important step in identifying people requiring further assessment and measuring improvements/decline in their risk of falling following interventions. A sensor-based risk assessment scale is preferable as it would ensure objective, repeatable and reproducible measurements. A first step in achieving this task is to objectively measure existing falls risk scales using sensors to identify which parameters give these scales their predictive strength. These parameters must be measured several times over a number of years in a large older cohort and an appropriate threshold measure must be identified at which further assessment of falls risk and supervised intervention will be required. These parameters must be incorporated into screening tools which are suitable for use by frontline healthcare staff. Early identification and treatment of falls risks might prevent a fall from occurring, thus preventing the physical, financial, and emotional costs of falling.

Self-management of falls risk will become more important as healthcare resources are increasingly stretched. A method of assessing falls risk and educating individuals on falls risk and interventions must be developed for the general population. In healthy individuals who are at low risk of falling, this system might be as simple as a factsheet\webpage that gives older adults a number of simple balance tasks to assess their own falls risk. If they are unable to perform these tasks, they should be prompted to seek further assessment by a doctor. For those who have been diagnosed as having an increased risk of falling, a tailored in-home intervention and monitoring package might be developed to measure individual risk factors, such as blood pressure, and interventions such as medication prompting may be supported. If this is a telemonitoring package, results from this monitoring and intervention package can be remotely viewed by a healthcare professional, who can intervene if an increased falls risk is detected.

Hybrid fall alarms, which combine automated fall detection and an alarm button, should replace manual alarm systems. Falls alarms are a vital tool for recurrent fallers; however their indiscreet design, limited coverage, and the incidence of false alarms affect compliance with these devices. Improved compliance is therefore dependent on practical and discreet design, support for mobile telephony, and improved algorithm development. Ideally, alarms could predict the onset of a falls event and warn the faller in real-time or near real-time of an increased risk of falling, thus allowing them to take protective measures and prevent injury. However, until the mechanics of falls are fully understood, through continuous recording of multiple parameters before, during and after a fall event, prediction of a falls event is still in the future.

CONCLUSIONS

Rapid global aging means that societies or economies can no longer afford "usual care". Technology can support and enable large scale studies required to answer outstanding questions about falls. As the ratio of clinical resources to older adults requiring those resources increases, technology will be necessary to streamline clinical assessments while maintaining quality of care. The aging baby-boomer generation will have the technical literacy and desire to educate themselves and self-manage their falls risks, but technology must be in place for them to do so. Front-line medical staff will require screening technology to identify those requiring a referral to specialist assessment centers. To achieve significant reduction in falls incidence, a holistic life-long approach combining cognitive, social and physical activities will be required. The challenges are significant; but with close collaboration between fallers, falls experts, and technical experts they are achievable.

REFERENCES

Alwan, M., Rajendran, P. J., Kell, S., Mack, D., Dalal, S., Wolfe, M., et al. (2006). *A Smart and Passive Floor-Vibration Based Fall Detector for Elderly.* Paper presented at the 2nd IEEE Information and Communication Technologies.

American Geriatrics Society, British Geriatrics Society, and American Academy of Orthopaedic Surgeons Panel on Falls Prevention. (in press). Guideline for the prevention of falls in older persons. *Journal of the American Geriatrics Society.*

Aminian, K., & Najafi, B. (2004). Capturing human motion using body-fixed sensors: outdoor measurement and clinical applications. *Computer Animation and Virtual Worlds*, *15*(2), 79–94. doi:10.1002/cav.2

Azkoitia, J. M. (2004). Mobile monitoring and automatic fall detection device for elderly people living alone. Retrieved February 23rd, 2009, from http://cordis.europa.eu/fetch?CALLER=FP6_PROJ&ACTION=D&DOC=1&CAT=PROJ&QUERY=011fa7ae372c:d909:4196ac8c&RCN=72186.

Barton, J., & Jung, E. (2009). Distributed, Embedded Sensor and Actuator Platforms. In *Ambient Intelligence with Microsystems* (pp. 105-129).

Besser, M. P., Selby-Silverstein, L., & Prickett, N. (2001). Predicting Fall Risk in the Elderly Using Temporal-Spatial Parameters of Gait. *Symposium of the International Society for Postural and Gait Research*, 70-73.

Bilney, B., Morris, M., & Webster, K. (2003). Concurrent related validity of the GAITRite® walkway system for quantification of the spatial and temporal parameters of gait. *Gait & Posture*, *17*(1), 68–74. doi:10.1016/S0966-6362(02)00053-X

BioMOBIUS. (2009). Retrieved February 15th, from http://www.biomobius.org.

Cappozzo, A., Della Croce, U., Leardini, A., & Chiari, L. (2005). Human movement analysis using stereophotogrammetry: Part 1: theoretical background. *Gait & Posture*, *21*(2), 186–196. doi:10.1016/S0966-6362(04)00025-6

Carnaz, L., Oliveira, A. B., Sato, T. O., Hansson, G. A., & Coury, H. (2008). Effects of sensor, trials and knee joint variables on electrogoniometric gait recordings. *Revista Brasileira de Fisioterapia*, *12*(6), 460–467. doi:10.1590/S1413-35552008005000008

Charnwood Dynamics Ltd. Codamotion. Retrieved February 24, 2009, from http://www.codamotion.com

Connect America. Medical Alarm and Medical Alert Systems. Retrieved February 23, 2009, from http://medicalalarm.com/.

Daniele, G. (2006). Investigation of fall-risk using a wearable device with accelerometers and rate gyroscopes. *Physiological Measurement*, *27*, 1081–1090. doi:10.1088/0967-3334/27/11/003

Doukas, C., & Maglogiannis, I. (2008). *Advanced patient or elder fall detection based on movement and sound data.* Paper presented at the Second International Conference on Pervasive Computing Technologies for Healthcare. Emporia Life Plus. Retrieved 15th January 2010, from http://www2.emporia.at/en/home/.

Finapres Medical Systems. *Finometer*. Retrieved January 2010, from http://www.finapres.com/site/page/2/10/Finometer_PRO/.

Giansanti, D., Maccioni, G., & Macellari, V. (2005). The development and test of a device for the reconstruction of 3-D position and orientation by means of a kinematic sensor assembly with rate gyroscopes and accelerometers. *IEEE Transactions on Bio-Medical Engineering*, *52*(7), 1271–1277. doi:10.1109/TBME.2005.847404

Gillespie, L. D., Robertson, M. C., Gillespie, W. J., Lamb, S. E., & Cumming Robert, G, & H, R. B. (2009). Interventions for preventing falls in older people living in the community. *Cochrane Database of Systematic Reviews*, 2.

Hendrie, D., Hall, S. E., Legge, M., & Arena, G. (2003). *Injury in Western Australia: The Health System Costs of Falls in Older Adults in Western Australia.* Perth, Western Australia: Western Australian Government. Intelesens. Vitalsens. Retrieved January, 2010, from http://www.intelesens.com/.

Kannus, P., Palvanen, M., Niemi, S., & Parkkari, J. (2007). Alarming Rise in the Number and Incidence of Fall-Induced Cervical Spine Injuries among Older Adults. *The Journals of Gerontology. Series A, Biological Sciences and Medical Sciences*, *62*(2), 180–183.

Lamb, S. E., Hauer, K., & Becker, C. (2007). Manual for the fall prevention classification system. (Publication. Retrieved January 15, 2010 from www.profane.eu.org/profane_documents/Falls_Taxonomy.pdf.

Lee, S. J., & Hidler, J. (2008). Biomechanics of overground vs. treadmill walking in healthy individuals. *Journal of Applied Physiology (Bethesda, Md.)*, *104*(3), 747–755. doi:10.1152/japplphysiol.01380.2006

Litvak, D., Gannot, I., & Zigel, Y. (2008). *Detection of falls at home using floor vibrations and sound.* Paper presented at the IEEE 25th Convention of Electrical and Electronics Engineers in Israel.

Lo, B. (2005a). *From Imaging Networks to Behavior Profiling: Ubiquitous Sensing for Managed Homecare of the Elderly*. Paper presented at the 3rd International Conference on Pervasive Computing.

Lo, B. (2005b). *UbiSense – Ubiquitous IR Sensing and Behaviour Profiling for the Care of the Elderly and Chronically-ill Patient.* Paper presented at the 2nd International Workshop on Body Sensor Networks.

Lord, S. R., Sherrington, C., Menz, H. B., & Close, J. C. T. (2007). *Falls in Older People: Risk Factors and Strategies for Prevention* (2nd ed.). Cambridge University Press. doi:10.1017/CBO9780511722233

Lorincz, K., Kuris, B., Ayer, S. M., Patel, S., Bonato, P., & Welsh, M. (2007). *Wearable wireless sensor network to assess clinical status in patients with neurological disorders.* Paper presented at the Proceedings of the 6th international conference on Information processing in sensor networks.

Mayagoitia, R. E., Nene, A. V., & Veltink, P. H. (2002). Accelerometer and rate gyroscope measurement of kinematics: an inexpensive alternative to optical motion analysis systems. *Journal of Biomechanics*, *35*(4), 537–542. doi:10.1016/S0021-9290(01)00231-7

McGrath D, Greene B, O'Neill R, & B., C. (2009). *SHIMMER: A new tool for long-term, extra-laboratory gait monitoring*. Paper presented at the European Society for Movement Analysis in Adults and Children 2009.

McGrath, M. J., & Dishongh, T. (2009). A Common Personal Health Research Platform - SHIMMER(TM) and BioMOBIUS(TM). *Enabling Healthcare in the Home*, *13*(3), 122–147.

Medtronic. Reveal® DX Insertable Cardiac Monitor. Retrieved January, 2010, from http://www.medtronic.com/physician/reveal/index.html.

Moe-Nilssen, R. (1998). Test-retest reliability of trunk accelerometry during standing and walking. *Archives of Physical Medicine and Rehabilitation*, *79*(11), 1377–1385. doi:10.1016/S0003-9993(98)90231-3

Monaghan, K., Delahunt, E., & Caulfield, B. (2006). Ankle function during gait in patients with chronic ankle instability compared to controls. *Clinical Biomechanics (Bristol, Avon)*, *21*(2), 168–174. doi:10.1016/j.clinbiomech.2005.09.004

Narayanan, M. R., Lord, S. R., Budge, M. M., & Branko, G. Celler, & Lovell, N. H. (2007). *Falls Management: Detection and Prevention, using a Waistmounted Triaxial Accelerometer.* Paper presented at the 29th Annual International Conference of the IEEE EMBS, Lyon, France.

National Institute for Clinical Excellence (NICE). (2004). *Falls. The Assessment and Prevention of Falls in Older People*. London: National Collaborating Centre for Nursing and Supportive Care.

Nurmi, I., & Lüthje, P. (2002). Incidence and costs of falls and fall injuries among elderly in institutional care. *Scandinavian Journal of Primary Health Care*, *20*(2), 118–122.

Nyan, M. N., Tay, F. E. H., & Murugasu, E. (2008). A wearable system for pre-impact fall detection. *Journal of Biomechanics*, *41*(16), 3475–3481. doi:10.1016/j.jbiomech.2008.08.009

O'Donovan, K., Dishongh, T., Foran, T., Leahy, D., & Ni Scanaill, C. (2008). *The Development of a Clinical Gait Analysis System*. Paper presented at the International Conference on Ambulatory Monitoring of Physical Activity and Movement.

O'Donovan, K. J., Greene, B. R., McGrath, D., O'Neill, R., Burns, A., & Caulfield, B. (2009). *SHIMMER: A new tool for temporal gait analysis*. Paper presented at the Engineering in Medicine and Biology Society, 2009. EMBC 2009. Annual International Conference of the IEEE.

O'Sullivan, M., Blake, C., Cunningham, C., Boyle, G., & Finucane, C. (2009). Correlation of accelerometry with clinical balance tests in older fallers and non-fallers. *Age and Ageing*, afp009.

Patel, S., Lorincz, K., Hughes, R., Huggins, N., & Growdon, J. H. Matt Welsh, et al. (2007). *Analysis of Feature Space for Monitoring Persons with Parkinson's Disease With Application to a Wireless Wearable Sensor.* Paper presented at the 29th Annual International Conference of the IEEE EMBS, Lyon, France.

Philips. (n.d.). Lifeline. Retrieved February 23, 2009, from http://www.lifelinesys.com/.

Philips. (n.d.). Philips Lifeline Tempo Watch. Retrieved February 26, 2009, from http://www.lifelinesys.com/content/lifeline-products/tempo-watch.jsp.

Piriyaprasarth, P., Morris, M., Winter, A., & Bialocerkowski, A. (2008). The reliability of knee joint position testing using electrogoniometry. *BMC Musculoskeletal Disorders*, *9*(1), 6. doi:10.1186/1471-2474-9-6

Profane. (n.d.). ProFaNE Clinical Assessment Tool (CAT) Publication. Retrieved January 15 2010 http://www.profane.eu.org/CAT/.

Rajendran, P., Corcoran, A., Kinosian, B., & Alwan, M. (2008). Falls, Fall Prevention, and Fall Detection Technologies. In *Eldercare Technology for Clinical Practitioners* (pp. 187-202).

Ross, A. C., Adam, L. B., Yonghao, P., Paul, M., Kim, B., & Michael, H. (2009). Validity and reliability of the Nintendo Wii Balance Board for assessment of standing balance. *Gait & posture*.

Sherrington, C., & Whitney, J., C., R. Lord, S., Herbert, R., D., Cumming, R., G., & Close, J. C. T. (2008). Effective Exercise for the Prevention of Falls: A Systematic Review and Meta-Analysis. *Journal of the American Geriatrics Society*, *56*(12), 2234–2243. doi:10.1111/j.1532-5415.2008.02014.x

Sixsmith, A., & Johnson, N. (2004). A smart sensor to detect the falls of the elderly. *Pervasive Computing, IEEE*, *3*(2), 42–47. doi:10.1109/MPRV.2004.1316817

The Economist Intelligence Unit. (2009). *Healthcare strategies for an ageing society*.

Tyson, S. F., & Connell, L. A. (2009). How to measure balance in clinical practice. A systematic review of the psychometrics and clinical utility of measures of balance activity for neurological conditions. *Clinical Rehabilitation*, *23*(9), 824–840. doi:10.1177/0269215509335018

Wang, L., Hu, W., & Tan, T. (2003). Recent developments in human motion analysis. *Pattern Recognition*, *36*(3), 585–601. doi:10.1016/S0031-3203(02)00100-0

Wherton, J., & Prendergast, D. (2009). Involving Older Adults in the Design of a Communication Technology to Support Peer-to-Peer Social Engagement. In *HCI and Usability for e-Inclusion* (pp. 111–134). The Building Bridges Project. doi:10.1007/978-3-642-10308-7_8

World Health Organization. (2008). *WHO global report on falls prevention in older age*. Geneva.

Zijlstra, G. A. R., van Haastregt, J. C. M., van Eijk, J. T. M., van Rossum, E., Stalenhoef, P. A., & Kempen, G. I. J. M. (2007). Prevalence and correlates of fear of falling, and associated avoidance of activity in the general population of community-living older people. *Age and Ageing*, *36*(3), 304–309. doi:10.1093/ageing/afm021

Zijlstra, W., & Aminian, K. (2007). Mobility assessment in older people: new possibilities and challenges. *European Journal of Ageing*, *4*, 3–12. doi:10.1007/s10433-007-0041-9

ADDITIONAL READING

Alwan, M., & Felder, R. A. (2008). *Eldercare Technology for Clinical Practitioners* (1st ed.). Humana Press. doi:10.1007/978-1-59745-233-5

Darowski, A. (2008). *Falls: The Facts* (1st ed.). OUP Oxford.

Lord, S. R., Sherrington, C., Menz, H. B., & Close, J. C. T. (2007). *Falls in Older People: Risk Factors and Strategies for Prevention* (2nd ed.). Cambridge University Press. doi:10.1017/CBO9780511722233

World Health Organization. (2008). WHO global report on falls prevention in older age. Geneva.

Chapter 5
The Use of Assistive Technology to Support the Wellbeing and Independence of People with Memory Impairments

Claire Huijnen
Smart Homes, The Netherlands

ABSTRACT

This chapter presents the research, results and lessons learned from a project to evaluate currently available assisted living technologies for elderly people with mild to severe memory impairments who want to age in place. During the project a number of households were equipped with assistive technology to enable the end users to better cope with the barriers and problems associated with their forgetfulness. End users were involved in different phases, starting with a problem and needs analysis and ending with an evaluation of the technology installed in their homes. It seemed that technology did have a positive impact on their lives as well as on the lives of the informal caregivers who often live with those who suffer from amnesia. This project gives insight into how we are coming closer to optimizing the positive effects which assistive technology holds for the elderly with memory impairments. Key insights are presented.

INTRODUCTION

In many European countries, including The Netherlands, the proportion of elderly people in the total population is growing rapidly. Simultaneously, care resources are shrinking. Many elderly people want to live independently in their own homes (age in place) for as long as possible despite the presence of age-related difficulties including memory impairments or early dementia. Low cost, low maintenance innovations are needed to enable people to retain their independence in a secure, safe and inclusive environment for as long as possible. A generally agreed upon vision is that assistive technology has the potential to make a contribution to the demographic challenges of the ageing population (Maciuszek, Aberg, & Shahmehri, 2005).

The study outlined in this chapter sought to empower elderly with memory impairments. The aim of the research was to gain insight into how to increase people's independence by assisting

DOI: 10.4018/978-1-61520-825-8.ch005

them to live in their own homes for longer periods of time. Assistive technologies were installed in homes and evaluated.

BACKGROUND

In common with other developed regions, the European Union is experiencing rapid growth among its ageing population. The European Commission's statistical reporting (2004) shows that in 2003 there were 74 million people aged 65 and over in the EU-25, compared with only 38 million in 1960. Life expectancy has increased considerably during the last 40 years, and by 2050 projections show that one third of Europe's population will be over the age of 60. Growth among the 80 years and older cohort will be particularly strong during the next few years. This unprecedented growth will have significant implications for the state of health of Europeans and pose distinct challenges to health and social care systems (European Commission, 2004). Moreover, in 2010, around one-third (32%) of the EU-15 elderly population (aged 65 and over) will be living alone. More than half (54%) will live with a partner (in a household that might also include children or adults). The remainder will live with children (or other relatives/friends) or in a home/institution. It is clear, however, that the demand for housing and care will continue to change considerably as people grow older.

Dementia is one of the diseases associated with ageing. Dementia is a brain disorder in which a progressive loss can be seen in affected areas, such as cognition, memory and learning, language and problem solving. Changes in personality are often reported as well. Dementia places a heavy burden on both the patient and carer. Typically, people with dementia are disoriented in time, place and person. They experience progressive cognitive impairments that start with working memory problems but can encompass speech production, planning, monitoring and visiospatial difficulties as the condition advances (Alzheimer Nederland, 2009).

The prevalence of dementia in Europe is around 2% for those aged 65-70, and doubles with every five year increase in age, reaching around 25-30% for all those aged 85 years and over (Lobo et al., 2000). In The Netherlands 250,000 people are suffering from dementia of whom 180,000 are actually diagnosed with dementia (Alzheimer Nederland, 2009). This means that there are estimated to be 70,000 people who experience symptoms and problems caused by dementia, but who have not yet been diagnosed with the disease. It is estimated that in 2020 there will be 350,000 people with dementia and in 2050 this will most likely increase to 580,000 people. Seventy percent of the people with dementia, in The Netherlands, live at home and receive care from family or close friends (Alzheimer Nederland, 2009).

However, another demographic trend, the decrease in the working population, compounds societal difficulties associated with the rising incidence of dementia and the burden of care faced by informal caregivers. In 2008 there were 57 potential working people for every demented person. In 2050 this number is expected to fall to 27 (Alzheimer Nederland, 2009). An almost inevitable consequence of this decrease is that there will be fewer qualified people to care for the increasing numbers of people who are in need of care.

Aging in Place

The home is an important symbol of a person's identity and personality. Oswald, Wahl, Naumann, Mollenkopf and Hieber (2006) note that older people perceive the danger of losing their homes as akin to losing an important part of themselves. They use the "environmental proactivity" hypothesis to explain the actions of older adults in adapting their homes to their changing needs, in order to maintain control and enhance competence in the house. For example, the residents themselves decide the preferred sites for positioning important objects in the home such as remote controls, TV, and telephone. Oswald et al. (2006) reinforce the point that with the aging process the home acquires other meanings and values due to the increased time spent at home, as well as the many activities that take place there.

People with early dementia clearly are confronted with considerable practical obstacles when it comes to aging in place. They face increasing difficulties in performing activities of daily living (Gill & Kurland, 2003) and may also experience diminished quality of life, poor self-esteem, anxiety and social isolation (Burns & Rabins, 2000). Any of these can result in their early relocation to residential care settings. However, they are also strongly dependent on others in the physical and psychological sense (Kitwood, 1998) and the strain imposed on informal caregivers can lead to the premature relocation of people with dementia to residential care settings. In the Netherlands 82% of all informal carers for demented persons report their burden of care is already too great or they are at high risk of becoming overloaded (Alzheimer Nederland, 2009). The inability of carers to cope is one of the main reasons for early institutionalisation of people with dementia.

Assistive Technologies and Aging in Place

People who suffer from dementia and who wish to age in place are often not well supported by technological products or services. Housing adaptation often goes only as far as structural or fixed adjustments such as ramps, accessible bathrooms or safer stairs. Examples of assistive environments exist, but they are mainly in experimental phases supported by universities or other institutions (Metsis, Le, Lei, & Makedon, 2008). High-technology has become pervasive in many hospitals, but domestic environments remain essentially low-tech and conventional, despite the care needs of the aging population who desire to age in place (Green, Walker, & Brooks, 2009). Where assistive technologies are used in the domestic environment they mainly involve commonly used products such as walking aids or personal alarms. However, there are many other assistive devices that have the potential to increase the wellbeing, safety and independence of people with dementia as well as their caregivers.

Assistive technologies have developed rapidly in recent years and it seems likely that they will play an important role in helping to address some of the challenges associated with an aging society. People who are aging cognitively often face a decline in their ability to perform activities of daily living, such as eating, cleaning, preparing meals and self-care. Assistive technologies can help people in these basic daily tasks, for example, "reminder devices" which provide cognitively impaired people with suitable prompts to help them with decision making and guide them through everyday tasks (Mann, 2004; Woolham & Frisby, 2002a). Astell, Ellis, and Alm (2004) showed that a touch screen could assist demented people to actively direct a conversation without having to rely on caregivers. Daniel, Cason and Ferrell, (2009) describe other devices which are able to safely prolong an elderly person's ability to live independently, or with minimal assistance.

A system such as the Gator-Tech Smart Home is a home that has a smart floor with pressure sensors in the floor that tracks the movement and location of the resident in the home (Johnson, Davenport, and Mann, 2007). The home triggers an alarm or queries when no movement is detected after a certain period of time. In a feasibility study in the UK conducted by Goodacre, McCreadie, Flanagan, and Lansley (2008), various adaptations were made to existing homes to increase the safety of seniors and thus allow them to remain in their homes longer. Based on individual needs, recommendations were made such as making personalized door handles, installing amplifiers on door bells and telephones, installing grab rails and handrails in appropriate locations, installing ramps, stair lifts, external lighting with passive infra-red, lowered light switches, raised electrical outlets, level thresholds, wider doors and corridors, and electric window and door openers. More examples of use of assistive technologies and related work are provided by Daniel, Cason and Ferrell (2009).

Hawkey, Inkpen, Rockwood, McAllister, and Slonim (2005) indicate that some of the assistive systems primarily monitor the elderly for safety and assurance purposes and that cognitive orthotic systems provide aids for people with reduced cognitive abilities such as dementia. Astell (2005) argues that technology can benefit people with dementia perhaps more than it can benefit people without cognitive impairments. It is important to note, however, that designing assistive technology for the home poses specific challenges. Bell, Blythe, Gaver, Sengers and Wright (2003) caution that workplace technologies that have been effectively introduced into the workforce to meet well understood principles and methodologies cannot simply be transferred to the domestic environment in the belief that they will be equally effective there. They describe the home as a private and intimate place where artifacts and technologies are "embedded within an ecology that is rich with meaning and nuance" (p. 1062). Therefore, issues such as emotion, affection, pleasure, and aesthetics must be considered if new technologies are to be effectively used in the home. These personal considerations about the home emphasize the importance of a holistic approach to assistive technologies in the home, an approach in which the user, the objects and the context of use are integrated into a network of actions and interactions.

Although people with memory impairments show a decrease in their learning abilities, they are still able to adjust to new objects or to learn some new things at the onset of memory impairment. Therefore, if the technology is to be effectively used to assist them to age in place, it is important that they become accustomed to its use, and understand the device or service before their memory becomes seriously impaired. In other words, efforts need to be made to bridge a grey digital divide that may be associated with new assistive technologies, early in the disease onset stage. The digital divide is not only about the possession of ICT but also the ability to use ICT. An assistive environment can be successful only if the target users are actually willing to adopt it (Metsis, Le, Lei, & Makedon, 2008).

PROJECT AIM AND MAJOR OBJECTIVES

Olivier, Xu, Monk and Hoey (2009) argue that the literature on assisted technologies contains many proposals for the use of technology to support people with dementia but few have been implemented as research prototypes, and none are in everyday use. With this in mind, the main aim of our project was to increase the understanding of how assistive technology and smart living can support people with memory impairments and their caregivers to maintain an independent and pleasant lifestyle in the home environment.

A number of main objectives were formulated to:

- Understand what appropriate technology is currently available for installation in people's homes, and learn more about how people with memory impairments and their formal and informal caregivers adapt to and use these products and services
- Assess whether installing technology in the early phases of memory problems results in retention of users' independence and common daily activities for an extended period and delays their hospitalization
- Gain more insight into the effects of assistive technology on informal caregivers, particularly whether they are able to extend the duration of their informal care.

MULTIDISCIPLINARITY AND PROJECT PHASES

The design of the study called for collaboration between a number of partners who would not normally work together in daily life. The partners consisted of researchers from an expertise centre for smart living and housing, a care provider, and two (technical) installation companies. This multidisciplinary team brought with them disparate areas of expertise that had to be integrated in an ethical and sensitive way throughout the course of the study. Areas of expertise included:

- Smart living, technology and physical housing adaptations
- Dementia and the consequences of this disease to daily living
- Installation of assistive technology in the home environments of the patients.

The project involved the following phases:

- selection of participants
- needs analysis and personalized selection of technology
- installation in homes
- explanation and training
- evaluation and assessment.

Each of these phases will now be discussed.

Selection of Participants

Forty participants with psycho-geriatric symptoms were selected to participate in the study by the care provider. Participants were selected on the basis that:

- they experience cognitive and memory impairments and restrictions in daily life and activities due to memory impairments
- they and their caregivers agreed to participate
- cognitive impairments were not caused by an acute disfunctioning of the brain.

These selection criteria allowed for people with dementia as well as people with mild cognitive impairment to take part in the study.

Needs Analysis and Personalized Selection of Technology

After the 40 participants had been selected, it became clear that all had memory impairments and cognitive problems in common. However, these impairments caused different impacts and problems in daily living for different people and so required different solutions. A needs analysis phase was conducted to get more insight into potential needs and solutions. Semi-structured interviews took place at the homes of the participants. An employee of the care provider led interviews with the participants and their informal caregiver. The main goal of these sessions was to determine in what domains of daily life the participants were impaired. These domains of daily life were categorized as:

- Independence. This entailed actions such as daily care and personal hygiene, the use of public transport, and communication activities. These included all kinds of actions that normally could be done automatically without too much effort in order to maintain the welfare and wellbeing of the participants.
- Productivity. This included actions that are carried out to enable people to make a contribution to society and/or their family.
- Relaxation. This entailed activities that people like to do, such as sport, games, parties and similar activities.

Every individual leads a different life and memory impairments cause different problems for different people. The results of the needs analysis

Table 1. Assistive technology categories and examples of devices

Category	Explanation
Automatic lighting	Lighting is triggered by sensors detecting movement and they automatically go out after a certain time. A toilet route can be established by placing the sensors and lights in such a manner that lights are automatically lit when the person walks towards the bathroom.
Sanitary	Examples are automatic flushing toilets, a shower with an automatic temperature setting, automatic taps, automatic air control in the bathroom and toilet.
Kitchen	Gas detection, smoke detectors, and automatic gas shut off in the hob.
Structure and day planning	Automatic medication box as a prompt to taking medication properly, calendar clock, whiteboards, computer programs for activity and day planning and overview.
Communication	Pictophone that provides easy dialling option, mobile phone designed for seniors, connection of phone to light signal in case of impaired hearing, video communication, memo recorder as memory aid.
Safety	Detection for wandering, electronic locks, GPS system.
Fall detection and social alarms	Fall detectors and alarms that people carry in case they are in need of help.

and interviews provided concise and personalized notes and alerts which were provided to all project partners. Where possible, the partners were also given notes that described participants' actions and the coping strategies they adopted. A personalized selection of appropriate technology was made in order to meet individual needs. The technology was chosen with the following criteria in mind:

- Physical, cognitive and social abilities of the participant
- Functioning in areas of independent living, productivity and relaxation
- Current areas of interest of both participant and caregiver
- Physical and social environmental aspects
- Burden on, and capabilities of caregivers.

A range of suitable technologies was identified through this process. The range included products which the user needed to learn how to use, for example an application on a computer with a diary function. There were also products that are triggered without the conscious action of the user. Examples of these are automatic lighting and automatic toilet flushing. Finally, there were products that stimulated actions stemming from habits and automatic patterns; for example, placing a ring in a particular manner would stimulate correct posture at the toilet..

Table 1 lists main product categories and examples used in this study.

Figure 1 shows the range and number of products installed and evaluated.

Installation in Homes

Once the needs analysis had identified the appropriate products and technologies, these could be ordered and subsequently installed in participants' homes. However, unexpected delays in delivery times of some parts or products led to practical difficulties with this phase. When dealing with persons with dementia, time can be of great importance because the disease often progresses rapidly.

When making appointments with the participants to install the products in their homes it was important that the installation personnel were sensitive to traits of the target group in general and the specific habits and requirements of individuals in particular. Attention was paid to the location and position of the devices as they were installed. Where possible, the end users decided on the location for the products so they would match their home and their habits. In addition, a number of practical aspects had to be taken into account.

Figure 1. Products that were evaluated, and number of users

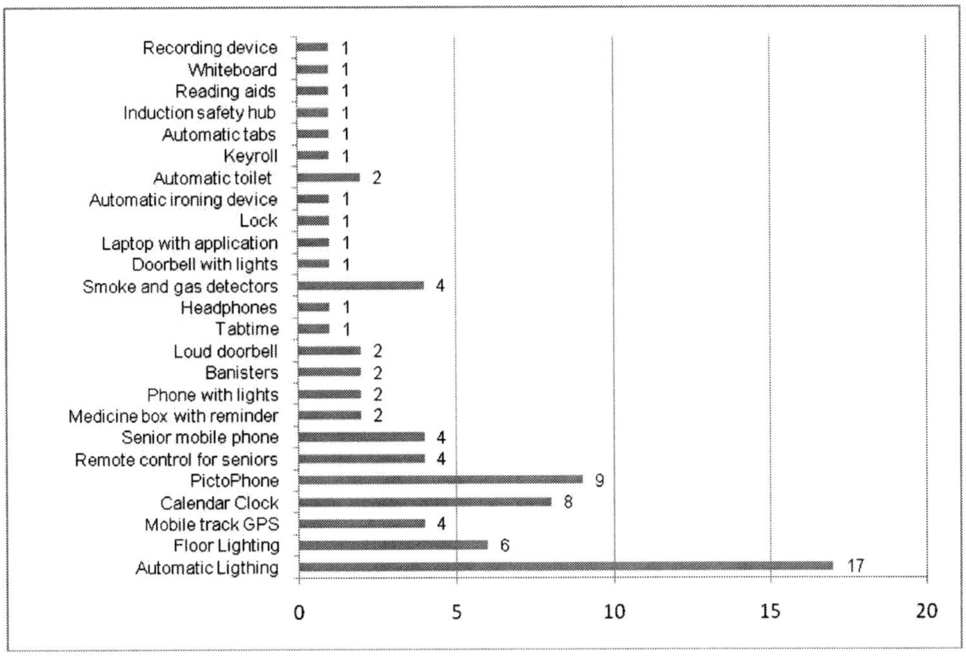

For example, many older people had several care moments during the day, or periods of rest during which they were not to be disturbed.

EXPLANATION AND TRAINING

As soon as the technology was installed, an appointment was made to explain the product and its use. Some training was given if needed. It was important to create a good first impression and dispel fears that participants might have about using the products. In a number of cases, additional support was needed, for example to make some adjustments in the home, or to answer questions about the use of the product.

The explanation given was tailored to the cognitive level of the participant, which required multiple visits for some. The repetition of information and the creation of many moments for practice were important. This was also of value to the researchers because, during the implementation phase, it was important for them to have a detailed knowledge of cognitive problems, communicative skills, learning styles and compensation strategies.

EVALUATION AND ASSESSMENT OF IMPACT ON LIFE

After a period of using these technologies, varying from a number of weeks to months, the use and experiences were evaluated in all households. Discussions and interviews were held with both the care recipient as well as the informal caregiver in order to get more information about people's opinions, attitudes and effects of the technology on their lives. A number of research questions were formulated during this evaluation phase:

- Is the assistive technology easy to use?
- What difficulties, problems, and barriers occurred?
- Did people use the technology regularly?

- What are the perceptions of both the person with memory impairments and of the care giver?
- What is the effect of the technology on people's independency, their wellbeing, their feelings of safety and quality of life?
- Does the technology promote a feeling of independent living?
- Did people stop using particular technologies, and if so, why?

At the start of the project 40 households participated in the project. By the time of the evaluation phase six households had withdrawn. The main reason for their withdrawal was related to health, for example, when participants' health had deteriorated significantly and they had to be hospitalized. Unfortunately one person died during the project.

The evaluations were undertaken by means of home visits and semi-structured interviews with the participants and their caregivers. During these home visits a short "home tour" was carried out to gain insights into how the users managed the installed technology.

When planning interviews we ensured that the person who would visit the participants during the evaluation phase was not the same person who had visited them during the needs analysis phase. This was to minimize the possibility of participants giving socially desirable answers to a person they believed to be in a position of responsibility for the project. Several times throughout the sequential phases we emphasized that the study was designed to test the technology and the products for ease and effectiveness of use, and we were not assessing the capacity of the participants to use the technology. That is, our aim was to help bridge the grey digital divide by improving the technology as opposed to skilling the participants.

We asked people to explain to us what technology they had and how and when they would use it. Furthermore, we asked them to tell us how it works. This gave further information into the difficulties and actual use in daily routines. Following these home tours, the interview took place focusing on the effect that the technology/products had on the daily lives of participants. To what extent did the aids contribute to their daily living, their perceived quality of life and their levels of independence? These effects and other results are described in the next section.

EVALUATION AND ASSESSMENT

One of the main objectives of the evaluation was to highlight the effects that technology had on users' daily lives. A second main objective was to obtain specific feedback on a number of issues, including product features. The main findings for both objectives will now be discussed.

Impact on Daily Life

A number of people mentioned that the effect on their lives was relatively small because the aids that they received could not make a difference to the lives of people with severe dementia. Others reported that they did experience some effects, and these are summarised in table 2.

The majority of the participants indicated that the support had the effect they had hoped for. A number of persons indicated that they expected more of the technology or were not able to use it. The following comments, which have been modified slightly during translation from Dutch to English, illustrate some of our findings.

- *"I think, generally speaking, that you need to start with these things earlier. Younger people (who are in their late fifties, early sixties) are much better with all these digital things. You see, he never had a computer and will never get one. All those kind of things are not interesting for him anymore. While if you apply smart living technologies to the group who are in their 60-65*

Table 2. Effect of technology on participants' lives

Effect of support on the life of the caregiver	Effect of support on the life of the person with memory impairments
Peace (at night in bed) and a feeling of increased control (for example, the carer knows that the light turns on automatically when the impaired person gets out of bed)	Less difficult to start to communicate (for some people making a phone call became increasingly problematic). With the images on the phone it is easier to call a person.
Convenience, less frustration and irritation, fewer confrontations (e.g. fewer questions about the time and day, or fewer actions needed to turn out the lights or turn off running taps)	Safer feeling, more prevention against falling.
Less inconvenience or annoyance for neighbours (e.g., due to noise produced by a TV that was too loud previously)	Independence, more autonomy, less dependent on caregiver (e.g. "I can look myself regardless of what time and what day it is")
Less need for checks (e.g. Are the lights and gas off? Is the tap still running?)	Fewer confrontations

they can learn to use it. Then you can have all kinds of practical solutions that are good for the caregivers and that can prolong independence."

- *"These are all small facilities, but every small thing can already make a contribution for me, these are amenities for me. I can imagine that this can be handy for healthy people as well, for example, a light that automatically turns on when you go to the toilet at night."*

The majority mentioned that the aids did have some contribution to their daily life. Their perceptions are summarized in Figure 2.

Many participants stated that the assistive technology had a positive influence on their independence and expressed the opinion that technology can prolong the period that people are able to live independently in their own homes. For example, automatic lighting decreases the risk of falling, which indirectly increases the chance that people can live longer at their home.

Participants also indicated that dementia is a severe and complex progressive disease that cannot be stopped by these aids. Having said this, many participants indicated that any help is welcome and appreciated. Some caregivers also observed that although products might be directed at the person with memory impairments they are, in fact, of more help to the caregivers (e.g., in terms of peace of mind, comfort, relief from the burden of care, less need for immediate action).

In the following section a number of specific technologies or products are discussed.

EVALUATION OF SPECIFIC TECHNOLOGIES OR PRODUCTS

We asked for participants' reactions to the frequency of use, the ease of use, the ease of learning to use the product, and the effect on the independence and quality of life of both the care recipient and the caregiver. The main points about three products are presented as follows.

Automatic Lighting

In total, 17 people reported their experiences with the automatic lighting. Sixteen out of 17 people used this device every day and night and most people had little difficulty learning to use it. One person had some difficulty which was caused by the fact that there was no manual switch available. At another household, the sensor was not installed properly in the bathroom. When the person with dementia was taking a shower, the sensor was not in range of the movements therefore the light switched off while the person was

Figure 2. Perceptions of the technology's assistance in daily life

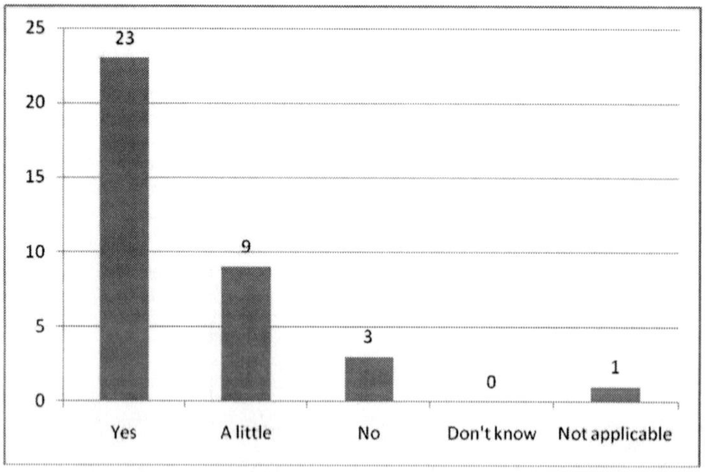

still in the shower. The person with dementia did not understand that this sensor could be manually adjusted and the caregiver had to help.

Another person was confused because he did not understand that he did not have to turn off the lights because of the automatic sensors. He did not want to leave the bathroom before the lights were off. During the project, we installed a manual light switch as well. If he remembered to turn off the lights he could do so, but if he forgot, the lights would automatically go out after a few minutes.

Half of the participants who used the lighting reported a positive effect on the independence of the care recipient and increased convenience for the caregiver. The other half mentioned that they did not experience an effect on their own independence, but could see benefits for the caregiver through less anxiety about checking whether lights were on or off.

Automatic Floor Lighting

The participants who received the automatic floor lighting used it daily. Because many people in care wake up during the night to go to the toilet, their caregivers experience poor quality of sleep. This is because caregivers are worried about the possibility of falls and they wake to help with turning on and off the lights. With this automatic floor light this becomes easier. One caregiver mentioned:

This is fantastic, because he gets out several times during the night. So then, the light automatically switches on. He walks very badly, so the lights in this room switch on and also in the hall." Another caregiver said: "before we had this I fully woke up, because I had to keep an eye on him, Now I am more at ease. I do still wake up, but am calmer now.

Calendar Clock

Eight persons reported their experiences with the calendar clock. Most of them used it at least once daily and usually more frequently. Even though this is a rather simple product showing the time, the day of the week, and the date, about half of the carers reported a positive effect on the independence and autonomy of the care recipient. Caregivers said that normally they would have to tell them the time and day several times a day. This can cause frustration and irritation which can be minimised when the calendar clock is used. One participant with memory impairments reported: "*I will forget the time and day in a few hours, but then I only have to look again*". A caregiver explained: "*sometimes she calls me to ask what time or day it is. This is not needed anymore with the clock*". Another informal caregiver observed: "*I cannot say that he really gets more independent, but it makes life more pleasant. He used to get up very early on a Sunday because he thought it was Monday and he had to go to day care. This does not happen now we have the new clock*". For half of the caregivers the burden has decreased. Two typical comments illustrate this point: "*It used to be frustrating sometimes because he had to ask so often that I thought to myself, 'I just told you that'* ", or another caregiver said about her husband: "*He became calmer, more at ease, and if he is at ease, I am as well*".

CONCLUSION

Reflecting on the outcomes of this project, a number of conclusions can be drawn.

Our study was not large enough to determine whether the assistive technologies definitively resulted in delays in hospitalization. However, a number of encouraging outcomes occurred.

The effect of the assistive technology on the independence and the quality of life varied considerably among participants and depended on the mental and physical condition of the person with memory impairments and the technology that was used. In a number of cases, the caregivers reported an increase in the autonomy, independence and quality of life of the care recipient and the caregiver. Moreover, in a number of cases, the informal caregivers reported that the use of certain aids led to a decrease in the burden and inconvenience of taking care of demented persons. In the cases where such an effect was not explicitly mentioned, people were positive about the support they got from the aids. In many cases people mentioned effects such as increased calmness, convenience, peacefulness and tranquility, minimization of dangerous situations, and feelings of decreased irritation and lessened emotional burden for both the care recipient and the caregiver.

These are positive signals. Most caregivers are very grateful for any kind of help or support that they can get in the difficult and emotionally charged situation that they are in when caring for a loved one. These are important findings for care recipients in particular; if the informal caregivers cannot cope anymore, then hospitalization is often the next step. It seems that certain assistive technologies are able to relieve some of the burden that carers experience and this may enable them to carry out their care tasks for longer and more effectively. The technology can support them in some tasks, freeing them to pay attention to others. For the wider society this can also have beneficial effects. Keeping people out of the formal system is much cheaper for tax payers,

Our findings suggest the need for additional research on the use of a number of specific aids which appear to have additional assistive potential. It was obvious that people were very keen on the automatic lighting functionalities. This function, which is triggered by unconscious movements/actions by people, helped participants a lot. The fact that the lights went off automatically also was a considerable help for some participants. The calendar clock meant a lot to a number of participants. Most of the remarks about this clock were positive in the sense that it provided substantial reassurance in the daily living of the person with dementia/amnesia. For the caregiver this was also beneficial because the care recipient did not ask so often for the time and day.

The "environmental proactivity" hypothesis discussed earlier (Oswald et al. 2006) makes it clear that older people need to be involved in the placement of everyday assistive technologies. For example, with the new clocks, our advice is to ask users where they would like their clock to be placed. They choose a familiar place where they are used to looking for a clock and therefore do not needlessly have to adapt to something new. Common sense actions such as consulting about the placement of assistive technologies are part of bridging the grey divide.

Although a number of aids were originally oriented or targeted for the person with amnesia, they seem to offer equally or greater support for the caregiver.

From the outset our team required a good understanding of the characteristics of people with dementia. As the study progressed it became clear that they also needed to be sensitive to the wishes and needs of caregivers. To generalize from our experiences, it seems important for other research groups who are working on similar problems, to establish open dialogue and communication both with the persons for whom the technology is primarily intended, and their caregivers. This is necessary in order to make certain adaptations that optimally tune the technology to the lives and habits of the people who are exposed to it. This is especially important in the case of dementia since many changes can occur during a month, both in the mental and physical skills of the users.

Taking into account the limited learning curve of people with dementia, it is essential that as much assistive technology as possible is installed when people are still in the mild cognitive impairment phase and able to adjust to new things. This may be easier said than done. The technical partners in this project reported that they needed considerable help and time to get used to, and familiar with, this target group. Normally, their clients know exactly what they want when they ask for their help in the area of smart living. Clearly our target group were not aware and independent, which required more time, patience and different expertise than the technical partners were accustomed to providing.

It seems likely that there are no standard solutions for people with dementia. Every household and every individual is different and the technologies and products have to be individualized in most cases.

In our study, a number of products did not seem to function as advertised. Moreover, it is clear that a number of problems cannot yet be solved by available technologies that purport to provide a specific solution. Technologically speaking, a considerable number of improvements and developments are still to be made. There appear to remain numerous opportunities for the development of products that help to bridge the grey divide in assistive technologies.

RECOMMENDATIONS

A number of recommendations which arise from this study can be made:

- Knowledge about the target group (patients with memory impairments and their caregivers) is crucial. This target group could possibly benefit from assistive technology in many different areas. It is important that a multidisciplinary team works together in order to arrive at useful solutions.
- Start as early as possible with raising attention in the wider community about smart living and assistive technologies. If this is done effectively people will become accustomed to the possibilities before they actually need it. Providing care personnel with knowledge of, and training in the use of new assistive technologies will aid in informing the end users and their informal caregivers about the benefits of these devices.
- Communication with the participants and their caregivers is crucial. Involve them in all steps of the process. Adjust the sensors / products as often as needed. This regular communication helps to ensure trust and adequate responses when needed.
- Minimize delays as much as possible (by better preparation, time management, communication, cooperation). Delays of some weeks can mean a totally new or different situation for a person with memory impairments.

FUTURE RESEARCH DIRECTIONS

Most of the participants mentioned that they were willing to make a financial contribution towards the aids used in this study if required. How much they would spend would depend on their income, current budget and price of the support. However, due to the relatively short duration of the project, there was no possibility of carrying out any cost / benefit analysis. In other words we cannot reach any conclusions about whether the psycho-social or health benefits that were associated with the products outweigh the costs. It might be the case, for example, that hospitalization can be postponed with assisted technologies thereby resulting in considerable financial savings to the public purse. The results discussed earlier make it clear that a number of people experienced an increase in their quality of life, even during the period over which the study was run. In addition, because people indicated that they would be willing to pay some of the costs themselves, it seems there is a latent market for these assistive technologies. The whole area of cost / benefit in relation to assistive technologies requires further research.

ACKNOWLEDGMENT

The work discussed in this chapter was partially funded by the program of innovative actions in Brabant; "Innovative Acties Brabant (IAB)". This program of the BOM (Brabantse Ontwikkelings Maatschappij) and the Province of Noord-Brabant (NL) aims to stimulate the innovation power of SME companies. The European Commission supports the IAB by means of the European Fund for regional development (EFRO). The author would like to thank the project partners and project team: Van Hout Elektroservice, Ad Soontjens Electrotechnische Installaties, Stichting Smart Homes and the care provider SVVE De Archipel. A special thanks to Ellen de Wit from SVVE and the participants in the study.

REFERENCES

Alzheimer Nederland. (2009). Cijfers en feiten over dementie, www.alzheimer-nederland.nl.

Astell, A. (2005). Developing technology for people with dementia. *Psychiatric Times, 22*(13).

Astell, A. J., Ellis, M. P., & Alm, N. (2004). Facilitating communication in dementia with multimedia technology. *Brain and Language, 91*(1), 80–81. doi:10.1016/j.bandl.2004.06.043

Bell, G., Blythe, M., Gaver, B., Sengers, P., & Wright, P. (2003). Designing culturally situated technologies for the home. In *CHI '03 extended abstracts on human factors in computing systems CHI '03*. Workshops.

Burns, A., & Rabins, P. (2000). Carer burden in dementia. *International Journal of Geriatric Psychiatry, 15*(S1), S9–S13. doi:10.1002/1099-1166(200007)15:1+<::AID-GPS160>3.0.CO;2-N

CBS. (2007b). *CBS Statline, Regionale kerncijfers Nederland, 2007-07-31*. The Netherlands: Voorburg/Heerlen.

Daniel, K., Cason, C., & Ferrell, S. (2009). Assistive technologies for use in the home to prolong independence. [Corfu, Greece.]. *PETRA, 09*(June), 9–13.

Dewey, M. E., & Prince, M. J. (2005). Cognitive function. In Börsch-Supan, A., Brugiavini, A., Jürges, H., Mackenbach, J., & Guglielmo Weber, S. (Eds.), *Health, ageing and retirement in Europe*. Mannheim.

European Commission (2004). *The social situation in the European Union.*

Gill, T. M., & Kurland, B. (2003). The burden and patterns of disability in activities of daily living among community-living older persons. *The Journals of Gerontology. Series A, Biological Sciences and Medical Sciences, 58A*(1), M70–M75.

Goodacre, K., McCreadie, C., Flanagan, S., & Lansley, P. (2007). Enabling older people to stay at home: How adaptable are existing properties? *The British Journal of Occupational Therapy, 70*(1), 5-15(11).

Green, K. E., Walker, I. D., & Brooks, J. (2009). ComforTABLE: a robotic environment for aging in place. *HRI '09: Proceedings of the 4th ACM/IEEE international conference on Human robot interaction*, March 11–13, 2009, La Jolla, California, USA.

Hawkey, K., Inkpen, M., Rockwood, K., McAllister, M., & Slonim, J. (2005). Requirements gathering with alzheimer's patients and caregivers. *Assets '05: Proceedings of the 7th international ACM SIGACCESS conference on Computers and accessibility*. October 9–12, 2005, Baltimore, Maryland, USA.

Johnson, J. L., & Davenport, R. & Mann. (2007). W. C. Consumer Feedback on Smart Home Applications. *Topics in Geriatric Rehabilitation, 23*(1), 60–72.

Kitwood, T. (1998). Toward a theory of dementia care: Ethics and interaction. *The Journal of Clinical Ethics, 9*(1), 23–34.

Lobo A., L. J., Launer, L., Fratiglioni, K., Andersen, A., Di Carlo, M. M. …A. Hofman. (2000). Prevalence of dementia and major subtypes in Europe: A collaborative study of population-based cohorts. *Neurologic Diseases in the Elderly Research Group*. Neurology 54 (11 Supplement 5), S4-9. Cited after Dewey & Prince 2005.

Maciuszek, D., Aberg, J., & Shahmehri, N. (2005). ASSETS'05, October 9–12, 2005, Baltimore, Maryland, USA.

Mann, C. (2001). Assistive technology and older adults. *OT Practice, 6*(10), 13–15.

Metsis, V., Le, Z., Lei, Y., & Makedon, F. (2008). Towards an evaluation framework for assistive environments. *PETRA '08: Proceedings of the 1st international conference on Pervasive Technologies Related to Assistive Environments*. July 15-19, 2008, Athens, Greece.

Olivier, P., Xu, G., Monk, A., & Hoey, J. (2009). Ambient kitchen: Designing situated services using a high fidelity prototyping environment. *2nd International Conference on Pervasive Technologies Related to Assistive Environments*, Workshop on Affect and Behaviour Related Assistance in Support for the Elderly. June, 2009, Corfu, Greece.

Oswald, F., Wahl, H.-W., Naumann, D., Mollenkopf, H., & Hieber, A. (2006). The role of the home environment in middle and late adulthood. In Wahl, H.-W., Brenner, H., Mollenkopf, H., Rothenbacher, D., & Rott, C. (Eds.), *The many faces of health, competence and well-being in old age: Integrating Epidemiological, psychological and social perspectives* (pp. 7–24). Heidelberg: Springer. doi:10.1007/1-4020-4138-1_2

ADDITIONAL READING

Badii, A., I., Etxeberria, C., Huijnen, A., Maseda, S., Dittenberger, A., Hochgatterer, D., & Thiemert, Rigaud, A-S. (2009). CompanionAble: Graceful integration of mobile robot companion with a smart home environment. *Gerontechnology (Valkenswaard), 8*(3), 181. doi:10.4017/gt.2009.08.03.008.00

Cuddihy, P., Weisenberg, J., Graichen, C., & Ganesh, M. (2007). Algorithm to automatically detect abnormally long periods of inactivity in a home. *HealthNet '07: Proceedings of the 1st ACM SIGMOBILE international workshop on Systems and networking support for healthcare and assisted living environments. HealthNet'07, June 11, 2007, San Juan, Puerto Rico, USA.*

Huijnen, C., IJsselsteijn, A., & Markopoulos, P., & Ruyter de., B. (2004). Social presence and group attraction exploring the effects of awareness systems in the home. *Cognition Technology and Work*, *6*(1). doi:10.1007/s10111-003-0141-z

Orpwood, R., Gibbs, C., Adlam, T., Faulkner, R., & Meegahawatte, D. (2005). The design of smart homes for people with dementia—user-interface aspects. *Universal Access in the Information Society, 4*(2).

Sixsmith, A., Meuller, S., Lull, F., Klein, M., Bierhoff, I., Delaney, S., & Savage, R. (2009). SOPRANO An Ambient Assisted Living System for Supporting Older People at Home. *ICOST '09: Proceedings of the 7th International Conference on Smart Homes and Health Telematics: Ambient Assistive Health and Wellness Management in the Heart of the City.*

Skubic, M., Alexander, G., Popescu, M., Rantz, M., & Keller, S. J. (2009). A smart home application to eldercare: Current status and lessons learned. *Technology and Health Care*, *17*(3), 183–201.

Wherton, J. P., & Monk, A. F. (2008). Technological opportunities for supporting people with dementia who are living at home. *International Journal of Human-Computer Studies*, *66*(8), 571–586. doi:10.1016/j.ijhcs.2008.03.001

Chapter 6
Meeting the Needs of Diverse User Groups:
Benefits and Costs of Pluggable User Interfaces in Designing for Older People and People with Cognitive Impairments

Gottfried Zimmermann
Access Technologies Group, Germany

Jan Alexandersson
DFKI GmbH, Germany

Cristina Buiza
INGEMA, Spain

Elena Urdaneta
INGEMA, Spain

Unai Diaz
INGEMA, Spain

Eduardo Carrasco
VICOMTech, Spain

Martin Klima
Czech Technical University Prague, Czech Republic

Alexander Pfalzgraf
SemVox GmbH, Germany

ABSTRACT

"Pluggable user interfaces" is a software concept that facilitates adaptation and substitution of user interfaces and their components due to separation of the user interface from backend devices and services. Technically, the concept derives from abstract user interfaces, mainly in the context of device and service control. Abstract user interfaces have been claimed to support benefits such as ease of implementation, support for User Centered Design, seamless user interfaces, and ease of use. This paper reports on experiences in employing pluggable user interfaces in the European project i2home, based on the Universal Remote Console framework, and the Universal Control Hub architecture. In summary, our anecdotal evidence supports the claims on the benefits, but also identifies significant costs. The experience reports also include some hints as to how to mitigate the costs.

DOI: 10.4018/978-1-61520-825-8.ch006

INTRODUCTION

Today, home devices and appliances come with user interfaces that are either built into the devices or are dedicated remote controls. For example, a washing machine has built-in dials and knobs to select the wash program parameters and start or stop the washing process. Additionally, a display may be integrated into the appliance to provide status information. All these controls are built into the washing machine - the user cannot take them away in order to control the appliance remotely.

Some home devices have a remote control in addition to a built-in user interface. This remote control is dedicated to the device or service it controls. For example, a DVD player usually ships with an infrared remote control, in addition to the buttons and small displays on the device itself. The user can choose between the dedicated remote control and the built-in user interface to control the DVD player. However, they cannot use the TV's remote control to play a DVD.

Universal remote controls are advertised for being the solution to the problem of having too many remote controls at home. Certainly, infrared-based universal remote controls are an improvement to dedicated remote controls since they allow controlling a variety of devices from a single ("universal") controller. However, universal remote controls have to be programmed prior to usage in order to know the infrared codes of a particular device. Moreover, they cannot provide feedback on a device's current state, such as whether it is currently on or off. Some advanced universal remotes, such as the high-end Logitech Harmony products, make guesses about the device state, but this is not always reliable.

Pluggable user interfaces allow the user interface to be adapted or substituted for one or multiple devices and services to be controlled. We refer to "pluggable user interfaces" as an architectural concept in device/service control that separates the user interface from the backend functionality in software, and sometimes in hardware (Zimmermann & Vanderheiden, 2007). An abstract user interface or "user interface model" is established as the dividing line between backend application (devices/services) and frontend application (user interface). In the area of user interfaces, the concept of "pluggability" at runtime is not present in today's typical design and development environments. Following the pluggable user interface approach, the user interface of a device or service is exchangeable, and can be attached or detached at runtime as appropriate. For example, for controlling a DVD player, one user might use a PDA with voice interaction, and another might use an infrared remote control for navigating the DVD controls on a TV screen.

The pluggable user interface concept supports a wide range of user interface needs and preferences. One device/service implementation, providing an abstract user interface, can host different versions of pluggable user interfaces, in order to serve different users in different usage contexts. This is particularly useful when designing user interfaces for elderly users and users with cognitive disabilities who represent diverse groups of users with regard to their user interface needs and preferences.

BACKGROUND ON HCI AND AGED USERS

There is a growing interest for designing and developing human-computer interfaces that fit the needs of the aged users. The interface's specific characteristics have to conform to the performance of older users. Design considerations include variations of the visual, auditory, cognitive and motor functions associated with the process of aging, but other considerations such as emotional, health and social aspects have to be taken into account as well.

It has been found that, related to aging, a decrease of human functions takes place. This includes a reduction of visual function, of sensibility to contrast, changes in the abilities to hear, smell and taste, as well as a decrease of the muscular mass (Witte, 1998). These aspects should be considered when designing user interfaces for the aged population, making deliberate decisions on the use of icons and graphics, text, font type and size, use of colors and screen titles, and audio feedback. In cognitive terms, some functions stay stable in the normal process of aging, such as automatic and well-learned responses, remote and semantic memory, and verbal reasoning and comprehension. In contrast, other cognitive functions decline, such as the information processing speed and the working memory. For older users interacting with computers, their cognitive abilities and disabilities can have more impact than sensory aspects. Therefore, the cognitive profile of older users is of crucial importance in the design of user interfaces.

Aging is a rather heterogeneous process, and it would be a failure to design user interfaces for the "typical elder user". The needs of the older users are diverse, following their varying physical, cognitive, social, and emotional requirements (Crossen-Sills, Toomey, & Doherty, 2009). There is no single user interface that can cover the needs of all older users. The challenge for the designer is to devise a variety of user interfaces, each tailored for the needs of a specific user group, taking into account physical, cognitive, and motivational aspects of older users.

It is the realization of a need for multiple user interfaces that motivates the use of a pluggable user interface framework in designing for older people and people with cognitive impairments.

BACKGROUND ON ABSTRACT AND PLUGGABLE USER INTERFACES

The idea of abstract user interfaces goes back to the "Seeheim model" (Pfaff, 1985) which defines an application interface model as the interface between an application and its presentation and dialog control modules. User Interface Management Systems (UIMS) implemented this model in the 80s and 90s, thus facilitating separate design processes for user interfaces and application functionality.

In the late 80s, the "Model-View-Controller" software design pattern was introduced by the Smalltalk-80 programming environment (Krasner & Pope, 1988). In the MVC approach, implementation responsibilities are clearly separated between the following components: The *model* contains the functional core of an application, the *view* displays information to the user, and the *controller* handles user input. The popular "Document-View" design pattern (implemented in many user interface toolkits today) is a variant of MVC in which view and controller are collapsed into one component.

Numerous projects and systems have explored the concept of abstract user interfaces, also often referred to as "model-based user interfaces". More recent examples include the SUPPLE project (Gajos & Weld, 2004) and the Web-based form technology XForms (W3C, 2007). SUPPLE claims to generate an "optimal" user interface for a specific user and their characteristics, employing a constraint-based optimization mechanism. XForms defines a set of "form controls" that can be used to specify abstract user interfaces for forms on the Web. The Pebbles project (CMU, 2009) at Carnegie Mellon University has investigated how handheld computers and smartphones can interact with personal computers and electronic devices such as a light switch, a photocopier, a stereo or a telephone. The "Personal Universal Controller" (PUC) (Nichols & Myers, 2003) generates a control interface on a PDA, based on the parameters of the controlled device, taking into account the properties of the PDA and user preferences. The control interface has also been demonstrated with an extension for speech input (Nichols et al., 2003).

These and other research and development efforts have shown the feasibility and utility of the abstract user interface approach. However, they focused on the generation or provision of user interfaces by a single party, typically the manufacturer of the device or service. What was missing was the explicit and practical capability for a user or a third party to substitute an existing user interface by an alternate or "pluggable" user interface based on a publicly acknowledged standard. To address these shortcomings, the Universal Remote Console (URC) framework (ISO/IEC, 2008) was developed and has been released as a 5-part international standard (ISO/IEC 24752) in 2008. It defines a "user interface socket" (termed "socket" in this chapter) as the interaction point between a pluggable user interface and a target device or service. In the context of URC, pluggable user interfaces are either generic, that is, generating a user interface based on any socket description, or specific to a socket, that is, relying on hard-coded knowledge about the socket.

The URC technology is an open user interface platform, allowing third parties to create a pluggable user interface and use it with any device/service that exposes its functionality through a socket. The framework includes a "resource server" as a global marketplace for any kind of user interface resources to be shared among the user community. It is expected that, supported by a growing community, this will eventually result in a global URC ecosystem, enabling open competition on user interfaces that will allow the user to pick the user interface that is most appropriate for their characteristics and particular context of use.

Work on URC started in the 90s at the Trace Center at the University of Wisconsin-Madison, with the "universal remote console communication protocol" (Vanderheiden, 1998), resulting in the creation of the V2 Technical Committee at INCITS in 2000. V2 developed the URC standards which were later released under ANSI (in 2005) and under ISO/IEC JTC1 (in 2008). Further work by Trace and the URC Consortium (URC Consortium, 2009) resulted in the development of implementation guidelines and other derivatives of the URC technology. The "Universal Control Hub" (UCH) is a profiling architecture of the URC framework, with the UCH acting as URC-conformant middleware between devices/services and controllers that do not support URC technology (Zimmermann & Vanderheiden, 2007). The UCH architecture has been adopted by multiple projects in Europe, including i2home (i2home, 2009). The architecture has already been implemented in a broad spectrum of applications, with the goal of making them accessible to all users. Implementations include areas such as mobile devices, consumer electronics, interactive TV (Epelde et al., 2009), and home security.

For a more thorough overview of abstract user interface approaches and their history, refer to Myers, Hudson, & Pausch (2000) and Trewin, Zimmermann, & Vanderheiden (2004).

BENEFITS AND COSTS OF PLUGGABLE USER INTERFACES

Pluggable user interfaces (which are based upon abstract user interfaces) claim to bring about benefits for system implementers, user interface designers and end users. Some of the benefit claims are:

1. **Ease of implementation of personal user interfaces.** Personalized user interfaces (that are a substitute for the "standard built-in user interface") can be implemented in virtually any technology, but the pluggable user interface approach is specifically designed with the goal of facilitating adaptation and substitution of user interfaces (Trewin, Zimmermann, & Vanderheiden, 2004). The effort for adding a personal user interface is relatively low since it is limited to creating a new pluggable user interface (frontend) for the abstract user interface; the implementation of the abstract user interface and its binding to the backend device/service is

shared by all pluggable user interfaces for a device or service.

2. **Support for the user-centered design process.** Due to separation of user interface and backend functionality, abstract user interfaces are well suited to be used in a user-centered design process (Trewin, Zimmermann, & Vanderheiden, 2004). Human factors experts and designers can create pluggable user interfaces, evaluate them and make changes on them based on early feedback from the users. Concurrently, device and service providers can implement the backend functionality in an incremental fashion.
3. **Seamless user interface, spanning multiple controlled devices and services, in heterogeneous device and service networks.** A pluggable user interface can span multiple devices and services since it is hosted on a remote device (controller) that is different from the devices and services that are being controlled (Zimmermann, 2007). For example, a pluggable user interface may offer a "watch DVD" task whose execution would involve multiple steps on various devices (which may require different control technologies such as infrared, serial or UPnP): Switch the DVD player on and play; switch the TV on and set input source to DVD player; switch the receiver/amplifier on and set input source to DVD player. In contrast, for built-in user interfaces (or remote user interfaces that are dedicated to one device), the "seam-full" user interface would consist of separate control interfaces for every device involved. In the example given above, there would be three separate user interfaces (one for the DVD player, one for the TV, and one the receiver/amplifier), and the user would have to switch between the interfaces (controllers) to execute the steps of the task.
4. **Ease of use of pluggable user interfaces.** Pluggable user interfaces have been shown to be easier to use than built-in or standard remote user interfaces (Nichols & Myers, 2003). This can be explained by the following reasons: First, a generic controller typically offers more screen estate and/or more and larger buttons than most devices and dedicated remote controls. Second, a pluggable user interface may be personalized to exactly fit the preferences and needs of a particular user group. Third, the separation of backend and frontend code facilitates a separation of programming and design activities (Zimmermann & Vanderheiden, 2007). Programmers can focus on writing the code for the device/service and its abstract user interface, and do not need to "mess up" with user interface functionality. Human interface experts can focus on good user interface design that does not require deep programming expertise and network-specific knowledge.

Obviously, the pluggable user interface concept also comes with costs, some of which are:

1. **Increased effort for first implementation due to technology learning curve.** It is clear that development efficiency is initially hampered by the modeling language and other implementation requirements of model-based user interface technologies (Myers, Hudson, & Pausch, 2000). However, it is expected that the time investment into the technology is recouped soon once the programmers and designers have understood and gained experience in its implementation. Also, the employment of suitable development tools, if available, should greatly expedite the introduction of the pluggable user interface technology in projects.
2. **Early freezing of user interface model.** Early in the development process, backend

programmers and frontend designers need to agree on the specification of an abstract user interface. (Note that this freeze applies only to the (abstract) user interface model, and not to the (concrete) pluggable user interfaces.) Changes to the user interface model at a later stage will trigger increased development costs. This can become a burden for projects using an iterative or agile development process. However, this problem is not necessarily unique to the abstract and pluggable user interface approaches. In general, changes to the backend will cause changes to the user interface, and the later the changes happen, the more expensive they will be.

PLUGGABLE USER INTERFACES IN THE I2HOME PROJECT

i2home ("Intuitive Interaction for Everyone with Home Appliances based on Industry Standards") is a three-year European project in the area of Ambient Intelligence, funded by the European Commission. Its goal is to make devices and appliances in the digital home more accessible to persons with mild cognitive disabilities and older people. i2home follows a user-centered design methodology, with a diverse set of users with regard to their age, region of living, abilities and user interface needs and preferences. i2home adopted Cooper's persona approach (Cooper, 1999) to represent users in various stages of the development process.

Technically, the project is building upon the Universal Remote Console (URC) framework (ISO/IEC 24752), and in particular on the Universal Control Hub (UCH) approach. This technical foundation has been chosen because of its perceived benefits with regard to a heterogeneous set of users. The URC/UCH technology was deemed to be suitable for designing very different user interfaces for different user groups, following a user-centered design process.

In the following, we describe the experiences of the i2home partners in using the URC technology for the design of user interfaces for (1) elderly people in Prague (Czech Republic), and (2) Alzheimer patients in San Sebastián (Spain). Following the Universal Design approach, we have also designed user interfaces for (3) middle-aged people with brain injuries (cognitive impairment) in Sweden. These people experience similar problems in using technology as older users do. In any case, it seems that a universal framework for the development of mainstream user interfaces should support the needs of all users, not only for the elderly. Otherwise it will likely not be adopted by industry.

The objective of these three reports is to reflect on the above benefit and cost claims of the pluggable user interface technology, with the background of experiences from a real project in applying the URC/UCH technology for different user groups. Note that these reports are based on subjective experiences and anecdotal data rather than hard metrics. This is due to the nature of the i2home project and its goal of developing most usable user interfaces in a three-year iterative process rather than doing a thorough comparison of software development strategies by running multiple complete development threads (which would also have been well beyond the project budget).

Elderly People in Prague

Introduction

At the Czech Technical University in Prague (CTU), several usability tests were conducted, all focused on the UCH technology and especially on the design and usage of user interfaces. The primary target group were seniors aged 65 or older. This group was comprised of several personas from which two were evaluated as the potential users of the system. The first persona called "Blanka" is a 73 year old woman who lives alone in a small flat. She has no experience with computers. Her performance with regard to memory, vision and hearing is in decline but she is nevertheless self-sufficient in her everyday life. She has major problems with new devices such as state-of-the-art TV remote control, DVD or digital radio.

The second persona "Arnost" is a 68-year old man who recently retired but still maintains his hobbies and keeps in touch with his colleagues from work. He has some experience with computers during his time at work. He wears glasses, can operate a cell phone and a PDA, but has minor problems with small fonts.

We designed two different user interfaces, one for each persona. While the user interface for Blanka is simpler and has only the basic set of functionalities, the user interface for Arnost is richer in terms of functionality and slightly more complex in structure. The interfaces were implemented as a combination of a Personal Digital Assistant (PDA) (see Figure 1) and a TV. For evaluation purposes, test participants were recruited for each user interface – 14 for the Arnost persona, and 14 for the Blanka persona. An evaluation of the two user interfaces was performed, based on objective observations and on subjective opinions of the participants.

Figure 1. User interfaces for Blanka and Arnost personas

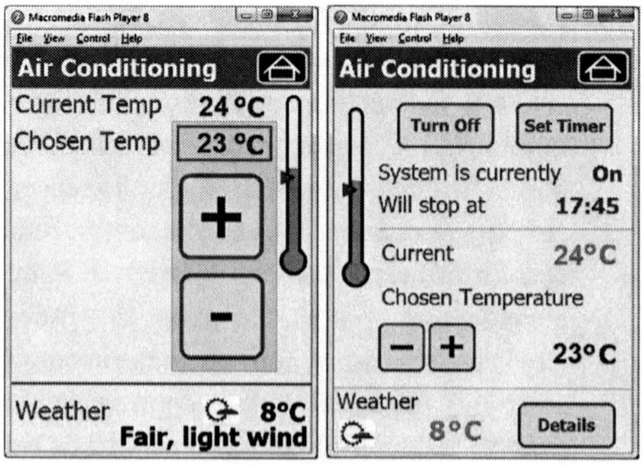

Experiences Regarding Benefits and Costs

Based on our experiences drawn from the implementation and evaluation of the pluggable user interfaces for elderly users, we can identify the following benefits and costs of pluggable user interfaces:

- The pluggable user interface architecture was a natural fit to the UCD approach involving personas. We were able to define the requirements of the two selected target groups, and implement them as pluggable user interfaces. In our experiments, we could easily interchange the user interface upon determining the most appropriate persona for a test user (Blanka or Arnost).
- The users appreciated the customized user interfaces with a selection of functionalities that matched their needs. For example, users conforming to the Blanka persona required only little functionality from the system.
- The given UCH architecture proved to be useful and appropriate for our implementation. This helped to speed up the development and testing process since we did not have to specify our own architecture. The architecture also contributed to higher stability of the application prototypes even in the early stages of development.
- During implementation, our developers gleaned knowledge of a device's capabilities by looking at its socket description(s). Thus they could easily check if the user interface covered the whole range of features offered by the device.
- Another benefit noticed was that the developers could utilize the socket description as semantic hints for user interface design. This could probably have been achieved

by other means of documentation as well, but it is an indication that the abstract user interface model is a useful basis for user interface development. In future, we would like to see tools for semi-automatic generation of user interfaces such as for wizards and visual control grouping.

- Learning the technology was a big challenge that was even more difficult because of the early development stage of the platform. Tools for the support of the design and development of user interfaces were not available. However, it should be easy to integrate the pluggable user interface architecture into development environments such as NetBeans or Eclipse.
- Suboptimal design of sockets can make the design and implementation of the pluggable user interfaces difficult for designers. In one case, the initial socket for the calendar system was poorly designed, and its revision resulted in a major effort on re-designing and re-implementing all related pluggable user interfaces.

Alzheimer Patients in San Sebastian

Introduction

Two research centers have cooperated in the following experiment. INGEMA, a research center on elderly and disabled people owned by Matia Foundation Group, has defined the user interface, conducted user tests, and evaluated a prototypical system on a group of 21 test persons with mild to moderate Alzheimer's disease. VICOMTech (www.vicomtech.org), a research center specialized in computer graphics and digital TV, has conducted the technical development. Both research centers work complementarily on finding new ways to better assist elderly people and especially those with cognitive problems such as Alzheimer's disease. Alzheimer patients, even in the first stages of the pathology, are not able to understand how to operate modern devices or services that could potentially benefit them. Intense research is being carried out in both institutions to identify and validate user interfaces that can be accepted by the target users.

In i2home, the characteristics of the targeted Alzheimer patients were summarized in the description of a persona named "Manuela". Manuela is 73 years old woman diagnosed with Alzheimer's disease three years ago who now attends a daily care center. Manuela usually forgets to take her daily medication but she is still able to perform simple tasks under supervision. She will become progressively more dependent. Manuela can answer the phone when she hears it, but as dialing causes her problems she tends to avoid it or wait for somebody to help her. Despite her anxiety about falling over, Manuela still goes out alone to do small amounts of shopping. However, she usually goes out with her daughter or grandson.

In our experiment, the user interface designed for this particular target group consisted of a realistic virtual character, also called an "avatar", rendered on a common television set (Figure 2). This virtual character plays the role of a virtual personal assistant conveying reminders and notifications to the user, and to engage in short dialogs with the user. Additionally, the television remote control serves as a return channel, capturing the user's responses to questions that the avatar raised (Carrasco et al., 2008).

The results of the evaluation show that, in the majority of cases, interaction with the avatar by means of a remote control was an easy task for the subjects to perform. Eighty percent of the users (n=12) responded to the avatar by voice, in addition to using the remote control, even though no directives were given to that regard. This reflects that this group of people with mild to moderate cognitive impairment were able to understand the avatar as an entity with which they could establish verbal conversation as a natural way of interaction.

Figure 2. Avatar on TV, interacting with Alzheimer patients

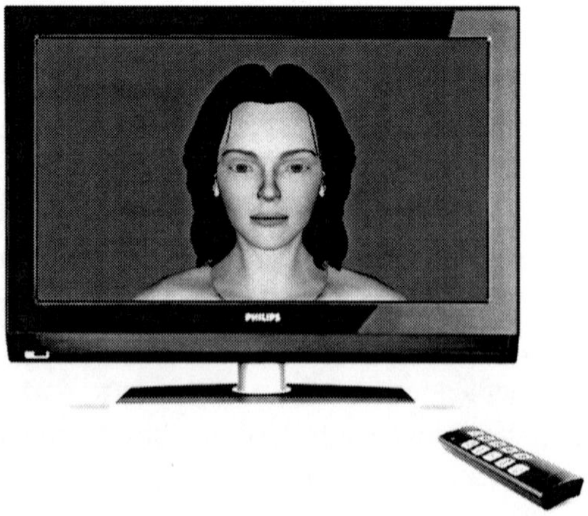

Experiences Regarding Benefits and Costs

Elderly people suffering from mild to moderate Alzheimer's disease are collectively excluded from participating in the information society. The main problem for them is that they do not understand how to use most of today's mainstream user interfaces. In this sense, as stated above, the paradigm of a speaking virtual character delivered on a television was perceived by the users as a natural interaction. Furthermore, the paradigm's usefulness in sending reminders, notifications and in conducting short simple dialogs with the users was demonstrated. The proposed user interface was demonstrated to be appropriate for these users, thus opening the door to a new world of services and assistance opportunities.

Technically, the URC technology and pluggable user interfaces provided a suitable platform in supporting the described user interface, and our experience was that most of the benefits mentioned above were met.

- Ease of implementation: The user interface was easy to implement because it was based on user interface sockets exposed by the UCH. Most importantly, it paves the way to a smooth replacement of the current user interface with other user interfaces. This feature is particularly interesting for Alzheimer patients because, due to their progressive decline of cognitive skills, different user interfaces (each matching a different stage of the disease) could be presented to them without the need for substituting the backend application(s).
- Support for the UCD process: The pluggable user interface approach was found to be suitable to bridge the gap between user needs and devices/services available, because it provides a framework that clearly separates frontend and backend through the definition of the user interface sockets. This division has allowed INGEMA and VICOMTech to concentrate on the definition, development and testing of the proposed "Avatar + TV" user interface, while having other partners in the i2home project work on the backend system and its complexity.
- Ease of use: The user interface proposed in this scenario has been tailored to our target users. In this sense, a simulation of natural interaction between humans was sought, and the results of the evaluations show that it has been readily accepted by mild to moderate Alzheimer patients. Furthermore, no complex information was given to the users through this user interface. Advanced device options or complex settings have been deliberately left out.
- An additional benefit of the URC technology is the reuse of existing user interfaces by other user groups, with possible variations and modifications to cater for subtle differences of users. Apart from Alzheimer patients, we have identified a wide range of other persons suffering from pathologies and conditions characterized by cognitive deterioration and disabilities, such

as stroke, vascular dementia, Parkinson-type dementia, and traumatic brain injuries that might benefit also from the existing pluggable user interface (avatar on TV) for Alzheimer patients.

Nevertheless, there are a number of important costs, including:

- Implementation was significantly harder than in a monolithic approach, mostly caused by the need for learning new technologies, and by the current absence of development tools for pluggable user interfaces and their sockets. On the other hand, this was our first experience with this particular technology. It is expected that implementation of further pluggable user interfaces in the project will be much faster due to the accumulated experience.
- The specification of user interface socket descriptions is a delicate task, and had to be done under supervision of an expert. This was to ensure that socket descriptions would not have to be changed often during the lifetime of the project, which would have triggered increased development costs.

People with Brain Injuries in Sweden

Introduction

For people with brain injuries in Sweden, the German Research Center for Artificial Intelligence (DFKI GmbH) and the Swedish Institute of Assistive Technology (SIAT) have jointly developed a user interface for younger and middle-aged persons with mild cognitive disabilities (Nesselrath et al., 2009). The typical characteristics of these persons were summarized as a persona called "Emma". Emma is 26 years old, lives with her boyfriend, and used to study at the university. Since a traffic accident which caused brain trauma,

Figure 3. User interface for persona "Emma" - multimodal interaction on a smartphone

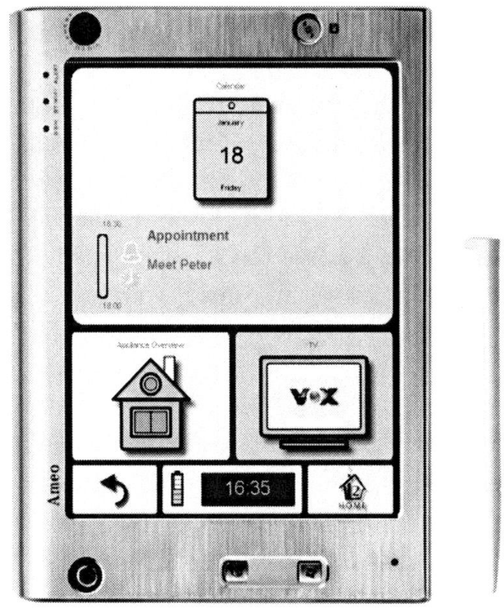

she has to deal with concentration problems and memory deficits. Emma is still very interested in technical devices and tries to use them in her daily life.

The user interface for Emma consists of a multimodal user interface implemented on an HTC advantage smartphone (Figure. 3). The user interface allows for interaction based on gestures with a finger or a stylus, and speech, or a combination thereof. For a description of the underlying technology, see Schehl, Pfalzgraf, Pfleger, and Steigner (2008). From a technical point of view, this user interface spans all available sockets that are exposed by the UCH (calendar, reminder, TV, and air conditioning). The main screen features a large pane containing the calendar application on the top. Underneath, a large button (showing a house icon) allows the user to access a list of available appliances; and another button allowing the user to go back to the previously used application (for example, the TV). The lower part of the main screen is common to all screens: On the left, the button with the curved arrow lets the user return to the previous screen; in the middle, the current time and the battery status is displayed; on the right, the i2home button allows the user to return to the main screen.

The user interface was evaluated by 10 test persons, all with cognitive disabilities caused by brain damage. Most of the participants rated the different visual parts of the user interface with "good" or "very good" (on a four-choice Likert scale ["bad", "less good", "good", "very good"]).

Experiences

It was possible to implement a user interface based on the URC technology and pluggable user interfaces meeting the majority of the requirements collected in the first phase of the user-centered design methodology. However, in our assessment we have to consider the whole user interface, which is not only composed of the visual display but includes other aspects of the device. With a weight of 355 grams, a size of 133 x 98 x 16 mm, and an LCD display with 640x480 pixels, the HTC 7500 Advantage[1] is quite large for a hand-held device. Although recognizing the advantage of a large screen, some of our participants found the device clumsy and too big for mobile use.

Regarding benefits and costs of the URC technology and pluggable user interface, we have found:

- User Interface Sockets and their descriptions are an effective and efficient means for separation of concerns. DFKI could focus on conceptual and user interface issues, and did not need to concerned with backend implementation and networking technologies such as for the control of consumer electronics and household appliances.
- The URC technology fits well with the user-centered design methodology, in particular with the creation of consistent user interfaces across all appliances and services.
- As soon as the socket descriptions were defined, it was possible to connect the user interface to simulated targets or services, even though these were not (yet) available. As a result, we were able to start end-to-end testing early in the development process, which clearly improved the quality of the user interface and saved time.
- The presence of a formal and explicit description by means of the socket description enables the automatic generation of call stubs. This enhanced the quality of the system particularly early in the development. In general, this increases the comprehensibility of target interfaces.
- The UCH approach allows for easy implementation of a user interface that lets the user control multiple devices and services in a seamless fashion.
- Finally, we found that the initial learning effort was significant. However, once the team had understood the concepts and details of the URC technology, the benefits were worth the effort.

CONCLUSION

Subjective evidence, based on our experience in the European i2home project, suggests that most of the claimed benefits of the pluggable user interface technology are evident. Most prominently, the implementers agree on the positive impact of URC technology on the user-centered design (UCD) process. Ease of implementation and its positive effects on development efficiency have been confirmed, in particular, where user interfaces had to be replaced swiftly. Further, the pluggable user interface technology is recognized to support the implementation of seamless user interfaces controlling multiple devices and services. In all cases, basic acceptance and usability of the resulting pluggable user interfaces has been confirmed by evaluation evidence. Additional benefits found include the reuse of existing interfaces across user groups, and the ability for early simulation of controlled devices and services.

On the cost side, our experience confirms that the initial overheads for learning new concepts and technologies are significant. One report mentions the absence of development tools as the main reason for this shortcoming. In this context, it should be noted that all three development teams had no prior experience and knowledge on the URC technology. Another problem identified was the expertise needed for the design of user interface sockets. Poor design decisions in the early phase did lead to an unexpected delay in the project in at least one case. This problem was compounded by the inherent need for freezing the user interface model early in the development process.

Further evidence should be sought for the reported benefits and costs, based on more formal evaluations and objective findings rather than subjective experience. For example, a formal comparison of abstract and non-abstract user interface approaches could be conducted to confirm or refute our subjective findings. However, objective studies may be hard to conduct, since parallel development of whole systems and the employment of a control group seems to be impractical for real projects in the size of i2home.

In this paper, we have reported on subjective evidence for the usefulness of the pluggable user interface approach and the URC technology in a user-centered design process. Much is still to be done, to make the pluggable user interface technology ready for take-up by industry in the development of real products. In particular, there is a strong need for better tool support, including design guidance, in the development and runtime process. Examples include a user interface builder for the development of abstract user interfaces and their pluggable counterparts.

ACKNOWLEDGMENT

This work was funded by EU 6th Framework Program under grant FP6-033502 (i2home); and by the US Department of Education, NIDRR, under Grant H133E030012 (RERC on IT Access). The opinions herein are those of the authors and not necessarily those of the funding agencies.

REFERENCES

W3C (2007). XForms 1.0 (Third Edition) as W3C Recommendation 29 October 2007. Retrieved February 18, 2009, from http://www.w3.org/TR/2007/REC-xforms-20071029/.

Carrasco, E., Epelde, G., Moreno, A., Ortiz, A., García, I., Buiza, C., et al. (2008). Natural interaction between avatars and persons with Alzheimer's disease. In *Computers Helping People with Special Needs* (LNCS 5105, pp. 38-45). Berlin/Heidelberg: Springer-Verlag.

CMU. (2009). *The Pittsburgh Pebbles PDA Project.* Human-Computer Interaction Institute, Carnegie Mellon University. Retrieved February 18, 2009, from http://www.pebbles.hcii.cmu.edu/.

Consortium, U. R. C. (2009). URC Consortium. Retrieved February 18, 2009, from http://myurc.org/.

Cooper, A. (1999). *The inmates are running the asylum.* Indianapolis, IN: Macmillan.

Crossen-Sills, J., Toomey, I., & Doherty, M. E. (2009). Technology and home care: implementing systems to enhance aging in place. *The Nursing Clinics of North America, 44*(2), 239–246. doi:10.1016/j.cnur.2009.03.003

Epelde, G., Carrasco, E., Zimmermann, G., Bund, J., Dubielzig, M., & Alexandersson, J. (2009). URC based accessible TV. *EuroITV '09: Proceedings of the seventh European conference on European interactive television conference* (pp. 111-114). New York: ACM.

Gajos, K., & Weld, D. (2004, January). *SUPPLE: Automatically generating user interfaces.* Paper presented at the international conference on Intelligent User Interfaces (IUI'04), Madeira, Funchal, Portugal. i2home (2009). Intuitive interaction for everyone with home appliances based on industry standards. Retrieved February 18, 2009, from http://www.i2home.org.

ISO/IEC. (2008). *International Standard ISO/IEC 24752. Information Technology - User Interfaces - Universal Remote Console (5 parts).* ISO/IEC.

Krasner, G. E., & Pope, S. T. (1988). A cookbook for using the Model-View-Controller user interface paradigm in Smalltalk-80. *Journal of Object-Oriented Programming, 1*(3), 26–49.

Myers, B. A., Hudson, S. E., & Pausch, R. (2000). Past, present and future of user interface software tools. *ACM Transactions on Computer-Human Interaction, 7*(1), 3–28. doi:10.1145/344949.344959

Nesselrath, R., Schulz, C., Schehl, J., Pfalzgraph, A., Pfleger, N., Stein, V., & Alexandersson, J. (2009). Homogeneous multimodal access to the digital home for people with cognitive disabilities. In *Proceedings of the second German Congress an Ambient Assisted Living.* Berlin, Germany.

Nichols, J., & Myers, B. A. (2003). Studying the use of handhelds to control smart appliances. *International Workshop on Smart Appliances and Wearable Computing (IWSAWC 2003) Proceedings of the 23rd IEEE Conference on Distributed Computing Systems Workshops (ICDCS'03)* (pp. 274-279). Washington: IEEE Computer Society.

Nichols, J., Myers, B. A., Higgins, M., Hughes, J., Harris, T. K., Rosenfeld, R., & Litwack, K. (2003). *Personal universal controllers: controlling complex appliances with GUIs and speech. Extended Abstract CHI'2003: Human Factors in Computing Systems (Demonstration Abstract)* (pp. 624–625). New York: ACM.

Pfaff, G. E. (1985). *User interface management systems.* Berlin: Springer-Verlag.

Schehl, J., Pfalzgraf, A., Pfleger, N., & Steigner, J. (2008). The BabbleTunes system - Talk to your iPod! In V. Digalakis, A. Potamianos, M. Turk, R. Pieraccini, & Y. Ivanov (Eds.), *Proceedings of the 10th International Conference on Multimodal Interfaces (ICMI 2008)* (pp. 77-80). New York: ACM.

Schulz, C., Neßelrath, R., & Alexandersson, J. (2009). Homogeneous multimodal access to the digital home for people with cognitive disabilities. In *Proceedings of the second German Congress an Ambient Assisted Living.* VDE, Berlin.

Trewin, S., Zimmermann, G., & Vanderheiden, G. (2004). Abstract representations as a basis for usable user interfaces. *Interacting with Computers, 16*(3), 477–506. doi:10.1016/j.intcom.2004.04.005

Vanderheiden, G. (1998). Universal design and assistive technology in communication and information technologies: Alternatives or complements? *Assistive Technology, 10*(1), 29–36.

Witte, R. (1998). Shrinkage, neuron and synapse loss: aging takes its toll on the brain. *Geriatrics & Aging, 1*(1), 14–15.

Zimmermann, G. (2007, September). *Open user interface standards - towards coherent, task-oriented and scalable user interfaces in the home environments.* Paper published at the Proceedings of 3rd IET International Conference on Intelligent Environments (IE07), Ulm University, Germany.

Zimmermann, G., & Vanderheiden, G. (2007). The universal control hub: an open platform for remote user interfaces in the digital home. In *Human-Computer Interaction. Interaction Platforms and Techniques* (LNCS 4551, pp. 1040-1049). Berlin/Heidelberg: Springer.

ENDNOTE

1 The HTC 7500 Advantage is sold in Germany by T-Mobile as the “Ameo” smartphone.

Chapter 7
A Robotic Arm for Electric Scooters

Samuel N. Cubero
The Petroleum Institute, UAE

ABSTRACT

This chapter describes the mechanical design, manufacture and performance of a three-degree-of-freedom manipulator arm and gripper that can be attached to a mobile vehicle or electric scooter. Known by the acronym "ESRA", or "Electric Scooter Robot Arm", this device can be remotely or automatically controlled to pick up and retrieve heavy objects, such as books or grocery products, from high shelves or difficult-to-reach locations. Such tasks are often considered to be arduous or even impossible for the frail elderly and people with disabilities. This chapter describes one example of how the combination of mechanical and electronic engineering technology can be used to perform physically strenuous tasks and enable the frail elderly and people with disabilities to enjoy a greater degree of self-sufficiency, independence and physical productivity. It includes the design process for robotic arm manipulators and actuators. It also provides a brief overview of existing "state of the art" robotic and machine vision technologies, and how these can be used to perform many everyday domestic or household chores.

INTRODUCTION

The population of elderly people is rapidly expanding worldwide. In developed countries, the large "Baby Boomer" generation (40-65 year old people) is approaching the age of retirement. Improvements in healthcare and food supplies over the last century have led to longer life expectancies. Currently, the population growth rate of people above 65 years of age is higher than the growth rate in any other age category in Australia (ABS, 2008).

The fastest growing population group is the cohort aged 80 years and older (ABS, 2008). In 2008, the life expectancy of Australian males was approximately 79.0 years, and for females, it was 83.7 years. There has been a rapid increase: In 1994-96, or a little over 10 years ago, the life

DOI: 10.4018/978-1-61520-825-8.ch007

expectancy for Australian males was 75.2 years, and for females, it was 81.1 years. Over the last 20 years, life expectancy at birth has improved by 6.0 years for males and 4.1 years for females. Hence, at present, life expectancy is increasing at approximately 3.6 months per year for males, and 2.46 months per year for females (ABS, 2008).

Chronic illness and disability tend to increase with age. Twenty-three per cent of people over 65 years of age in Australia have a profound or severe core activity limitation, and chronic illnesses are common conditions (AIHW, 2006). As the percentage of elderly continues to expand in the population, there is a growing need for tools and technologies to assist the frail elderly in completing day-to-day activities, such as shopping for groceries, completing housework tasks and performing heavy or strenuous lifting or other physical work.

The field of gerontology is the branch of medical science that deals with diseases and problems specific to the aged. Research in these fields continues to distinguish effects of disease from the effects of aging on the physical health and functioning of the elderly (Rowe & Kahn, 1987). The process of aging and its related physical and mental effects on the elderly are described by Moody (1998) and Ricklefs (1995). Aging studies, such as the one conducted by Rakowski and Hickey (1992), show that most of the elderly who were interviewed did not notice significant deterioration in physical health and ADL (Activities of Daily Living) over a period of one year. ADLs include daily activities such as dressing, bathing, using the toilet, eating, walking, getting outside and transferring (moving). However, other studies, such as those conducted by Parker et al. (2005) and Freedman et al. (2002) indicate that deterioration in quality of health and in ADLs are very noticeable over a much longer time period. Two large sample groups of elderly Swedish people, aged 77 years of age and over, were interviewed by Parker et al. (2005). Some of the health problems that were reported as becoming more severe over the survey period 1992-2002 included:

- Musculoskeletal pain: Shoulder pain, back pain, joint pain (in arms or legs).
- Functional limitations: Hearing, mobility, IADLs. (Instrumental ADLs include tasks such as house cleaning, shopping, and preparing food without help.)
- Nervous system / psychosomatic conditions: Dizziness, mental illness, depression, anxiety, sleeplessness, general fatigue.

Other health related problems reported were chest pain, heart problems, stroke and breathlessness.

Robotic or mechatronic devices can play a significant role in improving the lives of the frail elderly and people with disabilities by performing common daily physical manipulation tasks. Robotic and mechatronic engineering technologies can help the frail elderly and people with disabilities to regain some of their former physical functionality. The anticipated benefits and advantages of implementing such technologies are many and provide strong justification for further research into assistive robotic technologies:

1. **Psychological:** Frail elderly and people with disabilities people can regain a sense of freedom and independence by doing a number of physical tasks, such as heavy or strenuous work. Achieving a high degree of freedom, mobility, autonomy and self-sufficiency are all important for people to maintain personal pride, dignity and self-confidence. Robots can help the frail elderly and people with disabilities to feel more productive and physically capable. Gaining a high degree of independence will reduce the feeling of being an encumbrance on others. Being physically active and productive can also help people to feel more self-confident, positive and optimistic.

2. **Economic:** People equipped with assistive robotic technologies may choose to remain longer in or return to the workforce, perform manual labour work and improve their incomes. Robotic arms on wheelchairs and strength and endurance-enhancing exoskeleton power suits are two examples of robotic technology that can empower the frail elderly or people with disabilities to contribute useful physical labour to industries such as construction, transport, manufacturing, mining, agriculture, the military, security, entertainment and most service industries (Pons, 2008). Promoting assistive robotics technologies for automating or semi-automating household and domestic tasks also has the potential to create a number of high-skilled jobs for people involved in the design, manufacture, marketing, operator training and servicing of such hardware and control systems. Introducing such useful robotic technologies could lead to the creation of new markets and more export opportunities.
3. **Easier lifestyle:** The musculoskeletal pain and functional limitations often experienced by the frail elderly and people with disabilities, such as weak muscles, arthritic joints and low energy levels, can make completing ADLs and IADLs difficult and quite painful (Parker et al., 2005). Powerful and dexterous robotic actuators and manipulators, intelligent control systems and advanced sensors can assist in completing such activities (Alciatore & Histand, 2003). Such hardware and software can work synergistically and reliably enough to comprehend and interpret human instructions or intentions and perform actions necessary to carry out the commands and wishes of a human operator. As technologies and computers become more powerful over time, machines could one day become a natural "extension" of the human body and provide human operators with superhuman strength, indefatigable endurance and the ability to work many times faster or more productively than a person performing the same job.

Human guidance and supervision is still preferable to software instructions for controlling very complex machine operations and adapting to a wide variety of unusual operating conditions and unforeseen problems. The types of technologies and robotic machines developed from the field of assistive robotics research have the potential to be applied widely in industry for heavy lifting or physically onerous tasks. The core motion control, sensor and embedded computing technologies are already available. What is needed now is dedicated funding and a commitment to research appropriate devices to achieve these goals. The rewards and benefits gained from this kind of research and development work are many and worthy of pursuing.

BACKGROUND

Several different research groups have developed robotic manipulator arms for electric powered wheelchairs. For example, Martens et al. (2001) have developed a semi-autonomous robotic system called FRIEND which consists of an electric wheelchair with a robotic arm (called MANUS). This system utilizes a speech interface to control the MANUS robot arm. Other kinds of wheelchair-based robotic arms and convenient user interfaces have also been developed, such as the KARES 1 & 2 (Bien et al., 2003), the 'Weston wheelchair mounted assistive robot' (Hillman et al., 2002), a 'Brain-Controlled Robotic Arm for a Smart Wheelchair' (Fallon, 2009) and the USF 'Robotic chair arm' (Higgins, 2007).

In most "mission critical" applications, it is too dangerous and risky to fully entrust the safety and care of humans to fully automated computer control systems, without recourse to a "manual over-ride" of the controls, due to the ever-present possibility of a system failure or a complex series of unknown problems. Many microcontroller chip manufacturers print a liability disclaimer and a stern caveat on their user manuals or operator guides, warning engineers and developers that their products are not guaranteed or warranted for use in "mission critical" applications. These are applications that could endanger human life or cause serious property damage in the event of a hardware or software failure, such as life support systems or automotive control systems (Atmel, 2007). For example, human pilots are still needed for supervising the autopilot system for a commercial jet aircraft and for performing the complex manoeuvres of take-off and landing. Pilots are needed to over-ride the autopilot controller and take control of the aircraft in the event that flight control variables appear unacceptable or dangerous or need urgent correction. Serious problems can occur, such as a hardware failure or unpredictable or turbulent weather, which can create serious situations that a computer controller is unable to deal with, solve or avert successfully.

For the foreseeable future, human workers will remain superior to computers in terms of flexibility and adapting to and solving unexpected problems. This is because most computer controllers are very limited in functionality by their software instructions. Computers today are generally unable to imagine new solutions or formulate new strategies. Even the decision making abilities of highly flexible "Artificial Neural Network" learning control software (ANN) are very limited because procedural software is not capable of learning, adapting to and solving new problems with different kinds of control variables, since ANN software still requires a great deal of human training and human programming effort. At present, most computer controllers lack sensory input capability, and procedural control software is generally unable to emulate human-like intelligence, intuition or understanding. At best, procedural software programming tools and the code generated are tools that record and "play back" a limited number of human intentions, decisions and ideas, created by the programmer.

Despite these limitations, computers can direct robotic hardware to perform manual jobs that are repetitive, physically strenuous or laborious more efficiently, quickly and economically than human workers (McKerrow, 1991).

While many manipulator arm (and gripper) designs for wheelchairs and mobile robots are suitable for manipulating small objects such as cups, doorknobs and dinner plates, the majority are very expensive to manufacture. Due to many (often unnecessary) degrees of freedom, they require very complex and expensive controllers to operate, they are unable to reach distant positions (beyond 3 metres), and they are typically unable to carry loads above 20 kg (Martens et al., 2001). Although these robot arms were designed to help people with disabilities, especially those who are unable to use their hands, they are clearly not suitable for carrying or manipulating heavy loads over long distances, unless they resemble a forklift or an industrial "cherry picker" platform.

One growing trend is the use of 3 or 4-wheeled electric scooters used by many elderly and those who need assistance to carry their weekly groceries and shopping bags. While electric scooters are a convenient and cost effective method for giving the infirm elderly a greater sense of self-autonomy and mobility, they can be improved with the addition of robotic arms or manipulators to collect and retrieve heavy or unwieldy products in difficult-to-reach places. The electric scooter performs the functionality of human legs (i.e. transport and gross movement), while the robotic arm can perform most of the collecting and reaching work of capable human arms. Also, a mechanical arm can be designed to reach much further and carry heavier loads over longer periods of time than the arms of an average adult man.

ESRA – ELECTRIC SCOOTER ROBOTIC ARM

A final-year mechatronic engineering student, Mr Nyan Lynn Naung, at Curtin University of Technology (Australia), carried out a study to develop a general-purpose manipulator arm that could be easily fitted to any standard electric scooter (Naung, 2006). The goal of this project was to enable frail elderly or people with disabilities to collect and retrieve a selected shopping item located on a high grocery store shelf, and return it to a shopping basket. This section describes developments that have taken place since then. Figure 1 shows a drawing of the first ESRA prototype arm in the default "driving position".

Figure 1. Side view of ESRA – Electric Scooter Robot Arm (Naung, 2006)

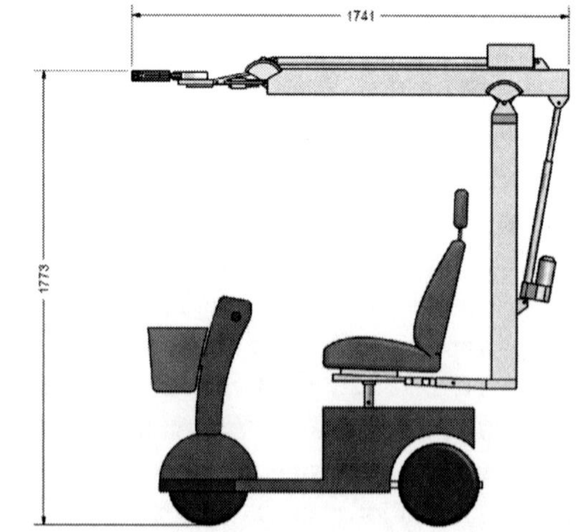

The ESRA is attached to the rear of the rotating "swivel chair" and uses this chair as one of its rotational degrees of freedom, namely, yaw rotation. Yaw rotation is similar to the kind of left-to-right or right-to-left rotation your forearm experiences when you wipe a flat table with a cloth. The actuator shown at the very right of Fig. 1 is the tilting actuator for the upper arm beam, which causes pitch rotation. Pitch rotation is an up-down or down-up rotation, similar to the kind of forward or backward rotation that an aeroplane fuselage experiences during takeoff or landing. The top actuator extends and retracts an internal telescopic tube which supports the "end effector" or gripper tool. This is known as a "translational" or sliding degree of freedom.

Several designs were proposed and analysed for the first ESRA manipulator arm; however, the most promising one appeared to be based on the popular telescopic Stanford arm design, as shown in Figure 2 (Klafter et al., 1989). This arm design was selected mainly because of its manufacturing simplicity, large spherical coordinate workspace and its relative compactness compared to other revolute-joint type robotic arms having the same maximum reach for the end-effector or gripper. (An "end-effector" tool fits on the end of the manipulator arm). To keep manufacturing and control complexity to a minimum, the wrist yaw and roll degrees of freedom were removed, and it was decided that the wrist pitch rotation should be controlled so that the gripper fingers always remain parallel to the horizontal plane.

The ESRA (Electric Scooter Robotic Arm) prototype arm shown in Figure 3 was designed and built on a modest budget of approximately $1800 AUD (materials and parts only). Aside from the location and direction degrees of freedom provided by the scooter, the ESRA has four manually controlled degrees of freedom, namely, chair rotation, elbow pivot (pitch rotation), arm translation (extension/retraction), gripper activation (open/close), and one passive degree of freedom (horizontal pitch rotation) to maintain a level orientation for the gripper at all times. Three electric ball-screw linear actuators were employed to drive the elbow pivot, arm extension and the gripper degrees of freedom. This particular prototype was designed with AutoDesk™ Inventor solid modelling software and was built using aluminium tubes and low-friction plastic for the bush bearings and slide guides. It weighs approximately 18 kilograms, including the masses of the linear actuators. Figure 3(b) shows the arm

Figure 2. Stanford robot arm

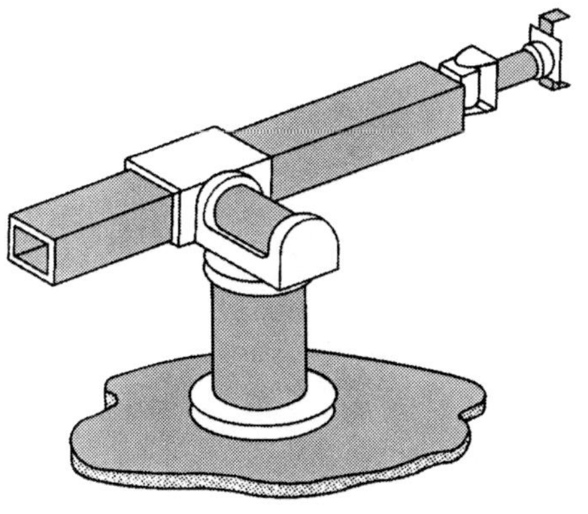

position during normal driving mode for the scooter. When the gripper is fully retracted, the user is able to reach forward easily with one or both hands to remove the retrieved object from the gripper's grasp, without leaving the chair.

At full extension, the gripper can reach objects within a distance of approximately 1.5 metres from the body of the driver, up to a height of about 3.3 metres above the ground. See Fig. 3(a). According to gripper and arm FEA computer simulations, the ESRA has a safe maximum gripper payload of approximately 20 kg without yield failure. (When materials fail by "yielding", they cannot return to their original dimensions.) The ESRA prototype shown in Fig. 3 has been able to successfully collect and retrieve 15 kg objects from the tops of 3 metre high shelves within one minute. This retrieval time is highly dependent on the ability of the operator to control and coordinate the movements of several actuators. At present, all the active degrees of freedom and all movements are push-button controlled, except for the chair and arm rotation, which must be performed manually by the driver. The arm points in the same direction as the rotating driver's chair. The chair can be rotated clockwise or anticlockwise and locked into position manually; however, this degree of freedom can be motor-driven in future versions of the ESRA system.

All actuators on the ESRA are manually operated with push-button controls on the hand controller, as shown in Figure 4. Simple relays are used to drive and change the polarity for each DC motor. Alternatively, an 'H-bridge' motor driver circuit could be used to drive each motor, using four switches, in order to achieve variable and bi-directional (two-way) speed and force control. PWM (Pulse Width Modulated) "on-off" signals from a microcontroller or control circuit can be used to control speed and force in the forwards or backwards driving direction for each actuator (Alciatore & Histand, 2003). The four switches could be MOSFETs (Metal Oxide Semiconductor Field Effect Transistors, which are low to medium current switches) or even IGBTs (Insulated Gate Bipolar Transistors, which are high current switches) arranged in an 'H-bridge' circuit which can change the polarity of the current passing through the DC motor driving each joint or axis (Braga, 2002). The gripper is attached to a "wrist" mechanism that always remains horizontal, or parallel with the ground plane, by means of a constant length cable that attaches the wrist's pitching joint to the base of the vertical tube, but wrapped around the elbow joint. The cable, shown in Figure 4, is always constrained by an outer tube. The length of this outer tube is not affected by the extension or retraction of the translating gripper position or the rotation angle of the elbow joint; this forces the gripper to remain level at all times without any need for an electronic controller or additional actuators for the wrist. The angle of the gripper is kept constant because the length of the cable remains constant, regardless of the shape or extension of the cable holding tube. Hence, this cable-restraining tube can fully extend when the gripper is at full extension, and it can curl up into a loop when the gripper is fully retracted, but the cable length, and hence, the gripper angle, both remain constant. Gravity acting on the gripper is used to maintain positive tension on this gripper orientation cable. The cable needs to be strong enough to hold up the weight of the gripper and

Figure 3. ESRA: (a) at full height and reach (left); (b) shown in driving position (right)

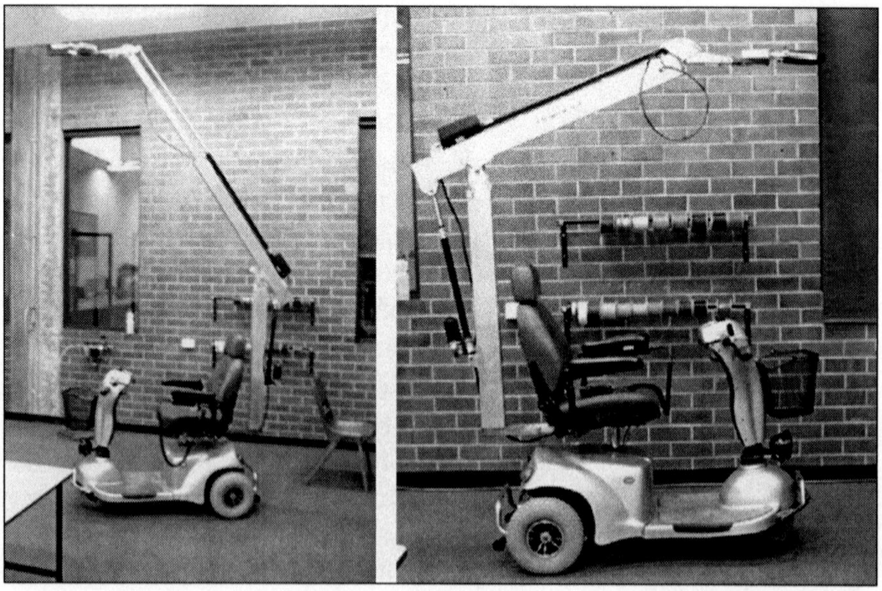

Figure 4. Control box and push-button control pendant (Naung, 2006)

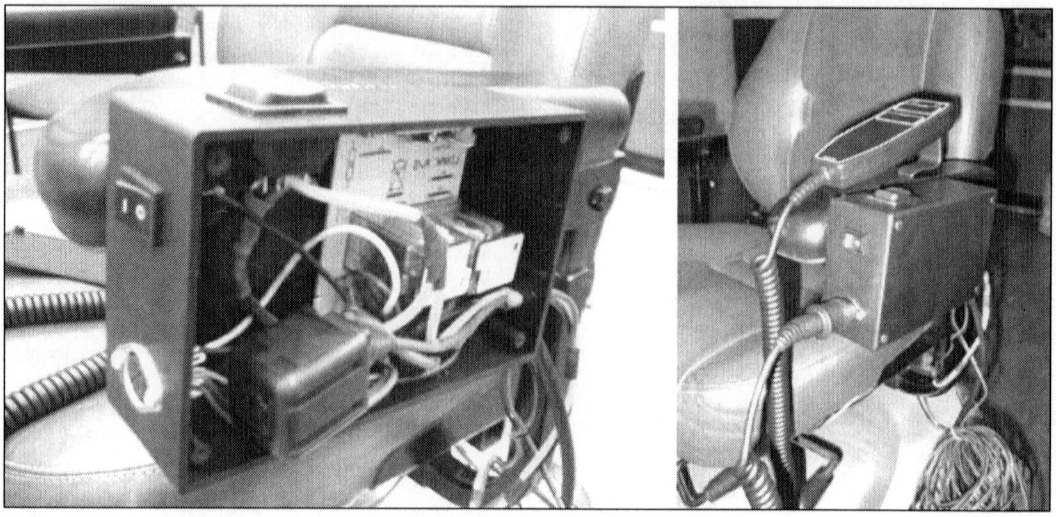

the maximum payload of 20 kg. This purely mechanical leveling system for the gripper is just one example of how good mechanical design can significantly reduce design and control complexity.

Figure 5 shows how a pivoting parallelogram mechanism is used for each finger to ensure that both fingers remain parallel to each other at all times as the ball-screw actuator drives it open or shut. All components and assemblies were designed and modelled using Autodesk Inventor™ solid modeling CAD (Computer Aided Design) software using standard 2D sketching and 3D modeling techniques (Banach, 2006). Inventor™ software can be used as a "virtual prototyping environment" because it enables designers to build geometrically accurate 3D models, identify and

Figure 5. Internal components of the 2-finger gripper (Naung, 2006)

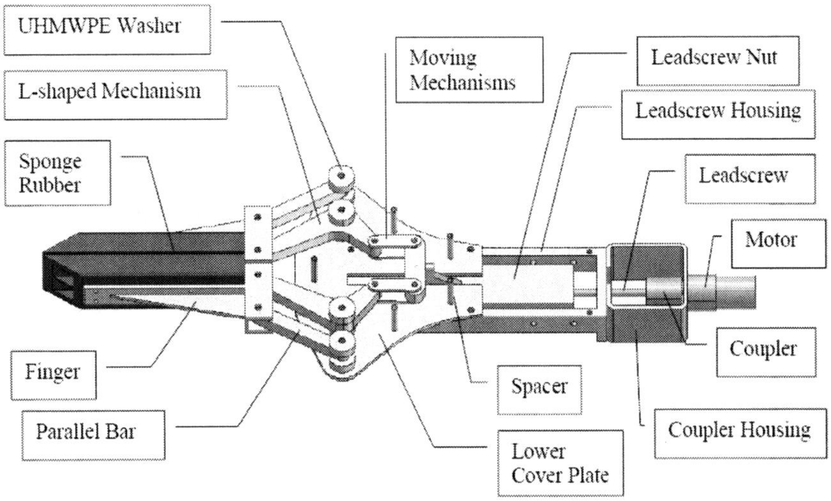

correct potential design problems and collisions, model and visualise the entire assembled product and create accurate dimensioned and toleranced drawings for all components. The ability to rapidly change and modify any geometric feature or dimension allows components and assemblies (or carefully arranged groups of components) to be designed quickly and usually successfully, the first time. Solid modeling CAD tools such as Inventor™, SolidWorks™, ProEngineer WildFire™ and IDEAS™ have similar features and functions. These software tools help designers to identify potential problems and reduce "trial and error" during the design process. They can also create top/front/side/section view drawings automatically from 3D solid models, thus speeding up the design and detailing process for creating manufacturing drawings.

Figure 6 shows the open and closed positions of the ESRA gripper. The generous 190 mm clearance allows the gripper to surround most vertical-standing bottles and boxes found on supermarket shelves, such as large 2 litre plastic bottles or metal cans of cooking oil.

Figure 7 shows one example of how equivalent stresses (or von Mises stresses) and deflections can be simulated immediately using a 3D model created within Inventor™ software, using the ANSYS™ FEA plug-in. Using a variety of different colours to represent different stress ranges, the FEA software reveals the most highly stressed regions that are most likely to yield or fail first based on the given external loads (i.e. applied forces and moments) and any fixed constraints (i.e. faces or features that do not move). Machine component designers and manufacturing engineers generally tend to add more material to or thicken the highest stressed regions in order to reduce equivalent stresses to well below the material's known yield stress (obtained from a simple tensile test). In this case, the aluminium used has a yield strength of approximately 70 MPa. In order to avoid breakage during operation of the gripper, it is possible to fit the fingers with strain gauges or force sensors to ensure that each finger does not exceed its material's yield strength. This would be especially useful during the closing operation, since the ball-screw drive is non-compliant and could easily damage the fingers, however, this is left for future work.

Figure 6. Fully assembled ESRA gripper (Naung, 2006)

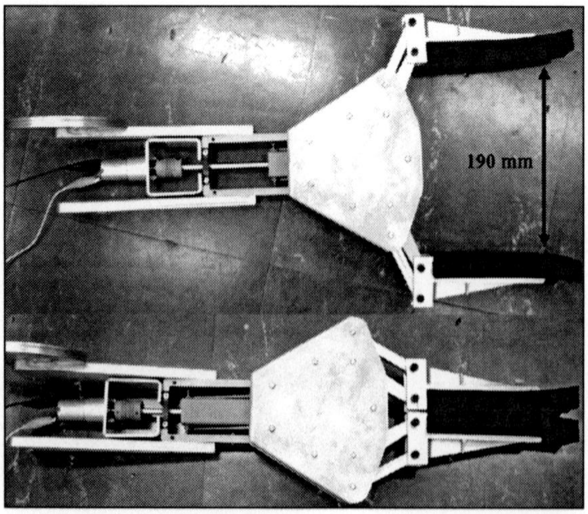

Figure 7. Simulating equivalent stress and deflections on a gripper finger using ANSYS™ FEA

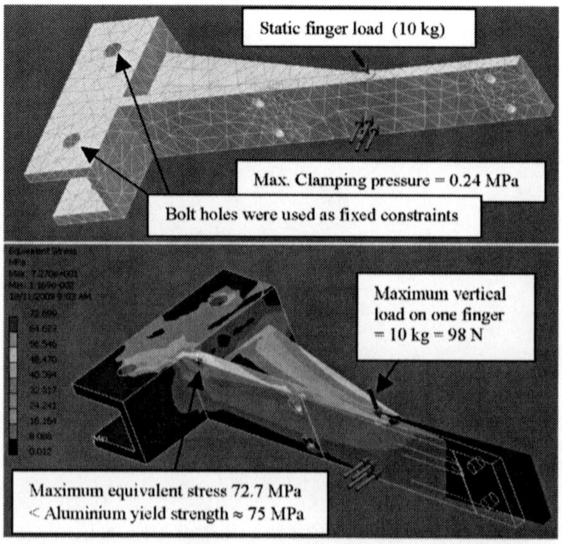

PERFORMANCE

The overall design of the ESRA manipulator worked exactly as planned; however, performance was a little slow because the traversal speeds of the Linak™ LA28 and LA30 linear actuators were the main limitations to speed of operation. The LA30 (elbow pitch actuator) had a top no-load movement speed of about 18.5 mm/sec and the LA28 (telescopic tube actuator) had a top no-load speed of about 46 mm/sec. While this is quite fast for ball-screw linear actuators, these traversal speeds are still slow considering that the stroke lengths for the LA30 and LA28 actuators are 400 mm and 900 mm respectively. In other words, to travel the full length of the stroke, the LA30 would take about 21.6 seconds, and the LA28 would take 19.5 seconds. These movement times can be significantly improved by using longer pitched thread for the lead screws, but at the cost of lower load carrying capacity for a given sized motor. At present, the total time it takes to move the gripper from the initial position shown in Figure 3(b), to pick up an object on the top of a 3m tall shelf (i.e. the fully extended position shown in Figure 3(a)), and finally to return to the finished 'unloading position' shown in Figure 8, is approximately 50 to 60 seconds, depending on the arm control skill and coordination of the operator. Admittedly, this total movement time is quite poor, and should ideally be around 10 to 15 seconds. However, slower speeds provide the advantages of allowing more time to make necessary movement corrections and, in general, lower risk of serious injuries to people.

Higher speeds could be achieved using pneumatic cylinders or even direct-drive DC motor powered linear actuators; however, these forms of actuation are inaccurate, fairly heavy and they do not provide high holding or stopping forces (Cubero & Billingsley, 1997). Additional gearing, brakes and hardware would be necessary to provide good holding forces and high load bearing capability. Pneumatic cylinders, for example, are very springy and poor in achieving accurate position control under heavy loads, and they require bulky onboard air tanks or a noisy compressor to provide high air pressure (Cubero, 1998). Direct drive DC motor mechanisms are typically very weak and compliant, just like air cylinders, and

Figure 8. Gripper position for collecting objects by hand

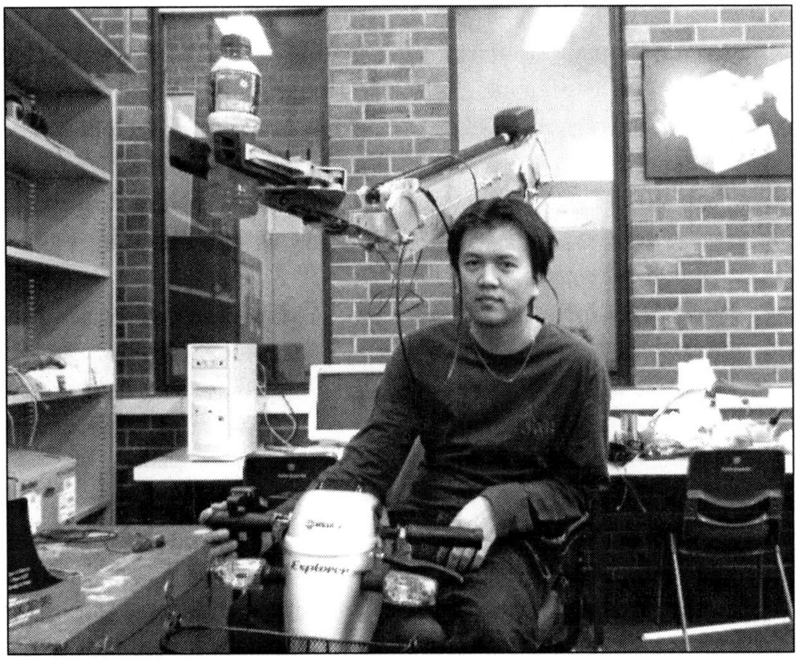

have no way of stopping quickly without stalling and overheating the DC motor, unless special brakes are fitted and carefully controlled (McKerrow, 1991). Lead screw actuators such as the Linak™, Thomson™ and Superjack™ brands of linear actuators typically cannot be 'back-driven' due to the very high gear ratio provided by the lead screw, hence, braking and holding a position without overheating or stressing the drive motor are easy to achieve (McKerrow, 1991). Unfortunately, lead screw actuators lack compliance or 'springiness' (i.e. lead screws are rigid and poor at absorbing shock loading or large position errors), and they are usually very expensive, typically costing around AUD $800 to $1200 each. An ideal actuator for the ESRA needs to employ larger pitched thread to provide much faster speeds, but still provide a high enough gear ratio to handle a maximum safe product load of about 20 kg. Such an actuator also needs to hold the entire gripper payload stationary, indefinitely, without being 'back-driven' by the weight of the arm and the payload and without overheating the drive motor. Unfortunately, it appears that no such actuator was commercially available while the first ESRA prototype was being developed.

FUTURE RESEARCH DIRECTIONS

Future research will focus on developing faster performing electric motor-driven linear actuators that can handle high loads and instant braking easily and reliably. Also, more work needs to be done on developing or implementing sensors for automated product retrieval, such as using 'machine vision' techniques to identify objects on shelves and automatically aligning the gripper's approach movement and positioning using automatic (feedback) control software (Davies, 2005). Users may one day be able to simply point at the product that they want to retrieve, as displayed on a 'touch screen' monitor showing an image from a digital camera, the vision recognition software will perform rapid edge detection to locate ideal finger placement points, and the control software will drive all the degrees of freedom for the arm simultaneously in order to guide the gripper fingers to the best grasping position around the object, without disturbing or knocking over other neighboring items on the shelf. Wrist orientation (roll and pitch control) may also need to be added and adjusted for achieving optimum gripper approach angles because there are cases where a horizontal gripper approach is unsuitable for grasping (e.g. the product might be too wide, or there could be an obstacle blocking the approach).

The large size and bulkiness of the current ESRA design could pose potential problems especially in cramped indoor environments. For example, if an electric scooter fitted with an ESRA needs to rotate on the spot in a small space, there is potential for the gripper to hit a wall or knock over objects inside the house. Therefore, it would be worthwhile to redesign the ESRA into a more compact and a more aesthetically pleasing package. Ideally, the ESRA should be hidden from view and unimposing, especially during driving or turning of the scooter. It could be possible to design a "snake-like" robotic arm that can curl up into a small compact arrangement (similar to a garden hose wrapped around a reel), for normal driving; however, due to the larger number of degrees of freedom and greater control complexity, such a design would be more expensive than the telescopic ESRA design. Materials and fabrication costs are typically proportional to the number of sensors, degrees of freedom and actuators used in a design.

Applications for the ESRA robot arm, or even several arms, include tasks such as house cleaning (window cleaning, mopping floors, dusting and wiping tasks), collecting and returning books on high shelves in a library, collecting products from grocery store shelves, wall and ceiling painting, car washing, building or construction work, or perhaps even gardening work, such as hedge trimming and tree pruning (where the gripper is replaced with appropriate end-effector tools, or tools that fit on the end of the manipulator arm). Different kinds of robotic manipulators may need to be fitted or mounted much lower on the scooter in order to reach low objects, touch the ground or even go below ground level, similar to a backhoe excavator arm. Different kinds of manipulators and end-effector tools need to be designed for specific household tasks to enable the frail elderly or people with disabilities to:

- Manipulate or wash dishes, cutlery, pots and pans, cups and other kitchen items in a sink and store them away in a dishwasher (for washing / drying) or placement into a cupboard
- Load and unload clothes and linen to and from washing machines and dryers
- Hang and retrieve clothes or linen on a clothesline, sort clothes into piles
- Vacuum floors, rugs and carpets; manipulate small furniture;, shake and move rugs
- Clean / wipe windows, toilets, bathrooms, benchtops; broom and mop floors
- Dispose of garbage, install new garbage bags; put garbage into a "wheelie bin" and manipulate or move the "wheelie bin" to the correct position for garbage truck pickup.
- Operate a lawn mower or a "whipper snipper" (grass trimmer) or an edge trimmer
- Cook or prepare food and operate a microwave oven
- Clean the "cat litter" by filtering out and collecting clumps of waste material every day, load new cat litter, and wash and dry the litter boxes regularly
- Perform simple gardening jobs, such as removing weeds, trimming hedges, planting, and many other kinds of household chores.

Unfortunately, at present there are no commercially available robots or machines that could adeptly perform even one of the above tasks as efficiently as an able-bodied human worker. However, the technology to do all of the above tasks using robots and machines exists today, and there is a strong possibility that the next generation of domestic robots and mechatronic devices will be able to efficiently perform such domestic chores and housework as quickly and as effectively as people, even under the guidance and supervision of a skilled operator.

CONCLUSION

The ESRA project is an example of how mechatronic hardware can simplify the task of retrieving a heavy or hard-to-reach object, and this is just one possible application for this manipulator arm. Although the linear lead-screw actuators of the ESRA are fairly slow, the entire manipulator arm performs its intended function reliably under manual control. The versatility and ease-of-use of the ESRA could be significantly improved through the use of additional hardware such as digital cameras for a machine vision system to guide the gripper, position controlled joints (requiring several microcontrollers and position sensors) and a more "user friendly" joystick or touch-screen user interface for controlling the gripper.

Robotic and mechatronic technologies similar to the ESRA have the potential to make life easier for the frail elderly and people with disabilities people worldwide. People with sound minds, good eyesight and good hand control can manually guide such manipulators or machines and live active and physically productive lives. Robotic technologies can help people to enjoy a greater sense of independence and the satisfaction and dignity of being able to continue working and contributing to the economy with minimum assistance from others. With the use of such technologies, the frail elderly and people with disabilities can feel more empowered and physically able to do many of the things that they would normally find tiring, painful, strenuous or impossible. Multi-purpose robotic arms, grippers and tools mounted on compact electric scooters can prove useful for doing many domestic and workplace tasks, and can benefit not just the frail elderly and people with disabilities, but also others who perform strenuous or physically difficult jobs.

REFERENCES

ABS. (2008). *Population by age and sex, Australian states and territories, Jun 2008. Document 3201.0,* Retrieved September 21 2009, from http://www.abs.gov.au/Ausstats/abs@.nsf/mf/3201.0.

AIHW. (2006). *Chronic disease and associated risk factors in Australia.* Canberra: Australian Institute of Health and Welfare.

Alciatore, D., & Histand, M. (2003). *Introduction to mechatronics.* USA: McGraw-Hill.

Atmel (2007). *ATmega640/1280/1281/2560/2561 datasheet.* Document number 2549LS–AVR 08/07 (p. 37). Retrieved on October 20, 2009, from http://www.atmel.com/dyn/resources/prod_documents/doc2549.pdf.

Banach, D., Jones, T., & Kalameja, A. (2006). *Autodesk Inventor 11 Essentials Plus.* USA: Autodesk Press.

Bien, Z., Kim, D., Chung, M., Kwon, D., & Chang, P. (2003). Development of a wheelchair-based rehabilitation robotic syem (KARES 11) with various human-robot interaction interfaces for the disabled. In *Proceedings of the 2003 IEEE/ASME International Conference on Advanced Intelligent Mechatronics 20-24 July 2003* (AIM 2003), 2 (pp. 902-907). Retrieved September 22, 2009, from http://ieeexplore.ieee.org/stamp/stamp.jsp?tp=&arnumber=1225462&isnumber=27509.

Braga, N. (2002). *Robotics, mechatronics, and artificial intelligence–Experimental circuit blocks for designers.* USA: Newnes.

Cubero, S. N. (1998). *Force, compliance and position control for a pneumatic quadruped robot*, Unpublished PhD dissertation, University of Southern Queensland, Australia.

Cubero, S. N., & Billingsley, J. (1997). Force, compliance and position control for a space frame manipulator. In *Proc 4th International Conference on Mechatronics and Machine Vision in Practice (M^2VIP)*, 22-24th Sep, 1997, Toowoomba, Australia: M2VIP.com.

Davies, E. R. (2005). *Machine vision: Theory, algorithms, practicalities* (3rd ed.). USA: Morgan Kaufmann.

Fallon, S. (2009). *Smart wheelchair features a brain-controlled robotic arm*. Gizmodo. Retrieved February 10, 2009, from http://i.gizmodo.com/5150632/smart-wheelchair-features-a-brain+controlled-robotic-arm.

Freedman, V. A., Martin, L. G., & Schoeni, R. F. (2002). Recent trends in disability and functioning among older adults in the United States. *JAMA, 288*(24), 3137-3146. Retrieved October 19, 2009, from http://jama.ama-assn.org/cgi/reprint/288/24/3137.

Higgins, S. (2007). *Engineers develop a 'helping hand'*. The Oracle (University of South Florida, USA). Retrieved December 6, 2007, from http://www.usforacle.com/2.6026/1.619334-1.619334.

Hillman, M., Hagan, K., Hagan, S., Jepson, J., & Orpwood, R. (2002). The Weston wheelchair mounted assistive robot - the design story. *Robotica, 20*(2), 125–132. doi:10.1017/S0263574701003897

Klafter, R., Chmielewski, T., & Negin, M. (1989). *Robotic Engineering – An Integrated Approach*. USA: Prentice-Hall International.

Martens, C., Ruchel, N., Lang, O., Ivlev, O., & Graser, A. (2001). A FRIEND for assisting people with disabilities. *IEEE Robotics & Automation Magazine, 8*(1), 57-65, Retrieved September 22, 2009, from http://ieeexplore.ieee.org/stamp/stamp.jsp?tp=&arnumber=924364&isnumber=19982.

McKerrow, P. (1991). *Introduction to robotics*. Singapore: Addison-Wesley.

Moody, H. (1998). *Aging concepts and controversies*. Thousand Oaks, CA: Pine Forge Press.

Naung, N. (2006). *Robotic arm for electric scooter*. Unpublished B.Eng. Mechatronic Engineering thesis, Curtin University of Technology, Australia.

Parker, M. G., Ahacic, K., & Thorslund, M. (2005). Health changes among Swedish oldest old: Prevalence rates from 1992 and 2002 show increasing health problems. *Journal of Gerontology, 60A*(10), 1351–1355.

Pons, J. L. (2008). *Wearable robots: Biomechatronic exoskeleton*. USA: Wiley. doi:10.1002/9780470987667

Rakowski, W., & Hickey, T. (1992). Mortality and the attribution of health problems to aging among older adults. *American Journal of Public Health, 82*(8), 1139-1141, Retrieved October 19, 2009, from http://www.ajph.org/cgi/reprint/82/8/1139.

Ricklefs, R. (1995). *Aging a natural history*. New York: Scientific American Library.

Rowe, J. W., & Kahn, R. L. (1987). Human aging: usual and successful. *Science, 237*(4811), 143-149. Retrieved October 19, 2009, from http://www.sciencemag.org/cgi/content/abstract/sci;237/4811/143.

ADDITIONAL READING

Bartlett, T. (2002). *Industrial control electronics: Devices, systems & applications* (2nd ed.). USA: Delmar / Thomson Learning.

Billingsley, J. (2006). *Essentials of mechatronics*. Australia: John Wiley & Sons. doi:10.1002/0471791539

Cetinkunt, S. (2007). *Mechatronics*. USA: John Wiley.

Cubero, S. N. (Ed.). (2007). *Industrial robotics: Theory, modelling & control*. Croatia: Advanced Robotic Systems International.

Culley, R. (2006). *Fitting and machining*. Australia: TAFE Publications / RMIT Publishing.

Holland, J. (2004). *Designing autonomous mobile robots*. USA: Newnes.

Klafter, R., Chmielewski, T., & Negin, M. (1989). *Robotic engineering – An integrated Approach*. USA: Prentice-Hall International.

Kuhnel, C. (1998). *AVR RISC microcontroller handbook*. USA: Butterworth-Heinemann / Newness.

Kuhnel, C. (2001). *BASCOM programming of microcontrollers with ease: An introduction by program examples*. USA: Upublish.com.

Paul, R. P. (1981). *Robot manipulators: Mathematics, programming and control*. USA: MIT Press.

KEY TERMS AND DEFINITIONS

CAD: (Computer Aided Design): Computer software that enables designers to quickly create 2D drawings and/or 3D solid models of mechanical or structural components and assemblies (ie. Groups of components specially arranged or connected at particular positions and orientations relative to each other to form a larger structure or a complete device, subsystem or machine.) Some of the most popular CAD programs in the world include AutoCAD™, Inventor™, SolidWorks™, ProEngineer WildFire™, IDEAS™ and ADAMS™. Most popular 3D CAD programs can export an STL (STereo Lithography) or similar 3D file for direct solid part creation with a 3D printer. Plastic and rubbery type (elastomer) parts, machine component prototypes and even casting patterns can be manufactured directly from the 3D CAD model using a 3D printer or Stereo Lithography machine. Useable metal components can now even be created or printed from a 3D file using a 3D sintering printer without any need to machine out metal parts using a conventional machining or cutting process, and without the need to cast molten metal in a foundry mould. Most modern manufacturing operations today involve the use of CAD software.

CAM: (Computer Aided Manufacture): A process involving the use of computer software to automate or semi-automate the manufacturing process using robots or CNC (Computer Numerically Controlled) machines. Typically, CAD software is used to generate detailed printed drawings, 3D pictorial views and animated simulations. Specially formatted files can be exported from CAD programs and used by CAM programs to generate machining programs (e.g. G-code) for automatically creating or sculpting solid components using 3D printers, CNC Mills, CNC Lathes, laser cutting machines, and many other kinds of manufacturing equipment. CAD/CAM software products, such as MasterCAM™ and AlphaCAM™, are used for editing and creating "tool paths" and generating machining programs for CNC cutting machines. A CNC milling machine or lathe is a special purpose robot fitted with cutting tools and a work-piece holder or clamp. CNC machines remove metal (or any material) from a starting blank work-piece (e.g. a solid block or a cylindrical round shape) to form a final object that matches the 3D CAD model.

Electric Scooter: A small battery powered motorcycle-like vehicle for transporting one seated human passenger. Typically, electric scooters have three or four wheels and are widely used by the frail elderly and people with disabilities for personal transport. Most operators of electric scooters are able to use both of their hands, since this is required for steering the scooter's handlebars. Electric scooters employ similar technologies used on electric wheelchairs and mobile robots (e.g. rechargeable battery power supply, speed and direction controllers, DC motors, etc.)

FEA: (Finite Element Analysis): A software method of analyzing simple or complex 3D geometry by subdividing a large 3D model into small primitives like cubes or pyramids. Boundary conditions and external loads or physical conditions are applied and algorithms are executed recursively in order to achieve a 'steady state' condition for the entire solid or volume being analyzed. (Typically uses the "Stiffness Matrix" method for solving unknown deflections or stresses). FEA can be used to simulate effective stress, deflections, temperature, and many other kinds of physical variables, at any location on the surface or inside the solid model.

Machine Vision: A form of sensing technology whereby a computer is programmed to identify patterns, shapes, edges, outlines, colours or features of recognizable objects from still images or video frames captured by an electronic CCD or digital camera (which is just a 1D or 2D array of optosensors behind a lens). Brightness and/or colour information for each pixel (photosensor) position on a CCD photosensor array are converted into numbers and these can be analyzed and processed by software algorithms to detect important features in a captured "image" frame, or an individual array of numbers representing a single frame or screen of pixel data. (Davies, 2005)

Mechatronic, or Mechatronic Engineering: This is a combination of the words "*mecha*nical" and "elec*tronic*", and is a general label for a machine or system that is comprised of mechanical and electronic components (and often software control code) which are all designed to work together to perform a function or task relating to motion control, actuator control, automation and the guidance or control of any physical work or process. Such components include products like motors (actuators), gears, structural supports, electronic controllers (chips, circuit boards), sensors, communication devices, user controls, displays, control panels and other forms of instrumentation. Mechatronic engineering is the field of study primarily concerned with machine design in the areas of manufacturing automation, motion control, robotics, industrial process control and automated machinery (e.g. CNC machines, NC lathes, etc.). Modern mechatronic devices usually incorporate an embedded microcontroller or microprocessor chip. Such a chip executes software code to process sensor information, make decisions based on preprogrammed rules or expert knowledge, and output necessary signals to force actuators or devices to make needed changes to controlled variables being monitored. (Billingsley, 2006) Industrial type controllers include PLCs (Programmable Logic Controllers, which are just dedicated computer controllers), networked SCADA systems, and industrial robot work-cell controllers. Such industrial controllers can be used for controlling all the motors, devices, robotic arms, pneumatic cylinders and hydraulic clamps and pistons in large factories, as well as monitoring and responding to most types of sensor output signals. (e.g. proximity sensors, position sensors, etc.)

Microcontroller: This is a very low-cost 'computer on a chip' and serves as the core component of an embedded system controller, typically costing less than $30 AUD each. It can be programmed to execute software instructions that can read sensor inputs, process control code and drive motors/actuators, display devices, communications hardware and other devices to perform desired tasks. The software executed by the microcontroller is the 'brains' responsible for controlling most embedded controller applications. Microcontrollers are commonly found in many modern devices and appliances, such as DVD controllers, air conditioners, water temperature controllers, garden sprinkler controllers, computer peripherals like printers and scanners, security alarm systems and engine monitoring systems for many automobiles. Microcontroller devices are supplied by several semiconductor device manufacturers (e.g. Motorola™, Atmel™, Microchip™, Intel™ and Phillips™.) For example, one of the most popular 8-bit families of microcontrollers in use today is the AVR ATmega family of chips. They can be programmed using a high level language like C or BASCOM, which is similar to BASIC or QBasic (Kuhnel, 2001), or low-level "machine code" type languages, like AVR Assembly language (Kuhnel, 1998). Microcontrollers can be used for controlling most kinds of small mobile robots, position-controlled actuators and very simple automation systems. Several microcontrollers can work cooperatively and communicate on a data 'network', and they can also work as dedicated 'slave' controllers, supervised and commanded by a 'master' computer or PC.

Robotic Arm: This is a special type of mechatronic device which serves as a multipurpose manipulator that can be programmed or controlled to perform a variety of different motion control tasks using an end-effector tool (e.g. a gripper), either automatically or via remote control. Individual links or joints of the robotic arm are linked in a serial 'chain' of links, where one actuator is used to drive each link or joint (ie. one translational or rotary type degree of freedom per link, or two rotary degrees for one spherical joint). The gripper (or end-effector tool) can be commanded to follow a desired trajectory or 3D path in cartesian space, and record and replay such movements. Automatic gripper or end-effector position and orientation control can be achieved by executing an "Inverse Kinematics" algorithm and feedback control code to control all actuators. The control software calculates the necessary joint angles or positions to achieve the desired trajectory, it outputs all motor or actuator control commands for all joints, and it uses sensor feedback to correct any errors, such as position, speed or force errors. Robotic arms and their end-effector tools can be controlled for variable position, speed, force and compliance, however, being machines, they do not tire out and can be designed to be much stronger, more reliable, more accurate and much faster compared to human workers. There are many different types of configurations and designs of robot arms, each best suited for particular applications.

Section 2
Innovations Supporting Engagement with Daily Life

Chapter 8
Thinking Outside the Box:
Novel Uses of Technology to Promote Well-Being in Older Populations

Nancy A. Pachana
The University of Queensland, Australia

Emma E. Poulsen
The University of Queensland, Australia

ABSTRACT

This chapter aims to examine the adoption of technology by older adults within a framework of current gerontological theories and research. Cognitive, physical, mental and interpersonal development and change later in life will also be described. Two main psychological frameworks for understanding successful ageing are briefly outlined and within these frameworks, the role of technology in enhancing the lives of older adults, regardless of the level at which they incorporate it into their lives, will be discussed. The chapter concludes with suggestions for removing barriers and enhancing uptake of technology for older adults, helping to bridge the grey digital divide.

TECHNOLOGY IN THE LIVES OF OLDER ADULTS

Parents-in-law Jack (83 yrs) and Jill (81 yrs) are mentally alert, have bustling social lives and are physically active. However the degree to which they incorporate and benefit from bringing technology into their lives is very different. Since his retirement as a civil engineer, Jack has increasingly explored technology as a recreational pursuit, as well as for financial gain and as a means of connecting with family and friends. He spends several hours each day trading stocks online, chatting to his overseas grandchildren on Skype, updating his Facebook page and trading and buying on eBay. Indeed, on a recent road-trip Jack became so engrossed in a new navigation application that he had downloaded for his iPhone, that Jill, baffled by such obsessions, snapped "No, I don't want to know how long it would take to drive from Brisbane to Broome!". While Jack has found another world of engagement in modern technology, Jill finds it a daunting and unconquerable environment.

Jill, a retired physiotherapist, does not own a computer and still records all important cor-

DOI: 10.4018/978-1-61520-825-8.ch008

respondence on carbon paper. She has a mobile phone at her family's insistence but rarely uses it and often only does so when sitting at her desk, following the instructions written down by her grandchildren. At one point she enrolled in a computer course at her local library but pulled out after deciding there would be little opportunity nor inclination to use those skills in her current life. Indeed, she sees little point in changing her routines to incorporate technology so long as the traditional systems are still working. While this attitude has merit, Jill often becomes frustrated operating in a modern world that relies on such technology, and doesn't effectively cater for individuals who do not wish to take on the same level of technology in their lives.

The case of Jack and Jill is not an uncommon one and represents two ends of a spectrum in an older cohort's attitudes towards technology and the extent to which it is incorporated into their lives. As the baby boomer generation continues to age, concepts of the grey digital divide continue to evolve. This is an issue which is very salient not only to individuals in society, but also to the business, education and social services sectors, along with governments and policy makers. As both the proportion of older adults in the population and the use of technology in everyday life increases, this is an issue that will assume increasing importance in the coming decades (McMurtrey, McGaughey, & Downey, 2009).

Recent research points to many factors which can have a profound impact on health and well-being in later life. Social network size (Bennett, Schneider, Tang, Arnold, & Wilson, 2006), continued exercise (Abbott et al., 2004), mental stimulation (Coyle, 2003) and pursuit of leisure activities (Verghese et al., 2003) have all been shown to have positive effects on morbidity and mortality later in life. Advances in medical technologies have contributed to increasing the lifespan (particularly for those over age 80), and assistive technology has improved daily functioning through improvements or augmentation of the senses, mobility and aspects of independent living. But perhaps the greatest growth (as well as potential growth) has been in the uptake of technologies related to use of leisure time, such as increased use of social networking sites to supplement and expand social networks, gathering information or even pursuing educational opportunities over the internet, the use of technology to organise and record personal documents/photos and use of e-book readers. An example of this latter innovation and its particular applicability to an older population is Amazon's Kindle program with its ease of manipulation and print-size adjustment functions (Robbins, 2009).

In many ways the incredible diversity of technologies on offer is in itself a good match for older adults. As a group older adults are more diverse than younger populations physiologically, psychologically, and socially; thus technology, as such a diverse medium in itself, seems to be ideally positioned to adapt to the older adult cohort (Hertzog & Light, 2004).

TECHNOLOGY ALLOWS PERSONAL GROWTH THROUGH LATER LIFE

Professor Gene Cohen, Director of the Center on Aging, Health and Humanities at George Washington University, author of the popular book *The Mature Mind* (2005), has put forward a theory of the developmental stages through which older adults progress later in life (Cohen, 2001). He labels these as *phases for human potential in the second half of life*. Technology can play a strong role in aiding an individual through these phases. Using Jack's case study as a discussion point, the way in which this can be done will be illustrated by further exploring his personal trajectory through the last four decades of his life.

According to Cohen, during the 40s to 50s there is a phase called "midlife re-evaluation" in which individuals search for ways to make life and work more gratifying and meaningful. Though often characterised (and caricatured) in the popular press as the "midlife crisis", such a phase can be productive and generative, resulting in enhanced relationships and productivity. Technology can be used as a means to assist or even enhance this period of self-discovery. Today, the internet can be used as a tool to research and pursue activities that bring value and gratification into an individual's life, helping to incorporate enjoyed pursuits with already existing commitments. In the case of Jack, the internet was not yet available in the 1960's, when he was 40 years old. Instead, it was the game of golf and golfing technology that sparked his interest. Having played the sport for a number of years, he began to enjoy it in earnest with new, high-tech "Ping" golf clubs that allowed him to drive his balls further and with less physical effort. The stereotypical action for a gentleman in this phase of life is to buy a sports car. For Jack, it was a golf buggy, a machine that made the sport faster, less physically exerting and more conveniently fitted in to the rest of his family and professional life.

The 60s and early 70s are described by Cohen as a phase of "liberation" in which creative pursuits are enhanced by a new sense of personal freedom and experimentation. In fact, Cohen (2000) argues that such an expansion in creative pursuits is also assisted by changes in the brain - a different message, surely, than familiar laments about the inevitable decline in brain functioning. Cohen describes how new neuroimaging technologies demonstrate that in some ways the ageing brain is more flexible than younger ones. In Jack's 60s, advances in computer technology were on the forefront of an explosive boom, about to be widely publically available and heavily relied on by business and education systems alike. Entering retirement age with less restriction on how the hours of each day must be spent, Jack was able to explore this new medium and gain knowledge and skill in a new and challenging field. He bought one of the first publically available Macintosh computers and before his retirement, incorporated high-tech IT systems into the designs of new oil refineries where he worked. Today, using technology can increase the accessibility of an activity or provide inspiration for a new pursuit that in turn, increases the likelihood of new discoveries and personal growth.

In the "summing up" phase (age 70 and above) (Cohen, 2000), there is a need to find meaning in life through summing up experiences and trying to pass on what one has learned to the next generation. This is a period when older adults may feel compelled to write their autobiography, volunteer with disadvantaged youth or engage in philanthropy. Indeed, during his early 70s Jack began to compile his memoirs, buying voice activated transcribing systems to recount his long professional career as a civil engineer. Having become familiar with the notion of computers in his late 60s (primitive machines by today's standards), he set about mastering the technology further to organise the large number of boxes containing copious hand written notes, that were to eventually become his written story. An unexpected by-product of this experience was that though using a computer to summarise his professional career, he became addicted to the efficiency of technology and became passionate about having mastery in the field. This in turn lead to him sharing his experiences with the rest of his family and in many cases, introducing them to and teaching them about a new program or function on their own computers.

In the phase that Cohen (2000) labels "encore", persons over age 80 feel the desire to make a final contribution or statement by which they might be remembered. At this time taking care of unfinished business is a high priority. According to Cohen, this is "motivated by a wish to affirm life and celebrate one's place in the family, community, and spiritual realm" (Cohen, 2001, p. 53). In the case of Jack, this became the organising of his affairs, particularly after the passing of his wife. Technology played an instrumental role in this process. He created spreadsheets to divide up family assets and those that were not claimed by any relative, he sold on eBay. He also set about scanning all of his old photographs onto the computer and converting his old photo slides into digital images, so that copies could be given to his family members. He also made a DVD photo slideshow, tracking his life to a soundtrack of meaningful songs, which was given to each grandchild at Christmas.

For Jack, technology was a useful medium that made existing hobbies easier to pursue (e.g. golf), acted as an avenue for discovering new passions (e.g. exploring a new computer), assisted Jack in completing his set goals (e.g. writing his memoirs) and connecting with his family (e.g. sharing photos and stories).

SELECTION, OPTIMISATION AND COMPENSATION

Across any stage of the lifespan, an individual will go though changes and will be required to adapt to those changes if they are to continue functioning at a high level. Paul Baltes of the Max Planck Institute in Berlin has contributed much to the literature on adult development and ageing. His well known theory of successful ageing, developed with his wife Margaret, is known as Selection, Optimisation and Compensation (SOC) (Baltes & Baltes, 1990). This theory can be used as a framework to discuss positive contributions of technology to successful ageing.

The SOC model attempts to describe lifespan development and ageing with the focus on successful adaptation to changing circumstances. The model takes the individual's gains and losses jointly into account. For example, while an individual may gain wisdom, material possessions or a wider social network with age, they may also experience losses such as physical functionality or adaptability to new situations. SOC considers these losses and gains and views eventual successful mastery of the individual's goals as the result of the interplay of three processes. These processes are selection, compensation, and optimisation. Here, selection refers to developing and choosing appropriate goals, optimisation of identified goal-relevant means, and compensation whereby there is a substitution of means when previous means are no longer available.

Consider the following example of Jill. While Jill refuses to incorporate the use of computers and mobile phones into her life, technology can emerge in many guises, some of which are less daunting and more familiar than others. Jill is a lifelong passionate gardener. In recent years she has lost some mobility and has difficulty getting up and down to the garden bed. This also meant that the lower section of her garden became inaccessible to her as it required a steep decent down a hill. The continued pursuit of the goal of gardening required a reassessment of her means. By choosing to pursue her goal (**selection**) after weighing alternatives and available resources, Jill took active steps towards realising her goal and continues to garden to this day. This process of selection for Jill was partly achieved through *researching options and information on the internet.* This was done on request by her daughter-in-law, an Occupational Therapist, who printed out a range of possibilities for her to consider and discussed possible alternatives in relation to raised garden beds and mulching systems to reduce hand watering needs etc. Mobility and strength, which had deteriorated due to age-related declines and diseases were **optimised** by using items of *assistive technology* (e.g. ergonomic gardening tools and kneeling pads with handles) that were found online by her daughter-in-law. Lack of means of maintaining her existing garden (lack of soil and space with the inaccessibility of her lower garden) was **compensated** for through making use of *further assistive technologies* (e.g. hydroponics and mechanised light and watering technologies in the rest of her garden). In this situation, the utilization of both modern internet and assistive technologies, both directly and indirectly, enabled Jill to adapt to her changing environment, realising her gardening goals. Despite having an aversion to using some technologies, Jill still benefited greatly from having technology aid her in the achievement of her goal. Being guided through the process by family members who were more familiar with where to look, what to look for, and how to access it made the journey far easier and more successful.

As is evident from Cohen's developmental life stage theory (2001) and Paul Baltes selection, optimisation and compensation theory (1990), technology and its application to older adults lives fits easily into the framework of current gerontological theories. Indeed, in many cases, technology can assist or even improve an older adult's transition throughout their later life stages. Current gerontological research in the field has further demonstrated this. In the sections below, studies showing how technology can positively impact on social interaction, cognitive functioning, physical ability and sense of self will be discussed.

SOCIAL INTERACTION, TECHNOLOGY AND SUCCESSFUL AGEING

In the Harvard Study of Adult Development, which followed a group of men over a period of 70 years, one of the most important variables for predicting future successful ageing (in terms of both health and economic factors) was whether these men had maintained close personal relationships over time (Vaillant, 2002). Greater social networks have been found to be associated with lower risk of psychiatric illness in later life (Bowling & Farquhar, 1991) and decreased the risk of dementia (Fratiglioni et al., 2000), and social networks have been found to enhance quality of life and well being later in life (Bennett et al., 2006).

Older adults, despite generally having smaller social networks than younger adults, nevertheless derive as much if not greater social support from their existing networks. (Carstensen, 1993). This is partly because these networks consist of close friends whose friendships have been retained and nurtured because they are such a strong source of social support (Carstensen, 1993). Despite the fact that a variety of factors might influence gains (e.g. grandchildren) and losses (e.g. death of spouse) in one's social network, the overall structure as well as subjective qualities of the social network (including both dependency and interdependency, closeness, and exchange of support over time) reflect the diversity of older adults themselves (Antonucci, 2001).

The internet is one tool that can be incredibly useful to connecting people. Many older adults look to the internet as a source of information, but a growing number of individuals are also exploring the internet's capacity to help them maintain and extend their social networks (Bargh & McKenna, 2004). Social networking sites can also be of great utility for older adults wanting to maintain relationships with friends and family who may have moved away. Such sites also offer the possibility of reconnecting with friends or family with whom contact has been lost.

These networking sites can also be used to discover new networks. As older adults are such a heterogeneous group, the internet can assist in making niche information and cohorts more accessible, and can assist in forming new relationships with spread-out factions (Bargh & McKenna, 2004). For example via the internet, Jack was able to connect with a local group called the ROMEOs (Retired Old Men Eating Out). Local neighbourhood groups accessed from these sites can help older adults find organised activities for those of a similar age and interest. Finally, older adults have also been increasingly participating in on-line dating services, locating like minded individuals interested in pursuing a more involved relationship (Silver, 2007).

As many of these sites are free, connecting in this way can often be a more feasible financial option, allowing greater levels of communication for those on a fixed income.

Telephone technologies are also enabling older adults to stay connected to their social networks. For example, new caller ID technology not only identifies who is calling but reminds the person taking the call of people whom he or she and the caller have in common as well as the subject of their last conversation. This is a way in which technology is actively supporting social network maintenance as well as assisting with any mild forgetfulness that might get in the way of maintaining robust social networks.

NOVEL USES OF TECHNOLOGY FOR PHYSICAL AND COGNITIVE ENGAGEMENT

As noted above, researchers have shown that keeping cognitively and physically active positively impacts the brain. These positive results on brain functioning have been shown at even advanced ages and also have been shown for people who already have some amount of cognitive decline or even who have already received a diagnosis of dementia. For example, computerised brain exercises have been shown to improve memory and lead to faster thinking in older adults as part of The Improvement in Memory with Plasticity-based Adaptive Cognitive Training (IMPACT) study (Smith et al., 2009). Access to the internet and opportunities for e-learning experiences provide an alternate avenue for cognitive stimulation as well as lifelong learning at all ages (Bakaev, Ponomarev, & Prokhorova, (2008). Supervised exercise programs have been shown to increase functional ability (Rolland et al., 2007) and decrease restlessness and agitated behaviours in persons with dementia in residential aged care facilities (Aman & Thomas, 2009). In fact, even in persons over age 80, a relatively small amount of physical activity can go a long way. In a recent study, modest exercise for as little as four hours a week was shown to have health benefits, including extending life by at least a few years (Stessman et al., 2009).

The latest trends in entertainment involve the Nintendo Wii – an interesting interactive gaming concept where people (including older adults) can test their hand-eye coordination by playing "virtual" games such as tennis. The device also has simple exercise and balance routines built in. The ability to maintain balance has been shown not only to reduce risk of falls but also to predict increased health outcomes (Low Choy, Brauer, & Nitz, 2007).

When physical functioning deteriorates, technology can provide an excellent avenue for further cognitive exploration. Computer games ranging from Sudoku to Solitaire help keep the brain active and engaged. Increased mental stimulation over time has been shown to reduce risk of dementia. Even using internet search engines has been shown to have measurable effects of the brain (Small, Moody, Siddarth, & Bookheimer, 2009). Combining mental and social stimulation (such as virtual contract bridge over the internet) helps improve social and cognitive status. A recent Scandinavian study demonstrated the largest health gains from leisure activities that combined at least two social, cognitive or physical activity elements (Karp et al., 2006).

TECHNOLOGY AS A TOOL TO PROTECT IDENTITY AND IMPROVE SENSE OF SELF

It is not uncommon for older adults to feel increasingly negative about their own selves as they age (Levy, 2003). Indeed, there is a large body of evidence that shows older adults are often explicitly and implicitly stereotyped as being less able and less credible than their younger counterparts. This occurs despite research that demonstrates it is not globally the case (e.g. Ostir, Markides, Black, & Goodwin, 2000) and that functioning in both mental and emotional spheres depends on a variety of factors (Pachana, 2006). When negative ageing stereotypes are allowed to persist, they can become internalised (Levy, 2003). This can have dramatic effects such as shortening the life-span and decreasing cognitive and physical functioning in addition to more specific deteriorations such as gait stability and handwriting. Improving these self-perceptions of ageing has been shown to significantly improve longevity, even after controlling for age, gender, socioeconomic status, loneliness, and functional health (Levy, Slade, Kunkel & Kasl, 2003).

Mentoring can assist in reducing the impact of this negative stereotyping by allowing the older adult to pass on valuable skills and knowledge. Studies have shown that older adults who engage in volunteer work, sharing and engaging their skills, have higher well-being than older adults who do not volunteer (Morrow-Howell, Hinterlong, Rozario & Tang, 2003). Cross-generation information transfer benefits not only the individual receiving the knowledge, but also the older adult who is given respect and a sense of worth through sharing the information. Indeed, intergenerational communication has become a topic of focus as companies and businesses alike recognise the value of merging extensive experience and with youthful drive and a new perspective (Lindenberger & Stoltz-Loike, 2005). Technology can play a role in the information sharing process through communication programs such as email, document share sites, online chat and website blogging. By increasing the accessibility of the information transfer, the likelihood of that transfer occurring is increased.

Studies have also shown that an individual's sense of self-worth and identity are linked to their place of residence, namely their home and the items within it (Cram & Paton, 1993). This is particularly the case in older populations where a residence may have been occupied for a number of years and is filled with treasured memories and keepsakes. Technology that assists older adults' social interconnectedness as well as physical and cognitive functioning results in increased likelihood of remaining at home, and thus is more likely to result in maintaining proximity to the material world that is so closely linked to their memories and self-identity. This not only benefits the individual, but also reduces the strain on the healthcare system by maximising the persons' happiness and independence, keeping them out of aged care where their condition may deteriorate further once removed from their familiar environment (Dishman, 2004).

Assistive technologies such as stair-lifts, level-access showers, bed-levers, raised lavatory-seats and social-alarms can greatly increase the functionality of older adults, giving them a greater chance at independently remaining in their homes (Tang & Venables, 2000). However, as technologies advance and designers become more creative, technologies are being implemented in ways that help older adults maintain independence in style. For example, the "House of the Future" occupies some 150 square metres of Lisbon's Museum of Communications in Portugal and features items made by multinational companies as well as prototypes still in development by local universities. A talking washing machine, mirrors that double as television screens and a virtual garden are among the gadgets on display; the home acts as a showcase for the latest technology aimed at helping older adults to live independently.

TIPS ON INTRODUCING TECHNOLOGY TO OLDER ADULTS

Often younger adults, who have had a seamless introduction to technologies via school or work, are frustrated at others' failure to take up what they may see as "essential" tools. But older adults are not only less familiar with many technologies as a rule, but also may have definite ideas on what sorts of activities they do and don't value. As a more heterogeneous group, technological devices or procedures that enhance specific valued activities are more likely to be adopted by an older adult (McCreadie & Tinker, 2005).

As a rule, older adults take longer to learn new routines compared with younger adults (Craik, 1994). This is particularly true with regards to technology, especially when experience with using a particular technology is low (Charness, Kelly, Bosman, & Mottram, 2001). However, having a broader context in which to embed new learning can offer some advantages to older learners (Small, 2002). Nevertheless, introducing a new technology at a comfortable pace for the older adult will also increase the chance it is successfully understood and applied (Convertino, Farooq, Rosson, Carroll, & Meyer, 2007).

Price can also be a concern. If possible, try to arrange for a trial of an item that may be of interest, before any actual purchase. In this way the relevance and any concerns about the device can be ascertained beforehand. This also helps to avoid the sense of frustration and failure when an expensive device remains unused but very much in the older person's mind as a costly mistake. Taking the time to understand how the use of some technology can cut down on costs may also help in the use of the product. For example, using email or online chat programs can quite significantly reduce the amount spent on postage and/or phone bills.

Allowing younger members of a family to teach their older relatives the ins and outs of technology has the added benefit of promoting intergenerational bonds. Such teaching may be more palatable for the older adult coming from one generation removed from them. Such contact has tangible benefits for both parties (Antonucci, 2001).

There is research demonstrating a tendency toward greater "computer anxiety" in current older adults compared to younger cohorts (Laguna & Babcock, 1998). This trend will likely change over time as subsequent generations become increasingly comfortable with computers, but for the moment it is a finding worth taking into account. Thus how and at what speed computer technologies are introduced to an individual is critical to successful uptake of this technology. Taking the time to introduce and explain how the new technology will benefit their immediate life is important for completely new users. When a first-time consumer is confronted with a foreign concept such as the internet, it can be very difficult to conceptualise how it works and how it can assist you. Being clear about the many different ways in which you can use the technology will reduce the risk of a product being rigidly used for only one function, when in reality it has many worthy applications.

Allow the older adult using the new technology to have ownership over it. The use of the technology has to be driven by the individual if it is to be effectively used and enjoyed as a tool to increase quality of life (McCreadie & Tinker, 2005). Forcing an unwanted technology into someone's life will often result in resistance to its use. However, it is also important to remember that technology cannot be taken up if insufficient access is an issue. When barriers to technology have been minimised and use of technologies such as computers has evolved more organically along with the needs and goals of older adults, positive results ensue (Carpenter & Buday, 2007; Naumanen & Tukiainen, 2007).

Finally, particularly if publicly available computers are used often, it is important for the older adult to be aware of the dangers of putting personal information on the internet. A general awareness of hoaxes or schemes to part older adults from their money is important if the older adult is new to computing.

CONCLUSION

There are many ways in which the grey digital divide can be bridged and the lives of older adults can be improved by incorporating technology into their daily living. Gerontological theories on phases for human potential in the second half of life (Cohen, 2005) and Selection, Optimisation and Compensation (Baltes & Baltes, 1990) were discussed in relation to two case studies involving the use of technology to varying degrees. Current research on cognitive, physical, mental and interpersonal development and change later in later life was also described, demonstrating the many successful ways in which technology has been used to improve outcomes in older adults. Lastly, a number of suggestions were made for removing barriers and enhancing uptake of technology for older adults, helping them to bridge the grey digital divide.

REFERENCES

Abbott, R., White, L., Ross, W., Masaki, K. H., Curb, J. D., & Petrovitch, H. (2004). Walking and dementia in physically capable elderly men. *Journal of the American Medical Association*, *292*, 1447–1453. doi:10.1001/jama.292.12.1447

Aman, E., & Thomas, D. R. (2009). Supervised exercise to reduce agitation in severely cognitively impaired persons. *Journal of the American Medical Directors Association*, *10*(4), 271–276. doi:10.1016/j.jamda.2008.12.053

Antonucci, T. C. (2001). Social relations: An examination of social networks, social support, and sense of control. In Birren, J. E., & Schaie, K. W. (Eds.), *Handbook of the psychology of aging* (5th ed., pp. 427–453). San Diego, CA: Academic Press.

Bakaev, M., Ponomarev, V., & Prokhorova, L. (2008). E-learning and elder people: Barriers and benefits. *Computational Technologies in Electrical and Electronics Engineering*, 110-113.

Baltes, P. B., & Baltes, M. M. (1990). Psychological perspectives on successful aging: The model of selective optimization with compensation. In Baltes, P. B., & Baltes, M. M. (Eds.), *Successful aging: Perspectives from the behavioral sciences* (pp. 1–34). New York: Cambridge University Press. doi:10.1017/CBO9780511665684.003

Bargh, J., & McKenna, K. (2004). The internet and social life. *Annual Review of Psychology*, *55*, 573–590. doi:10.1146/annurev.psych.55.090902.141922

Bennett, D. A., Schneider, J. A., Tang, Y., Arnold, S. E., & Wilson, R. S. (2006). The effect of social networks on the relation between Alzheimer's disease pathology and level of cognitive function in old people: a longitudinal cohort study. *The Lancet Neurology*, *5*(5), 406–412. doi:10.1016/S1474-4422(06)70417-3

Bowling, A., & Farquhar, M. (1991). Associations with social networks, social support, health status and psychiatric morbidity in three samples of elderly people. *Social Psychiatry and Psychiatric Epidemiology*, *26*(3), 15–126. doi:10.1007/BF00782950

Carpenter, B. D., & Buday, S. (2007). Computer use among older adults in a naturally occurring retirement community. *Computers in Human Behavior*, *23*, 3012–3024. doi:10.1016/j.chb.2006.08.015

Carstensen, L. L. (1993). Motivation for social contact across the life span: A theory of socioemotional selectivity. In J. E. Jacobs (Ed.), *Nebraska Symposium on Motivation: Developmental perspectives on motivation* (pp. 209-254). Lincoln, NE: University of Nebraska Press.

Charness, N., Kelly, C. L., Bosman, E. A., & Mottram, M. (2001). Word-processing training and retraining: Effects of adult age, experience, and interface. *Psychology and Aging*, *16*, 110–127. doi:10.1037/0882-7974.16.1.110

Cohen, G. (2000). *The creative age*. New York: Harper Collins.

Cohen, G. (2001). Creativity with aging: Four phases of potential in the second half of life. *Geriatrics*, *56*(4), 51–57.

Cohen, G. (2005). *The mature mind: The positive power of the aging brain*. New York: Basic Books.

Convertino, G., Farooq, U., Rosson, M. B., Carroll, J. M., & Meyer, B. J. F. (2007). Supporting intergenerational groups in computer-supported cooperative work (CSCW). *Behaviour & Information Technology*, *26*, 275–285. doi:10.1080/01449290601173473

Coyle, J. T. (2003). Use it or lose it - Do effortful mental activities protect against dementia? *The New England Journal of Medicine*, *348*, 2489–2490. doi:10.1056/NEJMp030051

Craik, F. I. M. (1994). Memory changes in normal aging. *Current Directions in Psychological Science*, *5*, 155–158. doi:10.1111/1467-8721.ep10770653

Cram, F., & Paton, H. (1993). Personal possessions and self-identity: The experiences of elderly women in three residential settings. *Australasian Journal on Ageing*, *12*, 19–24. doi:10.1111/j.1741-6612.1993.tb00579.x

Dishman, E. (2004). Inventing wellness systems for aging in place. *IEEE Computer Society,* 34-41.

Fratiglioni, L., Wang, H. X., Ericsson, K., Maytan, M., & Winblad, B. (2000). Influence of social network on occurrence of dementia: a community-based longitudinal study. *Lancet*, *355*(9212), 1315–1319. doi:10.1016/S0140-6736(00)02113-9

Hertzog, C., & Light, L. (2004). Methodological issues in the assessment of technology use for older adults. In Pew, R. W., & Van Hemel, S. B. (Eds.), *Technology for Adaptive Aging*. National Academies Press.

Karp, A., Paillard-Borg, S., Wang, H.-X., Silverstein, M., Winblad, B., & Fratiglioni, L. (2006). Mental, physical and social components in leisure activities equally contribute to decrease dementia risk. *Dementia and Geriatric Cognitive Disorders*, *21*(2), 65–73. doi:10.1159/000089919

Laguna, K., & Babcock, R. L. (1997). Computer anxiety in young and older adults: Implications for human-computer interactions in older populations. *Computers in Human Behavior*, *13*(3), 317–326. doi:10.1016/S0747-5632(97)00012-5

Levy, B. R. (2003). Mind matters: Cognitive and physical effects of aging self-stereotypes. *Journal of Gerontology: Psychological Sciences*, *58*, 203–211.

Levy, B. R., Slade, M. D., Kunkel, S. R., & Kasl, S. V. (2003). Longevity increased by positive self-perceptions of aging. *Journal of Personality and Social Psychology*, *83*, 261–270. doi:10.1037/0022-3514.83.2.261

Lindenberger, J., & Stoltz-Loike, M. (2005). *Why Mentor? Mentoring is a strategic business imperative*. Human Resources, The Lindenberger Group, LLC and SeniorThinking.

Low Choy, N. L., Brauer, S. G., & Nitz, J. C. (2007). Timed stance performances reflect differences in age, prevalence of comorbidities, medication use, fall history and activity level: Early screening for balance loss is indicated. *Australasian Journal on Ageing*, *26*(1), 29–34. doi:10.1111/j.1741-6612.2007.00202.x

McCreadie, C., & Tinker, A. (2005). The acceptability of assistive technology to older people. *Ageing and Society*, *25*, 91–110. doi:10.1017/S0144686X0400248X

McMurtrey, M. E., McGaughey, R. E., & Downey, J. P. (2009). Seniors and information technology: A potential goldmine of opportunity? *International Journal of Intercultural Information Management.*, *1*, 300–316.

Morrow-Howell, N., Hinterlong, J., Rozario, P. A., & Tang, F. (2003). Effects of volunteering on the well-being of older adults. *Journal of Gerontology: Social Sciences*, *58*, 137–145.

Naumanen, M., & Tukiainen, M. (2007). Seniors' club – Learning and blogging together. In P. Kommers & P. Isaías (Eds.), *Proceedings of the IADIS International Conference Web Based Communities* (pp. 312-316). Salamanca, Spain: IADIS.

Ostir, G. V., Markides, K. S., Black, S. A., & Goodwin, J. S. (2000). Emotional well-being predicts subsequent independent functioning and survival. *Journal of the American Geriatrics Society*, *48*, 473–478.

Pachana, N. A. (2006). Psychogerontology and cognitive disabilities related to ageing. In Morse, C. (Ed.), *The art of ageing in a global context: From theory and research to policy and practice* (pp. 435–452). New York: Baywood Publishers.

Robbins, S. (2009). Large print finds its mark. *Publishers Weekly.* Retrieved 17 September 2009 from http://www.publishersweekly.com/article/CA6658685.html?q.

Rolland, Y., Pillard, F., Klapouszczak, A., Reynish, E., Thomas, D., & Andrieu, S. (2007). Exercise program for nursing home residents with Alzheimer's disease: A 1-Year Randomized, Controlled Trial. *Journal of the American Geriatrics Society*, *55*(2), 158–165. doi:10.1111/j.1532-5415.2007.01035.x

Silver, S. (2007). "Internet Romance: How Match.com Found Love among Boomers; Dating Site Prospers Targeting Older Singles; The Body Art Question", in *Wall Street Journal. (Eastern edition)*, New York, January 27.

Small, G., Moody, T., Siddarth, P., & Bookheimer, S. (2009). Your brain on Google: Patterns of cerebral activation during Internet searching. *The American Journal of Geriatric Psychiatry*, *17*(2), 116–126. doi:10.1097/JGP.0b013e3181953a02

Small, G. W. (2002). *The memory bible.* New York: Hyperion.

Smith, G. E., Housen, P., Yaffe, K., Ruff, R., Kennison, R. F., Mahncke, H. W., & Zelinski, E. M. (2009). A cognitive training program based on principles of brain plasticity: Results from the improvement in memory with plasticity-based adaptive cognitive training (IMPACT) Study. *Journal of the American Geriatrics Society*, *57*(4), 594–603. doi:10.1111/j.1532-5415.2008.02167.x

Stessman, J., Hammerman-Rozenberg, R., Cohen, A., Ein-Mor, E., & Jacobs, J. M. (2009). Physical activity, function and longevity among the very old. *Archives of Internal Medicine*, *169*(16), 1476–1483. doi:10.1001/archinternmed.2009.248

Tang, P., & Venables, T. (2000). Smart Homes and Telecare for independent living. *Journal of Telemedicine and Telecare*, *6*, 8–14. doi:10.1258/1357633001933871

Vaillant, G. E. (2002). *Aging well.* Boston: Little Brown.

Verghese, J., Lipton, R. B., Katz, M. J., Hall, C. B., Derby, C. A., & Kuslansky, G. (2003). Leisure activities and risk of dementia in the elderly. *The New England Journal of Medicine*, *348*, 2508–2516. doi:10.1056/NEJMoa022252

Chapter 9
U3A Online and Successful Aging:
A Smart Way to Help Bridge the Grey Digital Divide

Rick Swindell
Griffith University, Australia

Peter Grimbeek
Griffith University, Australia

Jan Heffernan
Queensland University of Technology, Australia

ABSTRACT

Population aging is refocusing aging policy away from mainly remedial actions towards low cost preventative interventions that keep older people independent and participating in their communities for longer. The purpose of this chapter is 3-fold: 1) to outline the elements of the successful aging model; 2) to explain the worldwide, self-help University of the Third Age (U3A) adult education program as a very low cost, successful aging organization; and 3) to discuss findings from two related studies of older adults who were members of a virtual U3A called U3A Online. Considerable anecdotal evidence shows that U3A Online is particularly valuable for people who are isolated from their mainstream communities by circumstances such as illness, disability or care giving. An email focus group with nine participants from three countries was conducted over a two year period, using the successful aging model as a guideline to examine the characteristics of these older people who are attracted to online learning. Results based on the combination of automated computer text analysis and manual text analysis techniques supported a conclusion that the Internet was an integral part of the lives of these participants, particularly those with serious health difficulties or profound hearing loss. Outcomes also supported a conclusion that electronic communication can reduce feelings of isolation and provide stimulating and enjoyable pastimes with the potential to assist older people in aging successfully.

DOI: 10.4018/978-1-61520-825-8.ch009

INTRODUCTION

Faced with a bourgeoning aging population, governments in many countries are seeking creative ways for maximizing returns from relatively declining budgets and stretched social support services for the elderly. Inevitably the emphasis has swung from expensive, later life medical heroics to an approach that places increasing onus on aging individuals to take more responsibility for their own aging. Preventative rather than remedial interventions have become the major goal for addressing myriad social and economic challenges that accompany population aging.

Old machines wear out. However, with regular maintenance and timely expert mechanical intervention, old machines can continue reliably carrying out their designated functions for years. Something similar applies to older human machines. It seems that if people choose to adopt a few sensible lifestyle habits then they stand the best chance of maximizing their own longevity and independence. The key word in this is "choose". By choosing to follow a regular self-maintenance program throughout its life, the aging human machine is better able to carry on successfully to a ripe old age with far less reliance on expensive medical intervention needed to get it back on the road.

In this chapter, we first describe the successful aging framework and discuss its components and benefits. We then present information on organizations aimed to promote successful aging, with a particular focus on those that promote learning in older age with a goal of delaying cognitive decline and capitalizing on older citizens' cognitive resources. We then describe two related studies conducted with older participants in an online lifelong learning program called U3A Online. These findings are discussed in light of the successful aging framework.

BACKGROUND

Successful Aging

During the past two decades many studies have been carried out in an attempt to determine why some people in their 80s, 90s and older continue to engage optimistically and independently with everyday life, whereas others who are younger have already lost their independence. Successful aging, aging well, productive aging, active aging, healthy aging, and positive aging are among a number of closely related, evidence-based models that differ from each other in emphasis rather than absolute content (Friedrich, 2003). Regardless of which model is emphasized, each is about a quite small number of choices that older people should follow if they are to maintain a sense of control over their environment while balancing the gains and losses in later life.

The MacArthur Foundation Study of Successful Aging (Rowe & Kahn, 1999) illustrates the substantial gains in understanding of aging that can flow from a large, interdisciplinary research approach. The study, which was actually a coherent set of dozens of individual research projects led by 16 researchers from across the broad spectrum of gerontology, was the most extensive and comprehensive multidisciplinary study on aging in America. The successful aging model, which was an outcome of the collective findings, outlines three fundamental attributes of a successfully aging individual:

- low risk of disease and disease-related disability;
- high mental and physical function;
- active engagement with life.

Each of the three components of the model is important in itself. However they may be somewhat hierarchical in that the absence of disease and disability may make it easier to maintain mental and physical function. This in turn may enable, but not guarantee, engagement with life.

Low Risk of Disease and Disease-Related Disability

Many people consider that the risk of disease is entirely down to the lottery of genetics; did we choose our parents wisely? The role of genetics in successful aging is important but the influence has been considerably overstated. Family studies, population studies, adoption studies, and studies of twins, which were all components of the MacArthur Study, allowed the interplay between nature and nurture to be separated. For all but the most strongly determined genetic diseases, environment and lifestyle have a powerful impact on the likelihood of actually developing a disorder (Rowe & Kahn, 1999). Thus, decisions to cut out smoking; eat less fat and red meat; eat lots of fruit, vegetables and fish; reduce alcohol intake; lose weight; avoid over exposure to sunlight; and exercise regularly are some of the well-publicized environmental and lifestyle modifications that directly lower the risk of disease and disability.

However, even after health problems occur, older people can successfully continue to engage with life if they adopt health control strategies such as seeking help, devoting time and energy to addressing the challenges, and being committed to overcoming threats to physical health. For example, in a two-year follow-up study, Wrosch and Schulz (2008) found that elderly participants who were proactive and persistent in countering health problems showed greater physical and mental health benefits than those who were not. Their findings suggest that once disease strikes, active control strategies play an important role in the maintenance of older adults' physical health.

High Mental and Physical Function

Considerable evidence exists which demonstrates a link between cognitive stimulation and aspects of health and well being. Perhaps the most compelling recent summation came from The Foresight Project on Mental Capital and Wellbeing (Beddington et al., 2008) which took a whole-of-life approach in reaching its conclusion that countries must learn how to capitalize on their citizens' cognitive resources if they are to prosper. More than 450 experts and stakeholders from 16 countries were involved in the review of state-of-the-art scientific and other evidence to investigate the challenges and opportunities that lie ahead in the next 20 years. The recommendations regarding older learners are particularly noteworthy. The study recommended that "as people move into older age, learning should be encouraged and actively promoted, as this can protect against cognitive decline" (Beddington et al., 2008. p. 1058).

The benefits of exercise have been known for many years. Numerous studies continue to show that exercise reduces the risk of cardiovascular disease and overall mortality risk, as well as promoting psychological well-being. However, physical activity also improves brain function (Lautenschlager et al., 2008). Exactly why exercise has a positive effect on brain function is not yet known. One suggestion is that exercise helps to maintain the health of blood vessels in the brain, helping to ensure a steady supply of oxygen and nutrients to areas of the brain that are critical for thinking and memory. Physical activity may also help stimulate the release of factors critical for brain cell growth, increasing resistance to damage caused by dementia. Andel and colleagues (2008) studied exercise patterns in 50 year olds and followed up 30 years later. They found that exercise at midlife reduces the odds of dementia in older adulthood and concluded that exercise interventions should be explored as a potential strategy for delaying disease onset.

Active Engagement With Life

The successful aging model comprises two separate elements to actively engaging with life:

maintaining close social networks and doing interesting things.

The literature on social networks is extensive, and numerous research findings are linked with health outcomes (Bowling 1994). In fact findings about the fundamental importance of social networks have been sufficiently robust that more than twenty years ago a review of social network research prompted House, Landis and Umberson (1988) to conclude that a lack of social relationships constituted a major health risk akin to that of smoking. Recent findings continue to refine the specific benefits of social networks. For example, in a nationally representative study, Ertel, Glymour and Berkman (2008) provided evidence that social integration delays memory loss among elderly Americans.

The other element of actively engaging with life is doing interesting things. The domain of "interesting things" is subjective and open ended – in other words what is interesting for one older person may hold no attraction at all for another. Consequently, attributing a specific health and well-being outcome to a particular "engaging" activity requires targeted research. Volunteering is an interesting activity for many older people and volunteering continues to be widely studied. It seems that everyone can be a winner from voluntarism: participants, recipients of the services, and the wider economy alike. For the volunteers themselves, those who regularly engage in their voluntary activities enjoy better health and live longer thanks to the stimulating environments and sense of purpose engendered by the activities. Zedlewski and Butrica (2007) summarized the outcomes of 10 studies published since 1999 that documented the significant positive associations between volunteer activity and decreased mortality and depression, improved health and strength, greater happiness, and enhanced cognitive ability. Volunteers are doing themselves a considerable service while helping the wider community.

Successful Aging Organizations

The Rowe and Kahn (1999) model of successful aging has been criticized for being overly narrow despite their emphasis being on a lot more than physical health. For example, many older people rate their subjective health highly even though they have quite severe health problems of a kind which would earn them a "poor health" rating from a narrow medical model perspective. In addition, a more complete successful aging model must include recognition of existential aspects of life which are important to many older people, such as spirituality (not in the narrow doctrinal sense) (Glass, 2003). Despite criticism, however, the five elements which make up the three components of the successful aging model, namely:

- keep the mind active
- keep the body active
- maintain close social networks
- do interesting things
- take the necessary steps to avoid disease or minimize the consequences if disease occurs; form a simple evidence-based checklist by which older people can readily monitor their choices.

Earlier, it was noted that societies must learn how to capitalize on their citizen's cognitive resources if they are to prosper. The Foresight Project singles out the need to encourage and actively promote learning in older age as this can protect against cognitive decline (Beddington et al., 2008). In many countries, the latter end of the lifelong learning spectrum has been poorly supported by governments and policy makers. For the most part, any financial support for later life learning opportunities has focused on upgrading older workers' skills. For the very large and growing population of third agers who are no longer in the paid workforce, the benefits of later life learning have been largely ignored at the policy level. However, in spite of this lack of top-down support, a number of later life learning initiatives have prospered in many countries in answer to the grassroots groundswell of interest by many retired people in doing something meaningful with their minds (Swindell, 2009).

One of the most notable adult education success stories has been the rise and rise of the self-help University of the Third Age (U3A) model (Swindell and Thompson, 1995). The self-help idea has prospered without formal support because it is based on the fact that experts of all kinds retire with high level skills intact, and these are the best people to manage, teach and run educational activities for older people, on a purely voluntary basis. Everyone's a winner with the self-help approach. The volunteer teachers and administrators are advantaged by having meaningful outlets through which to apply and hone their skills for the benefit of an appreciative group of learners. The learners are advantaged by having access to a very low cost potpourri of intellectually and physically stimulating activities. And all members are advantaged by regular contact with like-minded others who like to do new things, and the allied possibilities for forming new social networks. Wider society is also advantaged by older people having a considerably increased choice of ways to engage in successful aging activities which maximize their chances for independence, with little or no implications for the public purse. Moreover, there is no need to base these learning organizations within former bastions of exclusivity and privilege such as universities. Effective learning and teaching programs can be carried out within the community in free or subsidized community facilities, even within members' own homes, at times and in formats which appeal to older learners. There are no entry requirements, no exams or awards, fees are very low because no one is paid, and learning takes place in an atmosphere and location that encourages participants to share their ideas. U3A is undoubtedly a smart idea for capitalizing on the mental wealth of older people.

There are many variations on the U3A approach worldwide which provide activities that encompass all or most of the five successful aging elements. Some approaches such as Lifelong Learning Institutes (LLI) in North America and Osher Lifelong Learning Institutes in the USA, or the French U3A model, followed in many countries, are based at universities or colleges (Swindell, 2009). Nevertheless, the teaching and program administration is mainly or solely carried out by skilled retirees, and the formal university system has little or no say over the educational content and process. In China, the Universities for the Aged use a combination of revered older teachers who are paid a stipend, and older and young unpaid volunteers, to teach a curriculum which covers compulsory subjects such as health and exercise plus a wide range of academic and leisure courses. In other countries different combinations of second and third age expertise provide popular programs for older people which encompass most or all of the successful aging model. Regardless of approach, the common-sense basis of adult education programs that empower older people irrespective of their prior educational backgrounds, has translated into very wide acceptance around the world (Swindell & Thompson, 1995).

It seems reasonable to describe these later life learning organizations as successful aging organizations. Unlike almost any other large, leisure time organization for older people, which may have its major focus on social or hobby activities, later life learning organizations embody all, or at least four of the five elements of successful aging. Classes typically include a panorama of intellectually, physically and socially stimulating options all prepared and run by retired people who are expert in their subject areas.

Older People and Novel Communications Technologies

Frequently, older people are isolated from their mainstream communities by a daunting array of constraints that make it difficult for them to continue to engage with life. Even in large, well resourced cities which offer many opportunities for older people to engage with life, abrupt changes to circumstance such as illness, incapacity, becoming a caregiver, giving up driving and so forth leave many older people with few compensatory options to choose from.

Communications technologies have considerable potential for motivating isolated older people to engage with life in entirely new ways. In the early 1990s, a series of studies was undertaken to investigate the possibility of setting up a virtual U3A for frail elderly people with sound minds. The studies showed that older volunteer teachers and learners alike are not averse to using novel technology to learn new things (Swindell & Mayhew, 1996; Swindell, Singer & Singer, 1994; Swindell, James & Mann 1992). In one of the studies 18 frail elderly people aged from 58 to 92, who were confined to their homes by illness or incapacity, showed measurable improvements in their quality of life over the course of an eight week educational program delivered by teleconferences run by volunteer U3A tutors. A trained nurse interacted with the participants throughout the study to monitor basic health data and record observations. The well-being of participants improved over the course of the study and several developed new social networks as a result of interacting with like-minded others within their virtual groups. They stated that the educational program was the catalyst that induced them to experiment with a novel method of communicating and exploring beyond their physically and socially constrained horizons (Swindell & Mayhew, 1996).

The Internet would have been a more flexible and cost-effective medium than teleconferencing for carrying out the above virtual U3A trials. However, in the early nineties, computers and the Internet were unknown quantities to the very large majority of older people. The situation is quite different today. Although a large disparity still exists between the numbers of older and younger Internet users, older people comprise the fastest growing group on the Internet in many countries, albeit from a low user base. The extent of this grey digital divide seems to depend on efforts made within various countries to provide older people with motivation, and assistance to learn to use the Internet. The World Internet Project (Pierce, 2008) reported that in New Zealand, Canada, Sweden and the United States at least 38 percent of the population aged 65 and older said they go online. In Australia, the number is substantially lower with 29 percent of the population aged 65 and older reporting that they go online. However, the Australian figure should show a marked increase from 2009 after the Australian Government Broadband for Seniors project begins a three year program of providing free Internet kiosks and tutoring provided by older volunteers, throughout the entire country (see http://www.necseniors.net.au/ for details). In contrast with the above "high" usage, other countries participating in the World Internet project like Macao, Hungary and the Czech Republic reported 10 percent or less of the over 65 population using the Internet. Even the "high" percentages listed above for the over 65 year group are disproportionately low when compared with total online usage within their respective countries.

Although a grey digital divide seems likely to persist for many years, perhaps until successive Internet-savvy cohorts have moved through the third age, the foregoing shows that many older people are happy to come to grips with technology that played little or no part in their earlier lives. The potential benefits of the Internet for all older people but particularly for isolated older people to engage with a virtual life seem limitless. Free Web 2.0 applications such as wikis, Skype and social networking sites, have considerable potential for widening the range of socially and intellectually enriching activities in the daily lives of older people, allowing them to communicate with like-minded others when and if they want to. However, using the Internet may have previously unrecognized direct health benefits for older "surfers" because the process may also help to exercise and improve brain function. Recent research with older people who surf the Internet shows that they trigger key centres in the brain involved in decision-making and complex reasoning when they make decisions about what to click on in order to pursue more information. This preliminary study, which used Magnetic Resonance Imaging to study brain activity in real time, showed that Internet searching engages a much greater extent of neural circuitry than reading does (Small, Moody, Siddarth & Bookheimer, 2009).

U3A Online

U3A and similar empowering adult education programs for older adults are widely available in many countries. As discussed above, however, the realities of later life are such that large numbers of older people are unable to engage with life within their wider communities. Circumstances such as being a caregiver, illness, disability and so forth isolate them from their social networks and opportunities for intellectual stimulation. As a consequence their health suffers.

By 1997 the Internet had become less of a novelty to growing numbers of retired people and the idea of using the Internet to deliver U3A services to isolated older people was discussed on an email list by a group of U3A enthusiasts from Australia, New Zealand and the UK. Their idea was to develop an electronic U3A without walls in which colleagues from any country could share resources with each other and provide intellectually challenging activities to older people wherever they lived, particularly for those who are isolated. In 1998, as part of the International Year of Older Persons celebrations in 1999, the Australian Government provided funding that led to the development of the first practicable, low cost, virtual U3A called U3A Online. From the outset the major objective of U3A Online was to develop and provide cognitively challenging activities which would be available through the Internet to all older people worldwide and to younger people with disabilities. Isolated older people were given first preference in the courses which had limited enrollments.

Just like any self-help U3A, all the administration and teaching within the world-first virtual U3A is carried out by retired volunteers. No one is paid. Governance and administration takes place through regular online meetings. Discussion and voting takes place by electronic forum, email and Skype. The annual general meetings, at which office bearers are elected, are also held online. In fact, it is not uncommon for volunteers to work closely together for many years, become close virtual friends, but never physically meet.

All courses are written and taught by retired experts with the assistance of volunteer online editors. At the time of writing this chapter in early 2009, 36 courses were available with another 18 in various stages of completion. Each course runs for eight or nine weeks and is offered once or twice a year when the volunteer course leader is available. Participants interact with the leader and with others in the course by forum. Live chat is not a mainstream communication mode for practical reasons. Because participants can come from any country it makes little sense to remove flexibility through scheduling live chat meetings at times that suit the tutors but few others. Another barrier to "chat" is that many older people are not skilled typists or have problems such as arthritis, which make keyboarding a burden. Attempts at keyboard chat have resulted in expressions of frustration by those who are left behind. Free voice-over-internet-protocol applications like Skype have considerable potential as an option, but because many older people with limited incomes use old hand-me-down computers and dialup modems which cannot run Skype, course communications must remain quite basic. An alternative mode of learning entailing self-paced study 365 days a year is more popular than the course led option. This appears to be because many older people have numerous activities in retirement and find it inconvenient to commit to a consecutive eight-week learning block. Others drop in and out of periods of ill health.

Griffith University in Brisbane Australia hosts the entire operation free of charge on university servers as part of its service to the wider community, and courses are delivered via the University online course delivery platform. The net result of running a learning organization in which overheads are negligible and no one is paid is that costs can be kept at an affordable level for retired people with limited incomes. For example, in 2009 the annual U3A Online membership fee was A$25 which entitled members to free access to all 36 courses, in self-study mode. Members pay an additional A$5 to take part in each course run by a course leader. (For comparison, in 2009 a movie ticket costs about A$13.)

SUCCESSFUL AGING CHARACTERISTICS OF OLDER INTERNET USERS

Little is known about older persons' learning via the Internet. Certainly, there are numerous examples of interesting and innovative computer courses for older people that are run in many countries, but almost all of these involve how to teach older people to use the Internet. What are the implications for further learning once this important but comparatively routine skill has been acquired?

U3A Online has been providing new, very low cost learning opportunities for older people for more than ten years and considerable anecdotal evidence shows that the process is making a considerable improvement to the quality of life of individual participants. For example, many comments like the following are accessible from the U3A Online home page:

I'll go as far as to say that being totally absorbed in my most recent online course has saved my sanity this year.

I care for my wife who has Alzheimers. Have done so for the last 8 years.

I am deaf – communicating online is wonderful for me. I am sure that is true for other people with disabilities of many kinds.

In light of the fact that the Internet is an integral part of the lives of most young retirees and is therefore destined to play an increasing role in the lives of growing numbers of older people, it is timely to seek answers to some basic questions about the characteristics and aspirations of older people who choose to learn via the Internet. For example, is it possible to identify some of the antecedents that might predict whether an older person chooses whether or not to take part in online learning? What modifications to personal learning styles might older learners need to adopt in order to compensate for aging-related decrements such as failing eyesight, declining short-term memory, and problems with mobility or health? How do older adults rate learning on screen versus the familiarity of the printed word? Can new, high quality social networks develop between older learners from distant places and different cultures, who can only ever meet in cyberspace? Do courses meet participants' needs and expectations or do they tend to sample and move to some other activity? What successful aging characteristics are exhibited by participants? Might the Internet be an effective medium for intergenerational cooperation between young people who are prepared to undertake short term voluntary projects and older learners? These and many other questions await answers in the comparatively new domain of cyberspace teaching and learning by and for older people. In the following section we describe two related studies that begin to reveal some of the successful aging characteristics of older Internet users.

Study 1

To begin the process of revealing some of the characteristics of older people who are attracted to online learning we initially considered sending an online questionnaire to a random sample of course participants. However we could find no prior studies of older persons' Internet learning to guide the framing of specific questions. Rather than inflict our agenda on the process we instead decided to attempt a virtual equivalent of a focus group in the belief that this approach could provide a grounded understanding of older online learners and their backgrounds. For our study, participants would be asked to respond in a stream of consciousness style by email to a sequence of open questions, each question to be structured on the basis of information gleaned from its predecessors, thereby building up a broad brush picture of participants' characteristics and aspirations, and engagement with life and online learning.

The task of finding suitable and willing participants who might take part in an email inquiry was considerably helped by having access to a pool of older learners who had already experimented with Internet learning via their U3A Online courses. In the last unit of every course, all participants are asked to voluntarily complete an online written evaluation form in which some of the questions ask for reflective or critical comment. The majority of participants ignore the request for detailed information but a few take the opportunity to provide thoughtful insights. The writers of these detailed evaluations were invited to take part in the online focus group in the belief that they would be more likely to be interested than those who had ignored earlier opportunities to give their opinions.

Initial screening identified a group of ten likely participants, all of whom agreed to take part. Seven were females; three were males. Seven lived in Australia, two in New Zealand and one in the UK. There had been no interaction between any members of the group prior to the study. Apart from that nothing was known about them or their backgrounds. To make it clear from the outset that participants understood that they were volunteering to do something that entailed reflective thought and writing, we suggested a guideline of three paragraphs as a minimum length for each email response from each of the ten.

We asked participants to respond to a series of questions/statements that were presented to them one at a time. This stepwise process was integral to our chosen method, which relied on analysis of preceding responses to inform the process of framing the next question. Replies to these were sent only to us. After we received all replies to a particular question, we removed the names and email addresses and replaced them with participants' nicknames. All ten responses, bearing only the nicknames as an identifier, were then consolidated into one lengthy email, often of six A4 pages or more, and sent to each of the participants, with an invitation to make additional comment on the replies of others or add more to their own reply. Any additional comments and responses were similarly emailed to all, and further comment invited. The composite responses and additional replies were then used to help structure a new question and the process repeated for a total of six questions.

Although grounded theory implies a clean mental slate to begin with, we came to this study with a certain mindset regarding the underlying constructs that might be elicited via this process of email inquiry. Bronfenbrenner's circles of influence model illustrates this mind set. Bronfenbrenner (1979) distinguished between immediate (personal) and increasingly remote (impersonal) spheres of influence, with the relationship between spheres depicted in the form of ever larger concentric circles arranged around a common central axis. Commensurate with Bronfenbrenner's taxonomy, we theorized that the content of participants' responses would move between immediate and personal versus remote and impersonal influences in such a way as to gradually reveal more about the person answering the questions. A further aim of the research then was to utilize the email messages generated by participants to chart and reveal the interplay of personal and impersonal circles of influence.

We avoided direct questions about age, personal circumstances, education, health, isolation and so forth because the intent was to build up a virtual group dynamic in which each individual would feel sufficiently comfortable that personal details would be revealed if appropriate, within the general course of email discussion. Our intended approach was to make the first questions as open as possible then to use participant responses to ask increasingly detailed and perhaps more personal questions that focused on the role of the computer and the Internet in participants' lives. Thus, the first discussion starter was "*Tell us something about yourself and how you came to the Internet*". This was intended to be a "comfortable" question, something like an icebreaker in a face-to-face focus group. The dual aim was to encourage participants to write freely about something that they were totally familiar with, namely themselves and their lives. As well, their initial responses would begin the process of the group getting to know each other. We hoped that throughout the study, participants would become increasingly comfortable with the idea of self-disclosure and feedback to a virtual group of complete strangers.

The inclusion of feedback was based on transformative learning principles derived from environmental education. That is, it was expected that in the process of responding to questions and then commenting on group feedback, individuals would be likely to become aware of, and perhaps comment on, the extent to which deeper-seated attitudes had undergone shifts occasioned by contact with a range of computer based communications systems. For instance, it seemed reasonable to expect that the need to allocate time to study online might have effects on the participants' social lives and that comments to this effect might color individual answers to questions and comments on group feedback, if not initially then later in the study.

The six questions (discussion starters) were:

- Tell us something about yourself and how you came to the Internet.
- What are the strengths and weaknesses of online learning? It would be helpful if you specifically focus at least some of your comments on U3A Online, including the all-important personal element.
- Personal history: What life events or personal qualities might have led you to take up computing and the Internet? (Note we are interested in your perception of self. We are not talking about technology and machines.)
- What changes have aging made to the way you work with information and ideas compared with how you used to work with information and ideas?
- What effect is the Internet in general having on you with respect to the following:
    - Time management
    - Daily routine
    - Personal life
    - Character
    - Social (how has this affected your relationship with other people? Has your circle of real friends changed?)
    - What are you becoming with your interest in learning via the Internet? Where are you going with all this?

Study 1 Initial Findings

From the outset it was made clear to participants that they were being asked to take part in a lengthy process that involved their doing a lot of thinking and writing. It was assumed that about half of the initial ten participants would pull out part way through the lengthy process. However, the only withdrawal was a male after the first question. The remaining nine replied to all six questions.

In conventional focus groups, a skilled moderator can pick up on comments made by individuals, and guide the group into discussion of specific points of interest, thereby yielding personal insights that might otherwise not surface. Initially our study attempted to introduce a similar element of group discussion by inviting participants to comment on responses from others, or by adding further to their own, but this idea proved to be impracticable. For various reasons including reflection on difficult questions, poor health, other commitments and computer problems, the time between sending a question and receiving responses was sometimes as long as three weeks and the envisioned six-week data collection time actually took 15 weeks. Therefore we chose not to press the idea of group discussion in the belief that the study might be jeopardized by participants becoming bored with the process and dropping out.

The richness, depth and variety of responses were surprising. As anticipated a few replies to the first question focused mainly on the safe technology-related issues. However, from the outset, other participants were unconstrained by the question or the process and wrote quite freely about themselves and their lives. Once the first composite responses had been sent to everyone, participants began to interpret the questions as though there were few boundaries on the kind of answer that was expected. In effect they began to respond in an open rather than technologically constrained way.

One of the major objectives of U3A Online is to encourage course participants to communicate with each other in the belief that isolated older people will benefit from social interaction with like-minded strangers. We were encouraged to find that the nine strangers in this study began to "bond" immediately after the first composite answer was circulated. A number of the participants asked for email addresses so they could correspond directly with some of the others. Another suggested exchanging photographs. We asked everyone who was comfortable with the idea to send us their photographs and to give us permission to send the photographs and email addresses to group members who asked for them. Six participants provided photographs and all gave permission for email addresses to be provided. We made no attempt subsequently to determine which members of the group contacted others.

At differing stages throughout the process, individuals outlined personal histories that helped the group to develop an understanding of the real people represented by the email nicknames. Individual responses of two or more pages were common and one response ran for more than three A4 pages. A number of participants indicated that they had difficulty in answering some of the questions and chose to set the question aside for a few days while they reflected on how they intended to answer. Nonetheless, they persevered with their interpretations of the questions and did not seek clarification. The imprecise nature of our questions and not wanting to place boundaries on responses was rewarded in terms of the patient, lengthy and insightful responses from all nine participants.

The questions revealed a lot about the participants. Some but not all revealed their ages. These ranged from mid fifty to the late seventies. Most appeared to be in their late sixties or early seventies. Two were profoundly deaf, three were managing serious health difficulties and four did not comment directly on their health. Illness prevented some from leaving their homes as often as they wished. All seemed optimistic about life despite various health-related problems and disabilities, and all had a wide range of regular leisure activities outside and/or inside the home. All had pursued a range of learning opportunities throughout life and considered learning via the Internet to be an absorbing continuation of a lifetime pattern of learning new things.

Our concerns about the process expanding from the envisioned six weeks to more than 15 weeks leading to participant fatigue and early withdrawal proved groundless. Participants remained supportive and interested throughout as typified in the following comments.

I understand this question is to be the last. How sad it is.

I have learnt something about myself through having to answer it. Thank you I'll be looking forward to the next challenge.

The series of six questions have been very stimulating. It has enabled me to be more focused and mentally alert.

I have really enjoyed being part of this survey and have not resented any of the time it has taken to answer each question, it has made me think a lot about myself and it has been most fascinating to read the other responses and to find out that others feel as I do on certain things. I have at times been a bit worried about putting my answers up, thinking that a particular thought might seem silly to others and then blow me down some one else has the same thoughts.

The process is interesting and useful as a means of self-discovery as well as providing interesting reading about the lives of fellow travelers.

Study 2

None of the initial questions specifically addressed the successful aging model. However, preliminary text analysis of the composite responses indicated that participants indeed exhibited most of the successful aging elements. They enjoyed mentally stimulating activity; they engaged with life by doing interesting things both on and off the Internet; they developed online social networks; and several spoke of managing health difficulties. Encouraged by the positive response to the first six questions we asked the nine participants whether they would take part in an extension to the study. All agreed.

In stage 2 of the study participants were asked a further series of five open questions that invited wide reflection. Most of the questions arose directly from the Rowe and Kahn model for successful aging. Our preliminary analysis suggested that they would amongst other things stress the importance of taking steps to maintain their health, developing new social networks, pursuing a range of hobbies, and enjoying doing new things.

With this in mind, all nine participants were asked the following five additional questions.

- We notice that some members of the group appear to be in good physical health while others are managing various diseases/disabilities. What are you doing to manage your heath (whether it is good or otherwise) and how have you attempted to maximize good health in the past and in the present?
- We notice that people are differently situated with respect to their group of close friends and acquaintances. Could we ask you to comment on your current network of friends, whether they are online or otherwise?
- Has participation in email and other Internet activities reduced any feelings of isolation or loneliness you may have experienced? If so can you tell me how?
- Can you please list your hobbies and interests, and tell me whether or not they influenced the courses you took.
- We think it likely that older people, who ventured into learning in cyberspace before the medium was well known by the wider aging population, must have an innate sense of curiosity and/or sense of adventure and/or are "risk takers". Please think about your entire life and describe

> what family or environmental circumstances may have shaped your willingness to venture into cyberspace.

Participant responses to the additional five questions were prepared for text analysis by collating these responses with responses to the first six questions to produce nine transcripts with responses to all eleven questions. The software package, Leximancer (www.leximancer.com) was used for initial screening for major themes. One thought here is that Leximancer automates the process of text analysis and can analyze vast amounts of text in doing so. This stands in contrast to manual methods (even those using Nvivo) that analyze selected portions of a text in some detail.

Leximancer computes the frequency with which each term is used, after discarding text items of no research relevance (such as "a" or "the"), and then computes the distance between each of the terms via computations equivalent to nonparametric factor analytic or cluster analytic procedures. As with other factor analytic procedures, there is no single solution and the quality of particular solutions is best judged in terms of interpretability.

The result of this computation is displayed in a two-dimensional spatial representation, illustrated in Figure 1. The user can set the percentage of terms on display; rotate the display to optimize the arrangement of terms, require that the software "learn", that is, re-compute the distances between terms based on the outcomes of previous computations, and explore the family of associations with any one term, including their sources in the source text.

Figure 1 displays the most frequently occurring terms retained in this analysis. The terms have been rotated so that the terms *home* and *online* align with the horizontal (x-) axis, and *computer* and *friend* align with the vertical (y-) axis. The intersecting axes partition the responses into four quadrants, which can help with identifying major themes that are common to participants' responses.

One way to interpret the above analysis is to consider the major partitions in which Leximancer has clustered participants' talk. To the right of the vertical axis the focus is on the technology and advantages of cyberspace. To the left the focus is on the other major domain of participants' interest, namely home life and personal history. Above the horizontal axis the focus seems to be on group activities "external to" the individual, whereas below the axis, the focus is largely on ideas "within" the individual. More specifically, in Quadrant 1 the analysis shows how the Internet has engaged participants with new ideas and activities involving other people (*group, U3A* [Online], *activities, email, world* etc). Below that, in Quadrant 4 the focus seems more on how the Internet engages the participants personally *(learning, study, read, information*). In Quadrant 2 the group focus is on social networks associated with home and personal history (*wife, school, family, friends*). The cluster in Quadrant 3 is the most difficult to interpret but responses appear to focus on a rejuvenated world of work in retirement, including creating a "going to work" environment via frequent, usually daily, visits to cyberspace.

In summary, the four quadrants of terms can be understood in terms of an aggregate discourse in which the term *home* serves to contrast the world of family and friends with the world of daily work, and the term *online* serves to contrast the world of new social networks with independent learning and ideas.

Text Analysis

In addition to the Leximancer screening the responses were analyzed using conventional text analysis techniques. The nine participants each answered 11 questions providing a total of ninety-nine responses which gave rise to a number of discrete themes discussed below.

Figure 1. Major themes identified by Leximancer

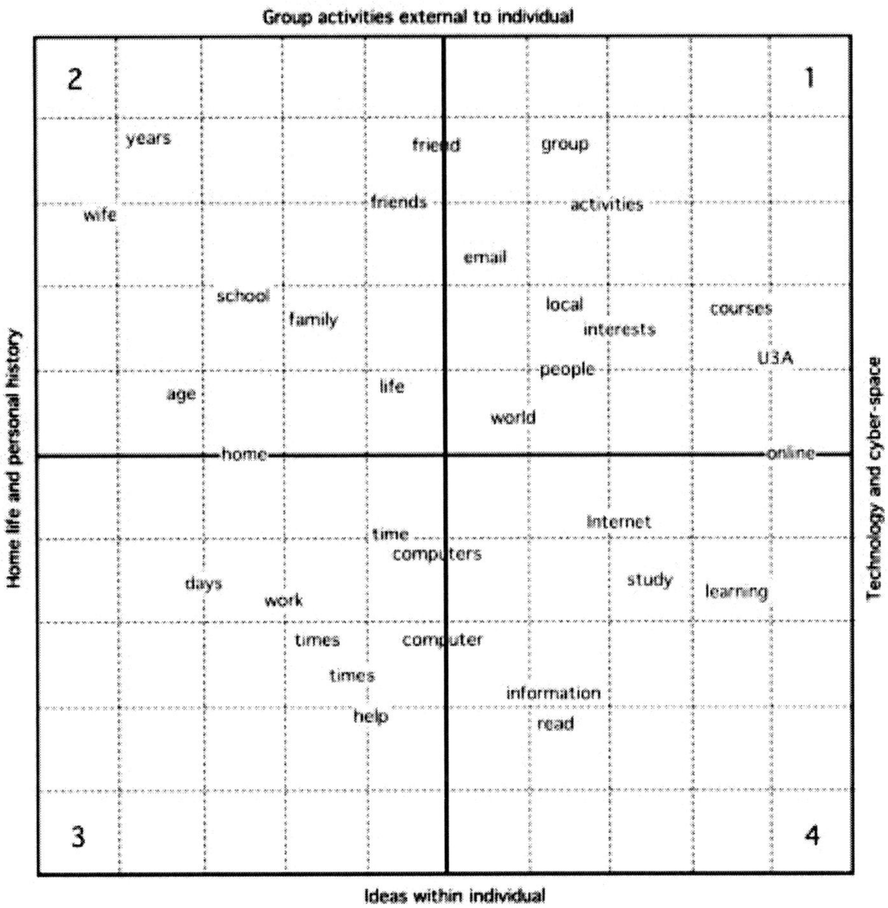

Catalyst for Involvement with Computers

The respondents described a range of personal, work related and education experiences that acted as catalysts for learning to use computers. With the exception of one, all participants had early contact with computers (1980s back to 1960s). Most saw the potential of computing for work purposes as well as for personal use and study, and actively set out to learn more. Several mentioned that their children's interest in computers gave them an interest. Those who bought computers in the early 1980s needed to persevere with unsophisticated programs and frequent changes in technology that necessitated frequent upgrades.

Most described two moves: firstly into computing and later into using the Internet, email and online learning. The transition from using a PC only to going online was prompted by a variety of circumstances: encouragement from others, work requirements, attraction of having vast amounts of information at hand, desire to preserve intellectual health and memory, potential for keeping contact with friends and relatives, the need to be current, and chance.

Health: Physical and Psychosocial

Physical and psychosocial health was a strong theme in responses in the two stages of the study, both when responding to the initial six questions where participants were not directed to disclose their health status and then later when a question was asked about how they maintained their health.

Three of the nine had serious physical health problems which were described in some detail, and another became seriously ill during the study. High importance was placed on electronic communication, online learning, and use of the Internet by the respondents who have conditions which keep them at home for long periods. They found the Internet a rich source of health information.

One participant who described experiencing difficulties and some near breakdowns found that online learning was one coping mechanism that she used to keep busy. This helped keep her mentally well. Two participants with profound hearing loss found email and online discussion very enjoyable as they could communicate in ways in which hearing is not important.

Three participants saw computing and Internet use as pleasurable experiences which provided fun, escape and relaxation. As well, five respondents described a reduction in feelings of isolation. Computing reduced geographical isolation and social isolation caused by ill health.

There was quite a clear distinction shown in responses between those who described themselves as in good health and with no physical limitations and those who were housebound and/or geographically isolated. There seemed to be strong evidence for the people in this study that electronic communication can reduce feelings of isolation and provide stimulating and enjoyable pastimes.

Self Image and Personality

Computing and electronic communication played a significant role in how the participants saw themselves. Most commented that computing had not changed their character; rather, their personality affected their approach. Two found that they could use the anonymity of online communication to experiment with different personas – to be bolder. Several noted that learning online and learning to master the new technologies revealed strengths they had been unaware of.

There was a very strong theme of 'keeping up with the times' and 'not getting left behind' and several revealed some one-upmanship over less computer literate friends and acquaintances. Two respondents noted that the anonymity of online communication was empowering in that those they communicated with did not necessarily know that they were older people. They could avoid the stereotyping of aging.

Responses provided glimpses of character traits which drove respondents into an activity which was very new, needed new skills, was peppered with technical difficulties, and was not something they could easily share with friends and family members who were not at that time interested in computing. To keep up with the speed of technological change, they showed resourcefulness, using a range of strategies: using more computer literate friends and family members, computing firms, online help, dogged persistence and experimentation.

Combined with this were personality and life experiences. All reported that they were curious people who were careful risk takers. They were widely traveled, including two who as 'alternative' tourists had travelled 'off the beaten track'. Most had lived in a number of different places, and two had migrated.

Three identified having 'something to prove' (to a mother [deceased], a father [deceased], and an ex-partner) as a strong impetus for mastering new technology.

Relationships and Friendships

Interest in computing and online activity had mostly positive influences on friendships and relationships although three respondents expressed concern that their time spent online and their interest in computing could impact on time spent with their partners.

Respondents reported the value of email to maintaining friendships and contact with relatives who lived at a distance, particularly in other countries. Those who had travelled extensively or worked in other countries mentioned the ease of email compared to the trials of third world postal and telephone systems. Email allowed friendships to develop where distance would not have allowed this, while other friendships had endured that once would have faded.

Attitudes to making new friends online fell into definitely yes and definitely no. However, the three who were most housebound through illness were the three who most valued new online friendships.

Approaches to Learning and Information

Respondents showed a deliberate or overt approach to learning as well as an understanding that learning can be incidental. Most had extensive tertiary education and strong links with learning institutions (an anthropologist, a teacher, two librarians, a school guidance officer, a university administration officer, and a member of the clergy). The participant who did not have a tertiary qualification had a long-term wish to complete a degree, which ill health had thwarted several times.

Several mentioned that online learning by its nature encouraged further learning because of the links contained in lesson material, and the awareness they gained of other fields of knowledge as they read through course descriptions. As well, they continually gained skills by having to keep up with computer technology and mastering new software.

Most respondents mentioned the scope of information available online and the need to be selective about how it is used given the little quality control over content posted on the Internet. Two mentioned that the amount of information can be overwhelming.

Two preferred print-based information and they downloaded and printed extensively. For one, this was because he experienced eyestrain; for the other, the cost of the Internet connection time had to be monitored carefully.

Role of Computing in Daily Routine and Time Management

Most participants had ample time for online activities with several mentioning that family did not live close by and they were not required to care for grandchildren. As well as participating in U3A Online courses, respondents described a range of practical uses for computers and the Internet which included sourcing information, for communicating, and storing data. Computers played an important role in day-to-day life such as shopping, banking, planning travel, research, email, and correspondence. The Internet was also seen as a very handy and important source of information to enhance enjoyment of hobbies and interests.

Three respondents usually had their computer turned on and connected from early morning until late in the evening while two worked mostly offline and connected for as little time as possible in order to save money and to keep the phone line free.

Computing and the Future

All participants made predictions that computers, online learning and the Internet would continue to play an important personal role and they encouraged friends and other acquaintances to become computer literate. They also predicted a looming equity issue for older people who did not use these technologies, noting that computer literacy was very important for full functioning in society.

CONCLUSION

We began by observing that governments everywhere are seeking inexpensive solutions to challenges associated with population aging.

Preventative approaches which encourage the population at large to adopt lifestyle choices which may delay or even prevent widespread reliance on expensive health and social support services in later life are both socially and financially sound ideas. The recent recommendation that "as people move into older age, learning should be encouraged and actively promoted, as this can protect against cognitive decline" (Beddington et al., 2008, p. 1058), further reinforces the "preventative" message.

U3A is a prime example of how the preventative approach might be effectively deployed on a much wider scale. For many years the very low cost, self-help U3A model has utilized the talents of retired volunteers to benefit the wider aging population. The approach has been a relatively long lived success because many of the rapidly growing population of retirees have the interest, expertise and time to volunteer for meaningful tasks. The do-it-yourself approach has rendered U3As immune to the vagaries of government funding and economic cycles. Experts of all kinds retire and research shows that if they are recruited into meaningful voluntary activities the volunteers, recipients of their services, and the wider economy alike, will benefit (Zedlewski & Butrica 2007).

More recently, U3A Online has also harnessed the talents of retired volunteers, but because the Internet has no boundaries the volunteers and participants alike can come from any country. All participants in our research shared an interest in lifelong learning and they believed their virtual activities in later life enriched their lives in many ways. As access by older people to the Internet continues to grow, the lives of increasing numbers of third agers are likely to be improved through participation in virtual learning communities which open new horizons for personal development and social networking. Information technology can expand the range of choices available to isolated older people in particular and compensate for some age related physical and social losses.

Our research points to the need for caution in placing too great an emphasis on the "low risk of disease and disease-related disability" attribute of Rowe and Kahn's (1999) successful aging model. Four of the participants in the online focus group would have failed the successful aging test in terms of a narrow clinical focus on disease. They were managing serious disease and one died during the last stages of the study. Another died several months later. However, as far as they were concerned they were aging successfully. They enthusiastically engaged with life, even if their outside lives were largely constrained to the Internet; they were adventurous in the way they leaped at new learning opportunities (such as taking part in, and persevering with the above study); they were quick to form virtual friendships (as demonstrated by the group bonding which happened after question one, and other outgoing virtual activities they were engaged in) and they were optimistic and cheerful throughout the lengthy course of the study. It would seem that the evidence-based models of aging may need to take account of subtle get-up-and-go characteristics of the aging individual as well as the more easily measurable characteristics.

U3A Online is a smart application of Internet technology for helping to bridge the grey digital divide and provide volunteers and participants, particularly those isolated from their mainstream communities, with meaningful activities which can improve their quality of life. The U3A approach, coupled with the considerable, low cost communication potential of the Internet, appears to offer considerable scope for policy makers to make much better use of the mental capital of its retired citizens than it has done to date.

REFERENCES

Andel, R., Crowe, M., Pedersen, N. L., Fratiglioni, L., Johansson, B., & Gatz, M. (2008). Physical exercise at midlife and risk of dementia three decades later: a population-based study of Swedish twins. *The Journals of Gerontology. Series A, Biological Sciences and Medical Sciences*, *63*(1), 62–66.

Beddington, J., Cooper, C., Field, J., Goswami, U., Huppert, F., & Jenkins, R. (2008). The mental wealth of nations. *Nature*, *455*(7216), 1057–1060. doi:10.1038/4551057a

Bowling, A. (1994). Social networks and social support among older people and implications for emotional well-being and psychiatric morbidity. *International Review of Psychiatry (Abingdon, England)*, *6*, 41–58. doi:10.3109/09540269409025242

Bronfenbrenner, U. (1979). *The ecology of human development: Experiments by nature and design*. London: Harvard University Press.

Ertel, K., Glymour, M., & Berkman, L. (2008). Effects of social integration on preserving memory function in a nationally representative U.S. elderly population. *American Journal of Public Health*, *98*(7), 1215–1220. doi:10.2105/AJPH.2007.113654

Friedrich, D. (2003). Personal and societal intervention strategies for successful aging. *Ageing International*, *28*(1), 3–36. doi:10.1007/s12126-003-1014-8

Glass, T. A. (2003). Successful aging. In Tallis, R., Fillit, H., & Brocklehurst, J. (Eds.), *Brocklehurst's Textbook of Geriatric Medicine and Gerontology* (6th ed., pp. 173–181). London: Churchill Livingstone.

House, J., Landis, K., & Umberson, D. (1988). Social relationships and health. *Science*, *241*, 540–545. doi:10.1126/science.3399889

Lautenschlager, N., Cox, K., Flicker, L., Foster, J., van Bockxmeer, F., & Xiao, J. (2008). Effect of physical activity on cognitive function in older adults at risk for Alzheimer disease: a randomized trial. *Journal of the American Medical Association*, *300*(9), 1027–1037. doi:10.1001/jama.300.9.1027

Pierce, J. (2008). World Internet Project International Report (2009). Retrieved September 19, 2009, from http://www.worldinternetproject.net/

Rowe, J., & Kahn, R. (1999). *Successful Aging*. New York: Random House.

Small, G., Moody, T., Siddarth, P., & Bookheimer, S. (2009). Your brain on Google: Patterns of cerebral activation during Internet searching. *The American Journal of Geriatric Psychiatry*, *17*(2), 116–126. doi:10.1097/JGP.0b013e3181953a02

Swindell, R. (in press). Educational initiatives for older learners. *Education Resources Information Center.*

Swindell, R., James, C., & Mann, M. (1992). *A study of teleconferencing as a medium for improving the quality of life of the frail elderly* (ERIC Document Reproduction Service No. ED 346 310.)

Swindell, R., & Mayhew, C. (1996). Educating the isolated ageing: Improving the quality of life of the housebound elderly through educational teleconferencing. *International Journal of Lifelong Education*, *15*(2), 85–93. doi:10.1080/0260137960150203

Swindell, R., Singer, L., & Singer, G. (1994). Teleconferencing as a medium for providing expert support to the isolated ageing. *Australian Journal on Ageing*, *13*(2), 93–94. doi:10.1111/j.1741-6612.1994.tb00651.x

Swindell, R., & Thompson, J. (1995). An international perspective of the University of the Third Age. *Educational Gerontology*, *21*(5), 429–447. doi:10.1080/0360127950210505

Wrosch, C., & Schulz, R. (2008). Health-engagement control strategies and 2-year changes in older adults' physical health. *Psychological Science*, *19*(6), 537–541. doi:10.1111/j.1467-9280.2008.02120.x

Zedlewski, S., & Butrica, B. (2007). Are we taking full advantage of older adults' potential? Perspectives on productive aging, *The Urban Institute. Number 9, December.* Retrieved September 19, 2009, from http://www.urban.org/UploadedPDF/411581_adult_potential.pdf

Chapter 10
Promoting Active Ageing through Technology Training in Korea

Donghee Han
Research Institute of Science for the Better Living of the Elderly, Korea

Kathryn L. Braun
University of Hawai'i, USA

ABSTRACT

By 2050, people aged 60 and older will comprise 33% of Korea's population, up from about 12% currently. In many occupational sectors, women retire at 55 and men at 60. This rapidly shifting demographic requires a new perspective on retirement and a better image of older persons in Korea. In line with the Active Ageing Framework of the World Health Organization, the Active Ageing Consortium in Asia Pacific (ACAP) advocates for changes to individual practices, social norms, and social policy to support the continued engagement of older adults as active contributors to society in the 21st century. Digital literacy is a critical element of Active Ageing, enhancing participation in today's modes of communication and social connectivity. To promote the concept of Active Ageing with Digital Ageing, Korea's Research Institute of Science for the Better Living of the Elderly (RISBLE) aims to increase Korean elders' access to information and their opportunities for communication and participation. RISBLE's programs—Cyber Family, Internet Navigator, and the 1080 Family Online Game Festival—help elders master new technology, strengthen intergenerational relations, gain leadership roles, and contribute as community teachers. This chapter reviews the Korean situation of ageing, outlines ACAP's commitment to Active Ageing with Digital Ageing, and presents information on three RISBLE programs. These "best practices" are shared in hopes that other communities can learn from RISBLE's work to reduce the ageing digital divide and promote digital life for older persons in South Korea.

DOI: 10.4018/978-1-61520-825-8.ch010

INTRODUCTION

In most countries, people are living longer and with less disability than ever before (Fries, 1980; U.S. Department of Health and Human Services, 2007; Wiener & Tilly, 2002). Concurrently, many families are choosing to have fewer children. Both trends are contributing to a worldwide increase in the proportion of older adults (Kinsella & Phillips, 2005; World Health Organization [WHO], 2002).

South Korea has realized significant economic growth since independence (1945) and the Korean War (1950-1953) and is now experiencing rapid population ageing. In fact, by 2050, people aged 60 and older will comprise 33% of Korea's population, up from about 12% currently. This compares to projections of 30% of the European Union population and 21% of the United States (U.S.) population (United Nations, 2002).

If Korea and other rapidly ageing societies are to survive, they need to find ways to tap older adults as social capital. Continued participation in society over the life course is one of the tenets of the Active Ageing Framework of WHO (2002). In an effort to promote Active Ageing in Korea, the Research Institute of Science for the Better Living of the Elderly (RISBLE) in the south-coast city of Busan, works to increase the digital literacy of older adults (http://www.wellageing.com).

In this chapter, we review Korea's changing demographics. We present WHO's Active Ageing Framework and the reasons for its appeal in East Asia. We discuss the role of informatization of older persons in Active Ageing and benefits associated with the ability to use digital technology. We then provide information on RISBLE's mission and describe three RISBLE programs that promote digital literacy. Specifically, we will summarize the history, procedures, and successes of RISBLE's Cyber Family Program, Internet Navigator Program, and 1080 Family Online Game Festival. These programs have helped older adults gain leadership roles, establish and strengthen existing intergenerational relations, and contribute as community teachers. We will conclude with suggestions for future programming and research into digital ageing in Korea.

BACKGROUND

Population Ageing in Korea

South Korea's incredible economic growth in the latter half of the 20th century has contributed to population ageing in this nation. Prior to 1945, Korea was forcibly occupied by Japan, which focused on extracting and exploiting resources. The Korean War (1950-1953) followed closely after independence from Japan, with extensive loss of life and property. Foreign aid helped Korea develop an industrial base, and spectacular economic growth has been fueled by the chemical, shipbuilding, automotive, and electronics industries. Today, South Korea is the 13th largest economy in the world, and per capita GNP exceeds US$20,000, compared to only US$100 in 1963 (U.S. Department of State, 2009).

Increases in industrialization, education, and income have been accompanied by improved environmental and healthcare supports, resulting in extended life expectancy (78.6 years in 2005), as well as declining birth rate, which stands now at 1.08 (Korean National Statistics Office, 2009; United Nations, 2002). Population also is shifting as young people leave the countryside for the city or pursue study and work opportunities abroad, resulting in senior populations of 30% or more in some rural areas.

Based on life spans of the past, the current retirement age in many occupational sectors in Korea is 55 for women and 60 for men (United Nations, 2002). Korea's pension system is relatively new. As older adults stay healthier and live longer post-retirement, concerns are being raised about the adequacy of the pension currently provided (Kim, 2000). In fact, many retired older adults in Korea do not have an income. Government and industry are working together to provide older adults with opportunities for employment post-retirement, and many older people are demanding that the government raise retirement age as a practical change to the social system.

Despite increasing knowledge about the many contributions elders make to society, older adults often are seen as vulnerable and in need of care. Over many centuries, Korea was an agrarian society. Families cared for elders within family homes, and feelings of filial piety were strengthened by Confucian values and behavioral expectations (Sung, 1995; 2001). Elders were respected, and caring for them was a family responsibility. Some negative stereotypes are associated with this perspective, for example an expectation for older people to retire and leave the workplace so that younger people can have their chance, a belief that older people cannot learn modern technology or have no interest in it, and a notion that older people do not have resources to cope with life, are vulnerable, and should disengage from society (Han & Kim, 1998; Han, 2006; 2007).

At the same time, modernization factors are weakening traditional values, and the values of individualism and independence have become prevalent themes. Elders are losing the protective shield of familism, which increases their risk of isolation and insecurity (Han & Kim, 1998). Unfortunately, despite a strong societal tradition of filial piety, reports of elder abuse are increasing in Korea (Han, 1998; 2008). Suicide rates among older adults have increased as well. Between 1995 and 2005, suicide rates have tripled for adults age 65 to 69 (from 19 to 63 per 100,000) and quadrupled for adults aged 80 to 85 (from 30 to 127 per 100,000) (Cheon, 2006).

With urbanization and population shifts, more and more elders are living alone. With increased life span and improved health, many elders have the energy and/or need to continue working and contributing to society. Many are exploring new relationships with family and new designs for their old age. Many are embracing opportunities to learn new skills, and many say they want to avoid or delay situations that suggest they are burdensome to their children and grandchildren (Han, 2007).

Active Ageing and its Appeal in East Asia

According to the WHO (2002), Active Ageing is "the process of optimizing opportunities for health, participation, and security in order to enhance quality of life as people age" (p. 12). The Active Ageing Framework was adopted by the UN following the 2nd World Assembly on Ageing held in Madrid in 2002.

Active Ageing includes, but is broader than, healthy ageing, successful ageing, positive ageing, the age-friendly community, and ageing in place. Healthy ageing refers to keeping as fit as possible throughout life, and thus better able to contribute and be less in need of health and social services (Fries, 1980; Peel, McClure, & Bartlett, 2005). Successful ageing, a term popularized by Rowe and Kahn (1998), is characterized by the avoidance of disease and disability, high physical and cognitive function, and sustained engagement in social and productive activities. Positive ageing is a term used in New Zealand to describe its framework for modifying policy to support improved opportunities for older people to participate in society (New Zealand Ministry of Social Policy, 2001).

Age-friendly communities are environments that "enable" people of all ages to continue to participate; these include accommodating workplaces, barrier-free access, walk-able streets and parks, programs that promote lifelong fitness and education, and opportunities to engage in civic and social affairs (United Nations, 2009). Recognizing that most people want to live in their own homes and communities until death, Active Ageing societies promote home and community care over institutional care, recognizing that home- and community-based care is often less expensive than institutional care and usually supports a better quality of life (WHO, 2002).

Active ageing also takes a lifecourse perspective on health development, as described by Halfon and Hochstein (2002), recognizing that health is a consequence of multiple determinants and the timing of beneficial and deleterious events. Thus, individuals become more diverse with age, reducing our ability to stereotype older adults. This perspective also recognizes the importance of maximizing opportunities for health, participation, and security throughout the life course if we are to assure that our older adults are ready and able to continue contributing their resources to families, communities, and society. Active Ageing policies must also consider the effects of culture and gender on opportunities for participation, security, and health, and they must promote intergenerational harmony, best supported through intergenerational exchange that is perceived as mutually beneficial. Finally, Active Ageing societies value social justice, striving to ensure that policies and programs uphold the rights of all people (WHO, 2002).

As a rapidly ageing and urbanizing nation, Korea is realizing that it cannot afford to think of elders as "non-contributors" or burdensome. Rather, older adults must be encouraged and supported to actively participate in life and continue to share their resources. This means that individuals and families need to prepare for long lives, staying healthy and engaged. Equally important, social policies must promote personal participation, health, and security throughout the life course. Policies based on the Active Ageing concept could help change views of elderly as "dependent" to views of elderly as essential contributors to society through paid employment or volunteer services (Carlile, 2007; Han, 2007).

The Active Ageing Consortium for Asia Pacific (ACAP) was established in 2005 to promote Active Ageing in the region. Current members include gerontologists, service providers, and policy makers from Korea, Japan, China, Mongolia, Malaysia, Indonesia, Hawai`i, and Canada. The mission of the group is to provide a forum in Asia Pacific for the sharing of research, policy ideas, and best practices for Active Ageing. Specifically, ACAP supports country and community representatives to increase local awareness of Active Ageing through lectures, conferences, and training. ACAP also contributes to global exchange of Active Ageing ideas through its website, through national and international conferences, and by collaborating on projects of mutual interest (ACAP, 2009).

Members believe Active Ageing requires an individual-family-social policy partnership (See Figure 1). Specifically:

- Individuals and families must prepare for old age and adopt positive practices for long life.
- Social policy must promote health and wellbeing and must encourage and reward participation of elders in work, education, volunteering, and family life.
- Social policy must support the building of age-friendly environments and must support home and community-based care (over institutional care) for people with disabilities, while maximizing their abilities to participate.

The Digital Divide and the Role of Informatization in Active Ageing

The term "digital divide" refers to the gap between those people and communities who have access to information technology (IT) and those who do not, as well as the disparity in the intensity and nature of IT use among groups (Aphek, 2001; Carvin, 2000; Jackson, Zhao, Kolenic, Fitzgerald, Harold, & Von Eye, 2008). IT includes computers, the Internet, the World Wide Web, mobile telephones, and even digital cameras and televisions.

Research has shown that disparities exist in the use of IT. Populations that have access to IT and the skills to use it tend to be younger, better educated, living in urban areas, and earning more

Figure 1. Active ageing: An individual, family, and social policy partnership (© 2009, Active Ageing Consortium Asia Pacific. Used with permission.)

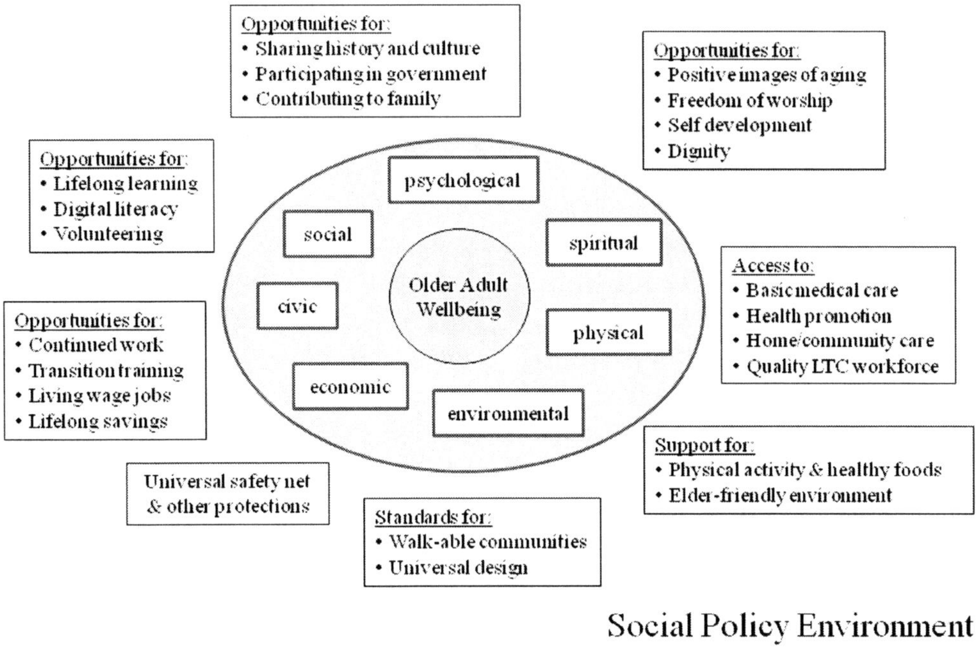

money than people without access and skills (Lorence & Park, 2006; Whaley, 2004). People who are not using the latest technology have reduced entrée to information, education, and jobs and fewer options for socialization and participation in society (Kuttan & Petters, 2003; Van Dijk, 2005). In short, independent functioning in today's society is increasingly difficult without IT skills.

Although the number of older adults online is increasing (White et al., 2002), they clearly face more barriers to IT use than younger people. Older people tend to be less educated, less wealthy, and less healthy than younger generations, and have fewer chances to gain computer skills and use the Internet. Even when older adults receive training, if they do not own a computer or have ready access to one, they cannot join the digital age and take part in cyberspace. These barriers may limit their access to news and health information, challenging their ability to stay abreast of global changes.

These barriers also may limit their options for social engagement, and a number of studies have found negative health and social outcomes associated with social and emotional isolation in older adults (White et al., 2002). The Internet, with its access to the World Wide Web and electronic mail, has greatly expanded our abilities to gather information, communicate, and stay connected. These technologies hold promise for preventing or reducing social, emotional, and informational isolation among older adults (Shapira, Barak, & Gal, 2007; Slegers, van Boxtel, & Jolles, 2008; White et al., 2002). In fact, Slegers and colleagues outline a number of potential advantages to being able to access and use the Internet (Slegars et al., 2008). For example, the Internet can:

- Facilitate communication and social interaction
- Expand access to entertainment and learning in the home

- Support autonomy
- Provide mental stimulation and challenge
- Decrease feelings of being left out of modern society
- Improve self-esteem and life satisfaction
- Improve access to health information and services

Specifically in the areas of health care, the Internet offers a number of advantages (Chang et al., 2004). For example, it offers access to information to help consumers and professionals gain knowledge and make decisions about care. It can be used to find health resources and link to support groups. When people have an Internet connection to a health care provider, they can be monitored and receive rapid feedback. A Cochrane review of the effectiveness of interactive health communication applications found them to significantly improve users' knowledge, social support, health behaviors, and clinical outcomes (Murray, Burns, See Tai, Lai, & Nazareth, 2005). The availability of health information and assistance over the Internet greatly expands health-seeking opportunities for people who live in rural areas, are unable to travel to health care sources, and/or want to receive healthcare advice in the privacy of their homes (Warmerdam, van Straten, & Cuijpers, 2007).

Other studies have examined psychological benefits among older adults with access to advanced technology. For example, Shapira and colleagues in Israel measured life satisfaction, loneliness, depression, and self-control in two groups of older adults in day care or nursing facilities; one group was provided instruction and technical assistance in computer operation and Internet use while the other group was not (Shapira et al., 2007). The researchers found significant improvements in the intervention group and deterioration in the comparison group. Other authors have reported more neutral findings. Using a randomized control design, Slegers and colleagues in Maastricht found no differences in everyday functioning, well-being, mood, and social networks of healthy individuals randomized into three computer-training conditions (Slegers et al., 2008). Using a quasi-experimental design, White et al. (2002) found that elderly participants in the trial successfully mastered use of the Internet and that measures of psychological impact trended in the positive direction; however differences were not significant, perhaps due to small sample size. These investigators advocate for continued research into the benefits of computer and Internet use, noting that digital literacy has the potential to improve participation and health-seeking, especially in groups with functional or social limitations (Shapira et al., 2007; Slegers et al., 2008; White et al., 2002).

The digital divide is not static or unbridgeable, and a number of programs have been tested to increase people's access to and use of IT (Kreps, 2005). Effective training programs for older adults must increase access to computers and must bring computers and seniors together with understanding teachers. In addition to training and access, older adults may require more senior-friendly computers, interface mechanisms, and software (Hutchison, Eastman, & Tirrito, 1997; White et al., 2002), readable and useable content (Selwyn, 2004), and an enabling environment (Namazi & McClintic, 2003). For example, attention must be paid to font size, colors of print and background, glare, and so forth, to compensate for visual changes that accompany normal ageing (Hooyman & Kiyak, 2005).

ACAP believes that digital literacy is a key component of Active Ageing, as technology increases one's opportunities to create a healthy and active later life (Han, 2006; 2007). As the world becomes more technological, it is imperative that older adults gain access to and skills in using IT to enhance their abilities to obtain information, address their own needs, communicate with others, and participate in society. We believe that full participation of older adults in the digital age will allow us to construct new models of social participation, health promotion, and safety. Full participation also will help us expand the ways in which families can demonstrate filial piety and strengthen intergenerational relationships. We believe that digital equality across age groups will reduce negative stereotypes about older people, facilitate intergenerational sharing and problem solving, and meet older adults' expressed desires to continue contributing to families and avoid or delay becoming burdensome to them (Han, 2007).

THE DIGITAL DIVIDE AND EFFORTS TO REDUCE IT IN SOUTH KOREA

Digital Divide in South Korea

South Korea is a world leader in the manufacture of IT. Commercial Internet services started in 1994, and regular surveys of Internet usage are sponsored by the National Internet Development Agency of Korea (NIDA, 2009). Current data suggest that 80% of households have access to a computer, and about 38 million Koreans (76% of the total population) regularly use the Internet (Internet World Stats, 2008; NIDA, 2008).

Cross-county comparisons of Internet use are facilitated by the Digital Opportunity Index (DOI), computed by the International Telecommunications Union. This index, which considers 11 indicators in 3 clusters—opportunity, infrastructure, and utilization—is a measure of the extent to which a country's residents have access to affordable interactive communication technology. In 2007, South Korea had the highest DOI in the world, at.80 (International Telecommunications Union, 2009).

Thus, Internet use is spreading to all parts of people's lives, creating a new kind of digital culture with the emergence of whole cyber communities. Digital culture presents new patterns of manageing life, different from patterns in the analog culture, which were more mechanical and less instantaneous. Digital culture is changing people's ways of thinking, working, relating, and enjoying life.

Because of its newness, however, many countries and communities experience a gap between residents participating in digital culture and those who are not. South Korea also has a digital divide, with greater utilization by men than women and by urban residents than rural residents. Differences among age groups are particularly striking. Although more than 90% of Koreans under age 30 are online, only 28% of 50-year-old and 16% of 60-year-old residents were online in 2006 (Table 1). Although still very low, the 16% use rate among seniors in 2006 is a large increase over the 3.3% rates found in the 2001 survey for this age group (NIDA, 2009).

How does older adults' use of the Internet in Korea compare with the U.S.? A number of surveys have included questions about Internet usage in Americans age 65 and older in 2005. Estimates range from 25% in the U.S. Census, to 41% in a national survey by the University of Southern California (AARP, 205). The same surveys estimated Internet usage by up-and-coming U.S. seniors (those 55-64) as 55-75%. Thus, Internet use among older adults in Korea appears lower than in the U.S.

It is not surprising that fewer older (vs. younger) adults are online. Van Dijk (1999) recognized four categories of barriers to IT that apply to older adults. First, many older adults have little or no digital experience. Some are not interested in the computer, some find the new technology unattractive, and some have anxiety about it (mental

Table 1. Internet Usage by Age Group. Source: National Internet Development Agency of Korea (2009)

Age group	10-19	20-29	30-39	40-49	50-59	60 and older
Internet usage	95.5%	90%	86.4%	58.3%	27.6%	16.2%

access). Second, few older adults own their own computer or have network connections (material access). Third, they may lack opportunities to use the technology (usage access). Fourth, they may lack digital skills (skills access).

All of these barriers still apply to some extent to older adults in Korea. Although Korea provides universal education in Korean and English, many older adults in Korea had limited educational opportunities in their youth. For example, those who were school-age during the Japanese occupation of Korea, when Japanese was the medium of instruction, did not learn to read and write Hangul (the Korean alphabet). Today's elders who were school-age during and immediately following the Korean War may have missed school altogether, because of the widespread destruction of infrastructure and the need to work to support themselves and/or their families (US Department of State, 2009). Most Korean older persons experienced a much poorer environment and lifecourse than today's young Koreans. Many have anxiety about technology. Few have had opportunities to own or gain skills with computers, palm-pilots, and other devices at which young people are so adept.

As a result, a cultural gap has occurred between generations that are familiar with the digital activities and those who are not. To overcome the cultural conflict between the analog and digital generations, addressing the digital divide has emerged as a core policy task. The current and anticipated growth in Korea's older population underscores the importance of integrating the older generation into digital culture and the information society (Son, 2007).

National Policies and Programs to Reduce the Age Divide

Korea is a leader in the electronics and technology industries. In fact, Korea aims to become the world's first ubiquitous society (Korea Ministry of Information and Communication, 2006). This phrase refers to a society that uses computers to monitor and improve daily living as well as education, medicine, and commerce. In a ubiquitous society, anyone can use the computer anytime. Tiny computers are embedded everywhere in the living space, for example in walls, appliances, and floors, and the technology allows them to communicate with each other to make the environment respond to human needs. For example, computers embedded in clothing can sense if a person feels chilled and can send a signal to a thermostat to increase the temperature of the room. Computers in street lamps, electric poles, and signs can make outside environments more responsive. Computers in stores can assure product freshness and track inventory. The goal is to create a more convenient society that increases the quality of life for all residents (Sakamura, 2008).

Thus, the Korean government has passed policies to reduce the digital divide with an aim of equitable information access regardless of age, physical abilities, economics, and region of residence. The lead agency to achieve this goal is the Korea Agency for Digital Opportunity and Promotion (KADO, 2008). To our knowledge, Korea is one of the few countries in the world to develop strong social policies promoting computer and Internet use among older adults. KADO is engaged in seven objectives:

- Information access environment creation
- Skills and content development aimed at bridging the digital divide
- Public education to upgrade people's IT literacy
- Promotion of public awareness of the digital divide
- Encouragement of productive information use
- Research and development on the digital divide and its bridging strategy
- International cooperation to narrow the global digital divide.

In 2001, the Korean government unveiled its first Master Plan (2001-2005) to close the divide and increase access by vulnerable groups to learning the computer, Internet, and other IT. By 2004, KADO had established almost 1,000 Local Information Access Centers around the country and facilitated the distribution of more than 60,000 used PCs to organizations and individuals in Korea. KADO helped disabled individuals obtain more than 6,500 devices and software programs to assist in their use of digital equipment. To expand Korea's pool of IT instructors, more than 2,400 volunteers had been trained to train others about computers and the Internet, and more than 200,000 had been reached by these volunteers. It opened a Center for Internet Addiction Prevention and Counseling, established a project to prevent cyber crime, and conducted surveys and research. KADO sponsors specific outreach efforts for individuals with disabilities and with older adults, often contracting with non-governmental agencies to extend its reach (Son, 2005; 2007). A second master plan (2006-2010) calls for the continued creation of policies and programs to expand computer use across society. KADO's objective for 2010 is to increase the informatization level of underprivileged groups (including older adults) to 80%. On the international front, 300 KADO internet volunteers were dispatched to 32 countries (for example Nepal, East Timor, Vietnam, China, Russia, and Kazakhstan) to provide IT training between 2001 and 2004 (Son, 2005).

Korea's Ministry of Education and Human Resources Development, along with its Ministry of Health and Welfare (2007), also has initiated a number of programs to support learning and activity. These include the Hangul (Korean) Education Program, the Silver Culture Program, and the Lifelong Learning Program. Other activities include volunteer training, program development, volunteer activity festivals, and the gold lifelong volunteer clubs. Since 2000, more than 10 million elders have been trained in computer use, and 40 IT volunteer teams are currently in action (Ministry of Health and Welfare, 2007).

KADO also calculates a Digital Divide Index for Korea, which is based on four factors—access, capacity, quantitative, and qualitative usage. In Table 2 are the digital divide index figures for individuals 50 and older in Korea. Overtime data suggest that the divide is declining relative to all factors, easing the gap between total population and persons age 50 and older. The general index combines access, capacity, and quantitative/qualitative usage factors. The index decreased by 4.2 points between 2006 and 2007, which means that the general informatization level of persons age 50+ compared to total population has risen from

Table 2. Digital divide index by factors and comparison level (%) for Koreans age 50+ (Source: KADO (2008), 2007 Annual Report of Digital Divide for People Age 50 and Older)

Factors	2004		2005		2006		2007	
	Divide index	Comparison level	Divide index	Comparison level	Divide index	Comparison level	Divide index	Comparison level
Access	33.7	66.3	26.5	73.5	17.1	82.9	9.9	90.1
Capacity	82.3	17.7	76.7	23.3	67.6	32.4	66.3	33.7
Quantitative usage	74.1	25.9	66.4	33.6	58.3	41.7	55.6	44.4
Qualtative usage	79.3	20.7	70.3	29.7	60.5	39.5	59.4	40.6
General usage	59.1	40.9	50.7	49.3	41.6	58.4	37.4	62.6

Table 3. Internet Usage Rate and PC Distribution Rate of the Primary Target for Policymaking (Source: KADO (2008). 2007 Annual Report of Digital Divide for People Age 50 and Older)

Groups	Internet Usage Rate (%)	PC Distribution Rate Per Household(%)
Less than 80%	0.3	54.8
Over 80%	99.5	98.6
Total	34.1	69.7

58.4% in 2006 to 62.6% in 2007. With respect to four factors individually, the access factor has shown the highest progress of all (Table 2).

When the general informatization level of Koreans age 50+ is examined by socio-demographic factors, the least digitalized groups are identified. These are termed the "less than 80% group." The main problems for this group are low capacity and usage factors. In other words, although 54.8%, of households of the most disadvantaged have personal computers, Internet use rate of older adults in disadvantaged households is only 0.3% (Table 3). So while public efforts to narrow the digital divide have proven successful in terms of quantitative expansion, more needs to be done to ensure the quality of IT use. The need to promote Internet training and computer education with isolated and disadvantaged older adults remains critical.

Programs of RISBLE

Localized outreach and training programs are the best mechanisms to reach isolated and disadvantaged older adults. The Research Institute of Science for the Better Living of the Elderly (RISBLE) is an organization in Busan, Korea that works on a number of fronts to promote elder well-being, including three programs aimed at reducing the age-based digital divide in Korea. Busan is a city of almost 4 million people on the south coast of Korea. It is Korea's largest port and its second-largest city (after Seoul).

RISBLE started in 1997 within Dong-In Hospital to explore best practices for elder care. In 2000, however, RISBLE was reestablished as a non-governmental organization (NGO) working in partnership with universities, government, and consumer groups. RISBLE's early programs included family and older adult counseling, and staff became concerned about the growing isolation of older adults and increasing reports of elder abuse and suicide. In 2000, RISBLE decided to expand its programs to promote the use of cyberspace by older adults to reduce isolation and increase quality of life. Funding to support RISBLE comes through grants and contracts from partners (especially governmental entities) and foundations. Staff size fluctuates based on funding and projects, and staff support is extended by a cadre of older volunteers. RISBLE also maintains an extensive Website with information on Active Ageing, digital ageing, dementia family support, and elder abuse (http://www.wellageing.com).

The use of the computer was not popular among older adults in Korea when RISBLE started to offer courses in 2000. Older people were not encouraged to try it, and many felt they were not able to learn. RISBLE began its courses with computers donated by IBM-Korea and classroom space donated by apartment complexes, public libraries, and other entities. Government funding became available to support this work in 2002, and KADO recognized RISBLE as a partner in IT education of seniors from this time.

Internet Navigator Program

RISBLE's Internet Navigators are older adults who have been trained to train others in the use of computers, the Internet, and various software programs. During RISBLE's first computer trainings offered in 2002, instructors identified older adults who demonstrated high comfort with and skill in the new technologies. Several of them were asked if they would like to become IT instructors for other older adults. These first instructors were trained as teachers and, in turn, they led IT classes for older persons in classrooms, community centers, post offices, and homes. When public computers were not available, an instructor might use his/her own laptop or borrow a laptop to teach computer skills.

By 2007, RISBLE was employing seven senior instructors who were leading classes for other older adults in Busan. Some instructors also offered classes in IT usage to other age groups. For example, one older man provided instruction in the use of digital cameras and PhotoShop to a group of disadvantaged youth in Busan. Others were developing new classes for seniors. In 2008, these seven instructors were asked to think about students who had potential to become IT instructors, and 20 more seniors were identified and trained.

RISBLE realized that the peer-education approach to IT training was working well, not only because the older instructors were skillful teachers, but also because they demonstrated that older adults could learn new things and enter new careers after retirement. Instructors found it best to work in teams, with a primary instructor and two helpers in a classroom. Besides teaching, instructors were providing individual technical assistance with computer-related questions. They also were asked about resources for older adults and caregivers, especially about informational and support resources available online. They also spent time responding to e-mailed and in-person questions on ageing, dementia, eldercare, caregiving, and family conflict. Because they were clearly more than teachers, the instructors renamed themselves Internet Navigators in 2008.

At the same time, Internet Navigation was seen as a new field of work for older persons, and government subsidies became available to provide stipends. Navigators were paid a small stipend from the Ministry of Health and Welfare for 20 hours a month of work, and some Navigators were able to leverage their training and practice to get other paying jobs.

In 2009, more than 150 older people applied to become Internet Navigators. Unfortunately, only 27 new Navigators could be accommodated, and RISBLE is seeking additional funding to support this expanded workforce to promote digital life for older adults. Currently, RISBLE also operates three "wellageing" centers where older adults can receive training and access the computer for education and personal use.

RISBLE staff members have heard many stories about how the Internet Navigator program has strengthened the self-esteem and self-satisfaction of older persons, as well as transferring to them useful skills. Several Navigators have said that this new role has helped bring new meaning to their lives and reduced feelings of isolation and depression. Trainees who have not become Navigators also report feelings of fulfillment and delight from being empowered with a new skill and means to stay connected with modern life. These stories attest to the power of digital education in preventing and reducing social exclusion of the elderly.

The Cyber-Family Program

The Cyber-Family Program was developed by RISBLE in 2005 with funding from the Korean Commission for Youth. It was designed in response to seniors' comments that it was not enough to learn IT skills. They also wanted more structured opportunities to use the Internet for personal development and to feel useful. Thus, older adults associated with RISBLE worked with young people to survey and comment on Web-based content targeted to young people. The students were identified in partnership with teachers of elementary and middle schools in nearby rural areas. This activity provided older people with reasons to engage in online dialogue with younger people and motivated them to expand their digital skills.

Once a year, Cyber-Family members were invited to participate in an "offline" gathering. At this day-long event, elders and youngsters who had communicated online engaged together in games and discussions. Pen-pals were happy to finally meet each other in person, and relationships were strengthened.

Soon, older persons were using cyberspace to exchange digital camera pictures, discuss good places to eat or travel, and share views on life. Some young people asked their new pen-pals for advice with academic concerns and adolescent relationships. As unrelated but concerned older adults, the seniors were good listeners and safe correspondents. Seniors, students, and teachers reported that the Cyber-Family Program generated warm relationships across the generations and allowed a sense of extended family relationships to spread throughout cyberspace. RISBLE published some of the senior-student stories in a book supported by the KT Cultural Foundation in 2007 (RISBLE, 2007).

The Cyber-Family Program (See Figure 2) represents another RISBLE effort to sponsor programming to overcome societal and family seclusion of older adults. First, the program helps seniors bridge the information gap experienced by not being online. It helps socially integrate older adults into families by offering new ways to interact among the generations, by teaching seniors IT vocabulary and concepts and giving them experience in e-mail relationships. Older people learn to express their own thoughts and better understand the young generation. It also helps socially integrate older adults into society by expanding their options for learning and participation. Finally, students benefit from getting to know elders outside of their own families and to see that they could be fun and helpful. This experience serves to break down stereotypes of older adults as "too old to learn" and "uninteresting."

Recognizing the significance of this program, RISBLE will continue to expand options for intergenerational digital engagement. Plans are underway to develop an International Cyber-Family program between young Koreans and older adults in foreign countries. As Korea encourages its young people to expand their foreign-language skills, especially English, Japanese, and Chinese, an International Cyber-Family program could offer Korean youth with opportunities to practice foreign languages while gaining respect for older adults through pen-pal friendships.

1080 Online Game Festival

Korea is a leading producer of IT and online games. In 2006, the combined revenues of some

Figure 2. Symbol of the cyber family program. (© 2004, Research Institute of Science for the Better Living of the Elderly, Busan, Korea. Used with permission.)

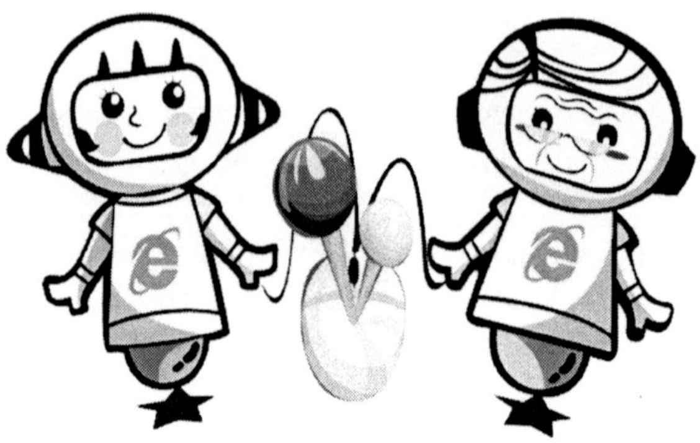

1,200 online gaming companies in Korea reached an estimated US$1.94 billion, up from US$1.54 billion in 2005, and it continues to grow (Business Week, March 26, 2007). To support the globalization of the Korea IT industry, Korea hosts an international Online Game Festival, an event in which online gamesters from around the world compete in Web-based games.

Most youngsters and young adults in Korea are extremely adept at online games. Older adults in Korea, however, are not as familiar with online games, and many seniors want to know more about them. A few IT companies are increasing their age-friendliness and developing online games that can be played by three-generation families. To expand opportunities for older adults to learn a new skill and participate in IT globalization, RISBLE began to think about ways to include older adults in online games.

Thus was born the 1080 Online Game Festival (See Figure 3). The 10 is the symbol of the young generation because it signals the beginning of adolescence and it sounds like "teen." The 80 is the symbol of the old generation and connotes longevity. In 2008, the Korea Association of Fame Industry (KAOGI) selected three partners in Korea to hold game festivals, and RISBLE was chosen as the Busan partner.

The first 1080 Online Game Festival was held in 2007 and the second in 2008. To be admitted to the Festival, young people had to bring a grandparent or other older adult. Each year, more than 200 families attended and competed in online games. Participants reported that they enjoyed the Festival and that it helped strengthen bonds within their families. Because of the festival, KAOGI realized the potential profit in developing more online games for older people and for multiple generations.

In the beginning, the possibility of online games as a new alternative for elder leisure activities seemed to be unlikely. However, as the 1080 Games Festivals have evolved, we see more and more elders express enthusiasm about participating in the games. We discovered that online games can point a new direction for achieving Active Ageing for older persons, especially those with physical disabilities and those residing in care facilities. There is potential for online games to facilitate enjoyment for older people, offering an option for spending time idly or in isolation.

As digital leisure is emerging as a major pastime of young people around the world, it becomes vitally important to promote cyberspace interaction between the younger and older generations. In this respect, the online game can be a very powerful tool for interactivity. Given global ageing, marketers should look more seriously at older adults as consumers of online games. Social norms about older adults also will change as they become a sector of the marketplace over which sellers compete.

Policy Development

In addition to program development and delivery, RISBLE works to influence social policy. RISBLE

Figure 3. Symbol of 1080 Games Festival. (© 2006, Research Institute of Science for the Better Living of the Elderly, Busan, Korea. Used with permission.)

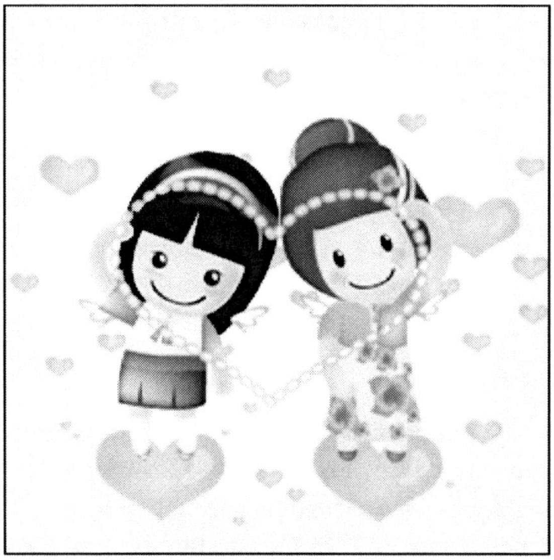

members attend professional and government meetings related to ageing, standing ready to advocate for policies and programs that promote elder health and wellbeing. The RISBLE director also represents Korea in international groups, such as ACAP and the International Network for the Prevention of Elder Abuse, a standing committee of the International Association of Gerontology and Geriatrics (IAGG). RISBLE members work to educate government and the public about elder abuse, dementia, family care, and digital ageing, and are often consulted by Korean and international media on these issues.

Several policy initiatives are evidence of RISBLE's commitment to eliminate the digital divide experienced by older adults in Korea. For example, in 2007, RISBLE organized the Namhae Active Ageing Conference in Asia Pacific, the third international conference of ACAP. This successful conference featured speakers from Korea, Japan, and the U.S., sharing best practices for increasing elder knowledge and use of IT. Conference participants signed the Namhae Declaration of Active Ageing, which includes recognition of the necessity of digital ageing in an Active Ageing society. The four resolutions of Namhae Declaration (2007) include:

- We recognize the need to empower the elderly as social capital (not as a burden).
- We commit ourselves to helping to create an age-friendly society, where healthy and active ageing is secured.
- We recognize the mutual relation between the healthy city and active ageing.
- We commit ourselves to integrate the elderly into society through digital ageing, which prevents elderly exclusion from information and raises the quality of life.

In addition to presentations made to Korean audiences, the RISBLE director has been an invited presenter on its digital ageing programs in Japan, China, the U.S., Canada, Europe, and South America, at conferences hosted by IAGG, ACAP, Senior Net, and other organizations. RISBLE now is supporting the Federation of Korean Gerontological Societies (FKGS) and IAGG in hosting the 20th IAGG World Congress. This congress will be held in Seoul in 2013, and the theme of the congress is Digital Ageing (http://www.iagg2013.org/eng/m11.php?menu=m11). The IAGG congress is the world's largest international meeting on ageing, attended by researchers, scholars, policy makers, program leaders, and activists in gerontology and geriatrics. It is anticipated that this gathering will further global awareness of and support of older adults' participation in digital life.

CONCLUSION

In this chapter, we reviewed information about ageing and the digital divide experienced by older adults in South Korea. We introduced the concept of Active Ageing and explained how digital ageing promotes Active Ageing. Information on three RISBLE "best practices" was shared in the hope that other communities can learn from RISBLE's work to reduce the ageing digital divide and promote digital life for older persons.

We have learned that older adults in Korea face many barriers to digital life. However, we also have learned that older people are willing to learn. When given access, provided with lessons, and given encouragement, older people can embrace IT and enhance their participation in life. They enjoy mastering new skills, creating new communities, and realizing new roles and avenues for themselves through digital participation. We have developed programs which are appreciated by older adults, and we are being challenged to increase the number of older adults we serve.

It is our belief that efforts to bridge the digital divide are important for the overall wellbeing of the elderly. Integration of older adults into the digital culture expands options for intergenerational communication and, hence, for family interaction and demonstrations of filial piety. It lessens isolation, which we hope will reduce the risk of elder abuse and suicide. Digital integration expands options for work and volunteering, creating new ways that older adults can support themselves and contribute to families and communities. Finally, it helps to create and improve images of ageing from those of today, which cast older adults as out-of-date, behind the times, and burdensome. We foresee new images of older people as active, able to grow, and willing to contribute their knowledge, skills, and wisdom through digital technology, as well as in person. We feel that the informatization of older adults can help eliminate prejudice and discrimination, as well as isolation.

The task ahead is to increase quality use of computers and the Internet by all older people, including those that are the most disadvantaged and isolated in today's society. To this end, RISBLE will continue to promote Internet Navigators in the local community and to sponsor digital opportunities for intergenerational exchange through our Cyber-Family and 1080 Games Festival programs. We will continue to speak to policy makers and gerontology colleagues about digital ageing and its importance in building an Active Ageing society, one in which everyone can contribute, regardless of age. Through these efforts, we will improve the overall quality of life of older persons in Korea. We also will continue to share our work with other nations, contributing our experiences so that others can learn from our challenges and build on our successes.

REFERENCES

AARP. (2005). *Doing the math. Older adults online 2005*. Retrieved from http://www.aarp.org/olderwiserwired/oww-resources/doing_the_math_older_adults_online.html.

Active Ageing Consortium Asia Pacific (ACAP). Retrieved March 9, 2009 from http://www.wellageing.com.

Aphek, E. (2001). Minimizing the digital divide and the inter-generation gap. *Ubiquity: An ACM IT Magazine and Forum*. Retrieved from http://www.acm.org/ubiquity/views/e_aphek_1.html?searchterm=aphek.

Business Week. (March 26, 2007). *South* Korea: *Video games' crazed capital*. Retrieved from http://www.businessweek.com/globalbiz/content/mar2007/gb20070326_937184.htm.

Carlile, L. (2007, May). *Active ageing: Theoretical background*. Paper presented at the Namhae Active Ageing Conference in Asia Pacific, Namhae, Korea.

Carvin, A. (2000). Mending the breach: Overcoming the digital divide. Edutopia. Retrieved from http://www.edutopia.org/mending-breach-overcoming-digital-divide.

Chang, B. L., Bakken, S., Brown, S. S., Houston, T. K., Kreps, G. L., & Kukafka, R. (2004). Bridging the digital divide: Reaching vulnerable populations. *Journal of the American Medical Informatics Association*, *11*(6), 448–457. doi:10.1197/jamia.M1535

Cheon, J. S. (2006). Suicide in the Korean elderly. *Journal of Korean Geriatric Psychiatry*, *10*(1), 14–19.

Fries, J. F. (1980). Ageing, natural death, and the compression of morbidity. *The New England Journal of Medicine*, *303*, 130–135. doi:10.1056/NEJM198007173030304

Halfon, N., & Hochstein, M. (2002). Life course health development: An integrated framework for developing health, policy and research. *The Milbank Quarterly*, *80*, 433–479. doi:10.1111/1468-0009.00019

Han, D. H. (2006). Digital silver for wellageing. [in Korean]. *Journal of Korean Geriatric Psychiatry*, *10*(1), 5–9.

Han, D. H. (2007, May). *The new strategy of social integration for older persons through Cyber Family.* Paper presented at the Namhae Active Ageing Conference in Asia Pacific, Namhae, Korea.

Han, D. H. (2008, February). *Perseverance to eradicate abuse of elderly women in Korea.* Paper presented at the Communities Working Together to End Violence against Women Conference, Ontario, Canada.

Han, D. H., & Kim, J. O. (1998). Elder abuse: Factors related to Korean elder abuse. *Journal of Asian Regional Association for Home Economics, 5*(1), 10–16.

Hooyman, N., & Kiyak, H. A. (2005). *Social Gerontology: A multidisciplinary perspective.* Needham, MA: Allyn & Bacon.

Hutchison, D., Eastman, C., & Tirrito, T. (1997). Designing user interfaces for older adults. *Educational Gerontology, 23*, 497–513. doi:10.1080/0360127970230601

International Telecommunication Union. (2009). Digital Opportunity Index. Retrieved from http://www.itu.int/ITU-D/ict/doi/index.html.

Internet World Stats. (2008). Korea. Retrieved from http://www.internetworldstats.com/asia/kr.htm.

Jackson, L. A., Zhao, Y., Kolenic, A., Fitzgerald, H. E., Harold, R., & Von Eye, A. (2008). Race, gender, and information technology use: The new digital divide. *Cyberpsychology & Behavior, 11*(4), 437–442. doi:10.1089/cpb.2007.0157

Kim, I. K. (2000, August). *Policy responses to low fertility and population ageing in Korea.* Paper presented at the United Nations Expert Group Meeting on Policy Responses to Population Ageing and Population Decline. Retrieved March 9, 2009 from http://www.un.org/esa/population/publications/popdecline/kim.pdf.

Kinsella, K., & Phillips, D. (2005). Global ageing: The challenge of success. [Washington, DC: Population Reference Bureau.]. *Population Bulletin, 60*, 1.

Korea Agency for Digital Opportunity and Promotion. (2008). *2007 Annual report of digital divide for people age 50+ and older.* Seoul, Korea (in Korean).

Korea Agency for Digital Opportunity and Promotion. (2009). About KADO. Retrieved from https://www.kado.or.kr/koil/aboutkado/.

Korea Ministry of Health and Welfare. KIHSA. (2007) *2006 national survey of living status and welfare needs of the elders and needs for the elderly welfare service.* Retrieved March 9, 2009 from http://www.kihasa.re.kr/html/jsp/ (in Korean).

Korea Ministry of Information and Communication. (2006). *U-Korea master plan: To achieve the world's first ubiquitous society.* Retrieved from http://www.ipc.go.kr/servlet/download?pt=/ipceng/public&fn=u-KOREA+Master+Plan+.pdf

Korea National Statistics Office. (2006). *Population prediction for Korea* Retrieved from http://www.nso.go.kr/eng2006/

Kreps, G. L. (2005). Disseminating relevant health information to underserved audiences: Implications for the Digital Divide Pilot Projects. *Journal of the Medical Library Association, 93*(4Supple), S69–S73.

Kuttan, A., & Peters, L. (2003). *From digital divide to digital opportunity.* Lanham, MD: Rowman & Littlefield Publications, Inc.

Lorence, D. P., & Park, H. (2006). New technology and old habits: The role of age as a technology chasm. *Technology and Health Care, 14*(2), 91–96.

Murray, E., Burns, J., See, T. S., Lai, R., & Nazareth, I. (2005). Interactive health communication applications for people with chronic disease. *Cochrane Database of Systematic Reviews*, (Issue 4), CD004274. doi:.doi:10.1002/14651858.CD004274.pub4

Namazi, K. H., & McClintic, M. (2003). Computer use among elderly persons in long term care facilities. *Educational Gerontology*, *29*, 535–550. doi:10.1080/713844391

National Internet Development Agency of Korea. (2009). Internet Usage Statistics. Retrieved from http://isis.nida.or.kr/eng/.

New Zealand Ministry of Social Policy. (2001). *New Zealand positive ageing strategy*. Retrieved from http://www.osc.govt.nz/positive-ageing-strategy/index.html.

Peel, N. M., McClure, R. J., & Bartlett, H. P. (2005). Behavioral determinants of healthy ageing. *American Journal of Preventive Medicine*, *28*(3), 298–304. doi:10.1016/j.amepre.2004.12.002

Research Institute of Science for the Better Living of the Elderly. (2007). *Cyber-family program*. Busan, Korea: Author.

Rowe, J. W., & Kahn, R. L. (1998). *Successful ageing*. New York: Pantheon Books.

Sakamura, K. (2008). *Ubiquitous ID technologies* 2008. Tokyo, Japan: YRP Ubiquitous Networking Laboratory. Retrieved from http://www.uidcenter.org/pdf/UID910-W001-080226_en.pdf.

Selwyn, N. (2004). The information aged: A qualitative study of older adults' use of information and communication technology. *Journal of Aging Studies*, *18*, 369–384. doi:10.1016/j.jaging.2004.06.008

Shapira, N., Barak, A., & Gil, I. (2007). Promoting older adults' well-being through Internet training and use. *Aging & Mental Health*, *11*(5), 477–484. doi:10.1080/13607860601086546

Slegers, K., van Boxtel, M. P. J., & Jolles, J. (2008). Effects of computer training and internet usage on the well-being and quality of life of older adults: A randomized, controlled study. *Journal of Gerontology*, *63B*, 176–P184.

Son, Y. (2005). *KADO 2004 annual report*. Seoul: Korea Agency for Digital Opportunity & Promotion.

Son, Y. (2007, May). Addressing the digital divide within the Korean ageing society. Paper presented at Namhae Active Ageing Conference in Asia Pacific, Namhae, Korea.

Sung, K. T. (1995). Measures and dimensions of filial piety in Korea. *The Gerontologist*, *35*(2), 240–247.

Sung, K. T. (2001). Family support for the elderly in Korea: continuity, change, future directions, and cross-cultural concerns. *Journal of Aging & Social Policy*, *12*(4), 65–79. doi:10.1300/J031v12n04_04

United Nations. (2002). *Population ageing 2002*. Retrieved from www.un.org/esa/population/publications/ageing/Graph.pdf.

United Nations. (2009). *Age-friendly cities*. Retrieved from http://www.who.int/ageing/age_friendly_cities/en/index.html.

U.S. Department of State. (2009). South Korea. Retrieved from http://www.state.gov/r/pa/ei/bgn/2800.htm.

U.S. Department of State and Department of Health and Human Services. (2007). *Why population matters: A global perspective*. Washington, DC: Authors.

van Dijk, J. (1999). *The network society: Social aspects of the new media*. Thousand Oaks, CA: Sage Publications.

van Dijk, J. (2005). *The deepening divide: Inequality in the information society*. Thousand Oaks, CA: Sage Publications.

Van Dijk, J. (2005, December). *From digital divide to social opportunities*. Paper presented at the International Conference for Bridging the Digital Divide, Seoul, Korea

Warmerdam, L., van Straten, A., & Cuijpers, P. (2007). Internet-based treatment for adults with depressive symptoms: the protocol of a randomized controlled trial. *BMC Psychiatry*, *7*, 72–78. doi:10.1186/1471-244X-7-72

Whaley, K. C. (2004). America's digital divide: 2000-2003 trends. *Journal of Medical Systems*, *28*(2), 183–195. doi:10.1023/B:JOMS.0000023301.09308.d9

White, H., McConnell, E., Clipp, E., Branch, L. G., Sloane, R., Pieper, C., & Box, T. L. (2002). A randomized controlled trial of the psychosocial impact of providing internet training and access to older adults. *Aging & Mental Health*, *6*(3), 213–221. doi:10.1080/13607860220142422

Wiener, J. M., & Tilly, J. (2002). Population ageing in the United States of America: Implications for public programmes. *International Journal of Epidemiology*, *31*, 776–781. doi:10.1093/ije/31.4.776

World Health Organization (WHO). (2002). Active ageing: A policy framework. Retrieved from http://whqlibdoc.who.int/hq/2002/WHO_NMH_NPH_02.8.pdf.

Chapter 11
Intelligent Transportation Systems for Older Drivers:
A Systems Approach to Improving Safety and Extending Driving Longevity

Christopher G. Hatherly
The Australian National University, Australia

ABSTRACT

This chapter covers current and future technologies relevant to older drivers. It does this using a systems framework, reviewing research and issues relating to older adults and technology at the level of the road user, the transport infrastructure and the vehicle. While most Intelligent Transportation Systems (ITS) currently exist at the level of the vehicle (technologies such as satellite navigation, collision avoidance, and hazard alerting systems), research and development at the infrastructure level also holds promise of significant improvements in automotive safety through the exchange and coordination of digital information between vehicles and the roads upon which they are driven. At the individual level, there are also increasingly sophisticated technologies being developed that aim to accurately identify potentially unsafe drivers, and to maintain and even enhance cognitive capacities that are critically important to safe driving. This chapter begins with a review of salient characteristics of older drivers, before discussing current and future technologies at each level of the adopted framework: the road user, the road, and the vehicle.

INTRODUCTION

In just over 100 years since the first Model T Ford rolled off the production line, there have been huge changes in all aspects of automotive transportation. Cars have become increasingly sophisticated, road networks have proliferated (from 230km of sealed road in the US in 1904, to over 9.2 million km today; Berger, 2001) and most of the Western population has come to rely on private vehicles for their everyday transportation needs. This century of change has had a profound impact on every aspect of society and culture, and it is likely that the continuing evolution of automobiles and automotive transport will have an even greater impact in the decades to come. This

DOI: 10.4018/978-1-61520-825-8.ch011

evolution will occur on two main fronts. On the one hand, the next 20 to 30 years will likely see a comprehensive shift towards environmentally friendly vehicles, with a majority designed for no or low emissions (Van Mierlo, Maggetto, & Lataire, 2006). On the other, and within the same time frame, there will be a growing technological revolution, with increasing incorporation of Intelligent Transportation Systems (ITS) into both vehicles and transportation networks enabling ever greater levels of driver convenience and safety. Reflecting on the probable future, US auto industry elder statesman Bob Lutz predicted that by the mid 2020s, there would be wide-spread implementation of fully autonomous vehicles (Lutz, 2004). The science-fiction future of clean, green self-driving cars may almost be here.

For this prediction to come to pass, however, the next 15 years will necessarily involve very rapid and very significant changes in vehicle design, technology and usage. These changes will naturally affect drivers of all ages, but for two reasons, the first and probably greatest impact will be felt by older drivers. First, older adults are the fastest growing segment of the driving population (NHTSA, 2006), with current and future cohorts of retirees driving more frequently and for more years than ever before (Molnar & Eby, 2008). In the face of age-related physical, sensory and cognitive declines, incremental advances in technology hold perhaps the greatest promise for enabling an extension of safe and independent automotive mobility that millions of aging baby boomers desire (Arentze, Timmermans, Jorritsma, Olde-Kalter, & Schoemakers, 2008). Second, technological innovations usually make their first commercial appearance in fully-featured or luxury model vehicles for which the largest market has always been older drivers (Choo & Mokhtarian, 2004; Coughlin, 2005). Together, these factors highlight the importance of understanding the nature of older adults' interactions with, and requirements for, ITS. Only with this understanding will policy makers and automotive technologists and designers be able to optimise future vehicles and transportation networks to maximise their safety, convenience, and usability for older drivers.

This chapter sets out to analyse issues surrounding older drivers and technology from a systems perspective, specifically, a system comprising three elements: the road user, transport infrastructure, and the vehicle. Research, issues, and current and future technologies will be examined at each level, before the concepts and discussions are drawn together with recommendations for consumers, researchers and policy makers regarding current technologies and the way forward. The analysis begins with an introduction to the characteristics of older adults as drivers of cars.

BACKGROUND

Older Drivers

Older drivers, typically but arbitrarily classified as those aged 65 and over, are the fastest growing component of the road user population (OECD, 2001). For instance, the number of licensed older drivers in the US increased by 17% between 1995 and 2005, in contrast to a rise of only 14% across other age groups (NHTSA, 2006). This growth is a result of several factors including population aging, increasing car ownership and usage rates, and a move towards increased social engagement and aging-in-place for many retirees (Smiley, 1999).

Whilst there is enormous variability between older adults across all aspects of ability and function, as drivers they do have several distinguishing characteristics. First, most of the sensory, physical and cognitive abilities that are required to safely operate a vehicle tend to decline with increasing age (Anstey, Wood, Lord, & Walker, 2005). For example, age-related structural changes in the eye result in a reduction of up to 90% in visual sensitivity and resolving power over a lifetime (Klein, 1991). However in other areas, age may be associated with improvements in abilities

Figure 1. Age and serious accidents. (Adapted from Li, Braver, & Chen, 2003)

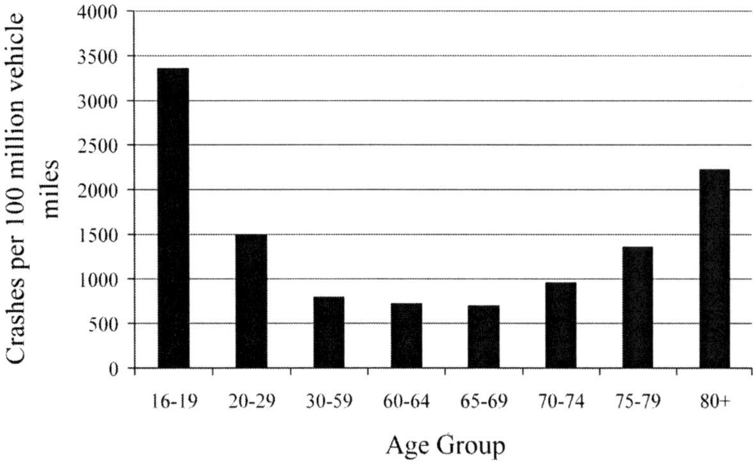

required for safe driving, anticipating hazards for example (Horswill et al., 2008) or having an accurate appraisal of one's own limitations and abilities (Marottoli & Richardson, 1998). Furthermore, there is evidence that many of the declining abilities associated with age can be improved or maintained, at least temporarily, with targeted training programs and interventions. Understanding these factors and the way they change with age is a vital first step to understanding potential benefits or problems in the interaction between older drivers and ITS.

A second characteristic of older drivers is the existence of a negative popular stereotype portraying them as hazardous and unsafe on the road. This stereotype is reinforced regularly in the media, highlighted occasionally by intensive coverage of horrific accidents involving elderly drivers (see, for example, Leduff, 2004). The general belief that older drivers are dangerous to themselves and others – often referred to as the 'older driver problem' (Smiley, 1999) – is pervasive and continues to influence public attitudes, policy decisions and research directions today. However the evidence supporting this belief is less clear and it appears that by many measures, older drivers are as safe as any other group of drivers on the road.

Older Driver Accidents and Risk

One of the most frequently replicated findings in the road safety literature is that of a U-shaped curve relating age to accident rates (see, for example, Liu, Utter, & Chen, 2007). This curve generally shows the greatest number of accidents per unit distance travelled for the youngest and oldest drivers, with a sharp decrease into middle-age (see Figure 1). The only significant change in this finding over many decades has been a steady downwards trend in the number of accidents per unit distance across all ages, and an upwards shift in the age at which accident rates begin to climb (Hakamies-Blomqvist & Henriksson, 1999). For example, in 1938, crash rates began to climb for 'older' drivers from age 48 (DeSilva, 1938) whereas today they are relatively stable from the early 30s to the mid-70s. It remains a fact, however, that older drivers are more likely to be involved in accidents than those in middle age. Furthermore, with the rapidly increasing proportion of older drivers, it has been predicted that by 2030, their rate of accidents and fatalities could increase by 178% and 155% respectively (Lyman, Ferguson, Braver, & Williams, 2002), whereas rates are expected to decrease for those aged under 65.

The fact that older adults are more likely to end up in accident statistics has important implications in the context of transportation technology and policy. However there are several important moderating factors that need to be considered when discussing the actual *danger* associated with driving in old age. First, due to reduced strength and increased physical frailty, older adults are inherently more likely to be seriously injured or killed in any given type of accident, and therefore to end up in the accident statistics than are younger drivers (Meuleners, Harding, Lee, & Legge, 2006). This finding is known as the 'frailty bias' and has been demonstrated on several occasions. Similarly, a 'low-mileage' bias, accounting for some of the apparent increase in crash risk for older drivers, has been identified by several researchers (see, for example, Janke, 1991). The assumption here is that low-mileage drivers (and this includes most older adults) do most of their travelling in high risk urban environments whereas those doing higher mileages – often younger and middle-aged drivers – travel more of that distance on safer interstate or highway systems. In studies conducted in Finland (Hakamies-Blomqvist, Raitanen, & O'Neill, 2002), Holland (Langford, Methorst, & Hakamies-Blomqvist, 2006) and the USA (Langford, Koppel, McCarthy, & Srinivasan, 2008), the low-mileage bias has been found to account statistically for all of the age-related increase in crash rates both with and without correcting for the frailty bias. Such research emphasises that older adults have an increased risk of accidents per kilometre travelled not necessarily as a result of driving dangerously, but simply because of a proportionally higher exposure to dangerous driving conditions.

A further important consideration, and one that is very rarely taken into account, is that of vehicle age. Specifically, several recent reports found that the risk of an accident increases by approximately 2% for every year of a vehicle's age (Blows et al., 2003; Poindexter, 2003). These studies did not look specifically at older drivers; however other reports find that while many older adults drive relatively new vehicles, a significant number also drive older cars (Federal Highway Administration, 1997).

Finally, a critical finding regarding older drivers' accidents is that they generally differ in cause and in type from those of younger drivers. Specifically, older drivers incur proportionally fewer accidents than younger or middle-aged drivers as a result of infringements (speeding or alcohol-related crashes for example), and proportionally more as a result of errors (for example, failing to give way, or misjudging gaps; Ryan, Legge, & Rosman, 1998). The location and type of accidents also differ between age groups. A relatively high proportion of the serious accidents of younger and middle-age drivers involve only a single vehicle; however, when older drivers crash, it is frequently with another vehicle (Haworth & Bowland, 2000; Ryan et al., 1998). Furthermore, many of these at-fault accidents of older drivers occur during right-hand turns (left turns in right-side travel jurisdictions) at non-signalised intersections, often as a result of failure to appropriately give way (Braitman, Kirley, Ferguson, & Chaudhary, 2007; Lord, van Schalkwyk, Chrysler, & Staplin, 2007; Oxley, Fildes, Corben, & Langford, 2006; Ulfarsson, Kim, & Lentz, 2006). For example, Lord and colleagues found that for drivers aged 80 and over, 55% of fatal accidents occurred at intersections, as opposed to only 23% for drivers aged under 50. Thus, while older drivers rarely speed or intentionally break the law, their accidents more frequently involve multiple vehicles, with high crash rates at intersections suggesting a specific age-related difficulty or impairment for some older individuals. These issues will be revisited in discussions on the driver, roadway design, and the vehicle later in this chapter.

Older Driver Vehicle Usage

During the middle of last century, suburbia in countries such as Australia and America was largely comprised of single-vehicle single-driver households (Nutley & Thomas, 1995). Men were predominantly the drivers, and in many cases, their wives never drove (Evans, 1991). Sometime after retirement, most older couples moved into smaller sized accommodation, often in centralised retirement or age-care facilities, and the necessity and frequency of vehicle usage declined (Cutler & Coward, 1992; Witkowski & Buick, 1985). Often, women would also outlive their husbands, and having never driven, would live their final decades with minimal use of cars (Hakamies-Blomqvist & Siren, 2003; Utz, Carr, Nesse, & Wortman, 2002).

Today, attitudes, expectations and practices have changed dramatically. Current retirees often own multiple vehicles and both men and women continue to use their cars for many years (Hakamies-Blomqvist & Siren, 2003). This is partly associated with a change in preferences for later-life accommodation – the phenomenon of 'aging in place' (Rosel, 2003) – but is also linked to increased rates of social and employment participation amongst older adults, generally necessitating longer and more frequent outings (Eby, Molnar, & Kartje, 2009). In addition, the majority of today's older adults have relied exclusively on private vehicles for transport for most of their adult lives (Chimpan, Payne, & McDonough, 1998), meaning that unlike previous generations who were generally more comfortable with lower mobility lifestyles and much more familiar with public or other transportation options, today's older adults will both need and expect to drive further, more often and for more years than did generations before.

Driving Behaviour

A second and related component of vehicle usage is that of driving behaviour. Generally speaking, older drivers are both more cautious and more alert behind the wheel than are younger drivers (Smiley, 1999). They are more likely to wear safety belts and less likely to take speed related risks (Yagil, 1998). They are also less likely to engage in potentially distracting dual-tasks such as talking on the phone or adjusting the radio while in motion (Bayly, Young, & Regen, 2009).

Older drivers are also generally aware of declining perceptual, motor and to some extent, cognitive abilities, and often take steps to minimise the impact of these changes on their driving (Smiley, 1999). Such changes include reducing distance travelled and/or frequency of trips (Ball et al., 1998), and avoiding difficult driving situations (such as wet weather, peak-hour traffic or low light; Brabyn, Shchneck, Lott, & Haegerstrom-Portnoy, 2005) and difficult driving manoeuvres (Ball et al., 1998; Hakamies-Blomqvist & Wahlstrom, 1998).

Future Cohorts of Older Drivers

Turning finally to future cohorts, if the prediction of autonomous vehicles by the mid-2020s comes to pass, tomorrow's older drivers may instead be older passengers of self-driving cars, and most of the issues discussed here might not apply. Until this point, however, designers, researchers and policy makers interested in this area should be aware of several important changes that can be expected in the older drivers of tomorrow.

First, as was mentioned previously, older drivers, particularly older women, comprise the fastest growing segment of the road-user population. As this proportion grows, the transport system will change too. No longer will the sight of an older driver moving slowly through busy traffic be unusual, and traffic flows in general will become better suited to older operators, generally slower and more forgiving (Hakamies-Blomqvist, 1999).

Second, older drivers in the future will have had, on average, better initial training and more years of driving experience in busier and more complex traffic conditions than older drivers in the past (Hole, 2007). This will result in better drivers who will be able to continue driving safely by relying on their expertise and adaptive strategies to deal with declining abilities. Finally, and of particular relevance to this volume, tomorrow's older drivers will have had a longer acquaintance, and therefore be more comfortable with certain types of technological aides than has been the case in the past (Coughlin, 2005). In contrast to their parents, older adults of the future will be much more accustomed to technologies such as communications devices and navigation aides, and as such will have very different aptitudes for, and attitudes towards, dealing with such technologies.

Road Safety Systems Framework

In previous decades, road safety researchers and policy makers tended to focus on specific aspects of road safety. In the case of older drivers, this focus rested upon age-related deficits of the individual, and possible safety implications of the road system and vehicles were taken largely for granted (see, for example, McFarland, Tune, & Welford, 1964). Today, most in the field have adopted a systems approach (Evans, 1991; Langford & Oxley, 2006). This system, depicted in Figure 2, comprises three elements, specifically: the *individual*, including the behaviours, attitudes and abilities of the road user; *transport infrastructure*, incorporating roadway design, traffic management, and regulation; and the *vehicle*, focussing on safer cars. Most of the automotive technology within this system currently exists at the level of the vehicle, and much of the discussion in this chapter will focus there. However the future development of integrated infrastructure-based ITS will dramatically increase the level of technology present in the roads themselves, and as time passes, such systems will likely result in new safety and traffic network systems

Figure 2. Safe Systems framework for road safety. (Adapted from Langford & Oxley, 2006)

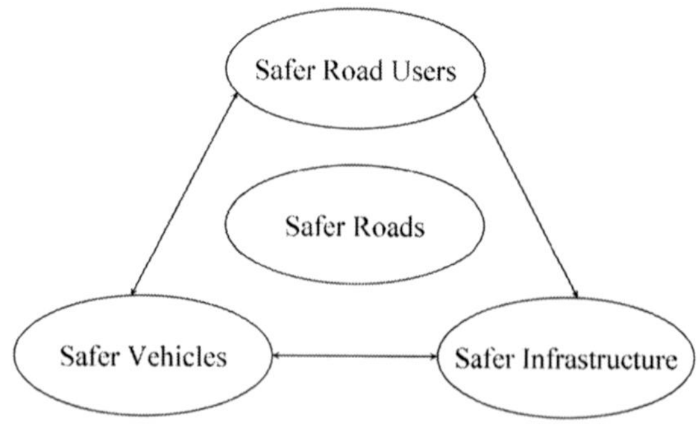

(as well as lifestyle and commercial applications) that can scarcely be imagined today. There are also technologies relevant to older drivers that are being developed at the individual level, with increasingly sophisticated screening measures and technology-driven interventions.

The following sections will address each component of this system in turn, starting with the individual.

ROAD USER

The first and most fundamental component of the safe systems approach is the road user. Regardless of the quality or technological sophistication of roadway design or the safety features built into cars, it is the driver who has ultimate control over the movement of their vehicle. Numerous studies have documented age-related changes (generally declines) in a range of fundamental sensory, physical and cognitive abilities, both in general and in relation to driving. These factors are reviewed comprehensively elsewhere (e.g.; Birren, Schaie, Gatz, & Salthouse, 2006), and will not be dealt with here. Instead, this section will first summarise a framework proposed by Anstey and colleagues (2005) for understanding the factors that lead to safe driving behaviour amongst the elderly, before outlining how technology is being

Figure 3. Model of factors enabling safe driving behaviour. (Source: Anstey et al., 2005. ©2005, Elsevier. Used with permission)

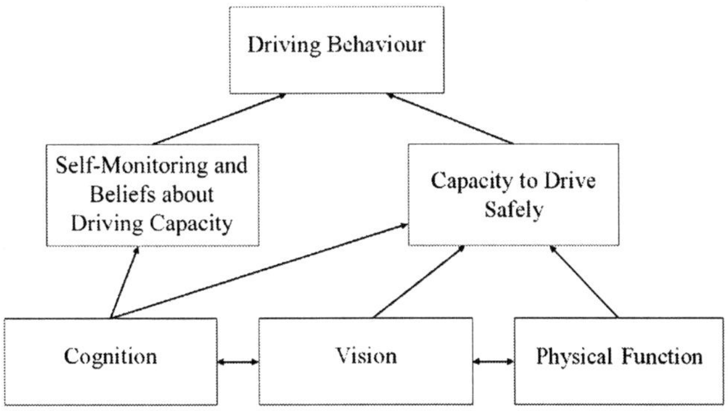

used to develop more reliable screening measures and interventions for use with older drivers.

Framework for Understanding Factors Affecting Driving Behaviour

Many studies have investigated the impact of age-related declines in basic sensory, motor and cognitive abilities on the capacity of the driver to safely control their vehicle, however few have addressed the role of higher order cognition (e.g., self-monitoring) in older driver safety, and fewer still have succeeded in taking account of the various factors in a comprehensive model. Recently however, a hierarchical model of safe driving behaviour has been proposed (Anstey et al., 2005). This model comprises sensory, cognitive and physical abilities at a basic level which contribute to both an individual's capacity to drive safely and to their beliefs about their capacity. These factors, in turn, determine driving behaviour, safe or otherwise (see Figure 3). Returning to the discussion of accident rates at the beginning of this chapter, it has been suggested that the fact that older adults do not demonstrate a significant increase in driving risk with age (after adjusting for a variety of known biases), despite the decline in abilities such as vision, reaction time and physical strength and flexibility, could perhaps be explained by an associated increase in accurate self-monitoring, resulting in more conservative and safer driving behaviour (Langford & Koppel, 2006; Pachana & Petriwskyj, 2006). In turn, such a model may partly explain why the youngest drivers, generally with excellent visual, physical and cognitive function, have the highest crash rates; they may lack the experience to know the limits of their capabilities and as a result, engage in riskier driving behaviour (Ulleberg & Rundmo, 2003).

Returning to older drivers, this higher level of self-monitoring ability also has important implications for age-related cognitive impairment. Sufferers of Mild Cognitive Impairment (MCI) or dementia for example often experience declines in the ability to self-monitor, generally significantly overestimating their performance (Graham, Kunick, Doody, & Snow, 2005). This in turn is likely to have a detrimental impact on their ability to adjust their driving behaviour to better fit their abilities to the task demands (Brown, 2004).

While models such as these reflect an increasing understanding of the role of higher-level cognition, self-monitoring, and behavioural modifications in safe driving, these factors have not yet appeared in the technological realm. Instead, technologies at the individual level are currently being developed that target capacities, specifically in regard to screening and intervention.

Screening Measures

Efforts to identify potentially unsafe older drivers date back to the middle of last century (see, for example, Johnson, 1946), and research into this area has developed significantly over the past 20 years. Screening is also one of the most controversial areas in older driver safety circles, with significant recent debate about necessity, ethics, methods and consequences (Hakamies-Blomqvist, 2006). Despite these issues, screening instruments abound, some validated, and some not, and most jurisdictions in the developed world insist on some form of mandatory age-based screening (Subzwari et al., 2009). In Australia for example, six out of eight states and territories require mandatory periodic vision and medical screening by a health practitioner for relicensing after a specified age such as between 70 and 80 years (Austroads, 2004). The problem however is that except in cases of severe impairment, there is very little association between these measures and safe driving behaviour. An early prospective study of 10,000 drivers by Johnson and Keltner (1983) found that only those older drivers with severe binocular visual field loss had accident or conviction rates higher than those of controls. Reduced visual acuity, the usual visual screening method, has similarly been found to have a relatively weak association with on-road safety (Hills, 1980; Rubin et al., 2007; Wood & Owens, 2005).

Despite the low correlations between clinical visual measures and road safety, however, both anecdotal, such as self-reported driving difficulties (Kosnik, Sekuler, & Kline, 1990) and circumstantial evidence such as patterns of intersection accidents (Preusser, Williams, Ferguson, Ulmer, & Weinstein, 1998) point to some form of deficit with vision; vision does after all account for about 90% of the external information available to the driver (Hole, 2007). As such, recent research has focussed on developing alternative laboratory based predictors of road safety targeting cognitive rather than sensory aspects of visual perception.

The most significant measure developed by this research effort is the Useful Field of View test (UFOV®; Ball, Beard, Miller, & Roenker, 1987; Ball, Roenker, & Bruni, 1990; Sekuler & Ball, 1986). The UFOV® test has evolved through several different versions since it was first reported in the late 1980s, initially assessing detection of rapidly presented targets across the central 30° of vision (i.e., a circular field with a diameter of 60° of visual angle, centred on the point of fixation). The early version of this instrument required specialised equipment and near viewing distances to assess performance across the requisite visual field, and it was defined as "the visual area in which information can be acquired within one eye fixation" (Ball, Beard, Roenker, Miller, & Griggs, 1988, p. 2210). More recently, the UFOV® test has evolved to assess presentation speed thresholds for dual-targets at fixed positions across a restricted field of view using sophisticated psychophysical estimation software. It is now conceptualised as a measure of visual processing speed for complex targets rather than an assessment of a functional field of view per se (Edwards, Vance et al., 2005), and is administered using standard desktop computer equipment. Importantly, the UFOV® has been shown to be one of the best lab-based predictors of driving safety available (Ball, Owsley, Sloane, Roenker, & Bruni, 1993; Owsley et al., 1998; Owsley, Ball, Sloane, Roenker, & Bruni, 1991; Sims, McGwin, Allman, Ball, & Owsley, 2000). It has also recently undergone a large-scale field test as part of a short screening battery for older drivers (including physical, and other cognitive measures) across Department of Transportation offices in Maryland, USA, and was shown to be predictive of crashes over the following 4-5 years (Ball et al., 2006).

Given the multitude of abilities involved in the driving task, other recent screening measures have adopted a multi-domain approach involving brief measures of several abilities across cognitive, physical and sensory domains (Edwards et al., 2008; Wood, Anstey, Kerr, Lacherez, & Lord, 2008). Most of these demonstrate high sensitivity and specificity in distinguishing safe from unsafe older drivers on a range of outcome measures. In addition, several studies have started using new computational techniques and recent display technology to investigate extensions to the UFOV® paradigm. The object of these studies is to assess performance in the far periphery of vision (a concept similar to early versions of the UFOV®), where evidence from intersection accidents suggests that some older drivers may have particular difficulty. Such methods, strictly in the research phase at this stage, use novel displays – in some cases large custom built LED arrays (Rogè, Pèbayle, Aurèlie, & Muzet, 2005), and in others, large LCD or plasma touchscreens – to present scenes and targets across a wide-visual field. One of these methods builds upon both the UFOV® methodology and an established body of research in the fields of cognitive psychology and perception, using sophisticated real-time model fitting algorithms to estimate both spatial and temporal components of visual processing efficiency across an 80° diameter visual field (Hatherly & Anstey, 2008). Work is currently underway to validate this screening measure against on-road performance of older drivers.

Interventions to Improve Older Drivers' Capacity

One of the major dilemmas with off-road screening tests is what to do in the case of a fail (Hakamies-Blomqvist, 2006). The best approach is follow-up assessment by qualified driving assessors or occupational health and safety professionals; however, assessments are time consuming and resource intensive. On the other hand, restriction or cancellation of driving rights without such assessment procedures is very rare, and in most cases unwarranted (Cole, 2002).

An alternative that has gained significant attention in recent years is intervention, the goal being to improve or maintain the skills and/or behaviours of potentially unsafe older drivers in order to keep them driving safely for longer (Vance et al., 2007). Several types of interventions have been trialled, the most common being education programs. Studies of such programs show promising results in relation to certain aspects of the driving task, for example increased awareness of, and adherence to merging or give way rules, or more frequent checking of mirrors (Owsley, McGwin, Phillips, McNeal, & Stalvey, 2004). However, these improvements have not translated into reduced accident frequency in longitudinal follow-up, possibly due to relatively small sample sizes and the rarity of accidents in general driving. Furthermore, one study reported an *increase* in accident rates following an education intervention for male drivers aged 75 and older (Nasvardi & Vavrik, 2007). Education programs that have combined classroom education and on-road training by a qualified instructor demonstrate stronger effects on driving performance (Marottoli et al., 2007), indicating that such methods might be most useful.

The second class of intervention are those targeting basic cognitive processes thought to be essential for safe driving. Cognitive intervention has become increasingly technologically sophisticated, and has seen the rapid parallel expansion of both research and consumer 'brain training' products aimed at children and older adults (McCurry, 2006). Studies on cognitive training for older adults have also coincided with the growing understanding that cortical plasticity (the ability of the brain to adapt to change) extends right into later life (Colcombe et al., 2004), and such methods aim to capitalise on this ability in order to arrest or reverse age-related sensory and cognitive declines (Edwards, Wadley et al., 2005; Roenker, Cissell, Ball, Wadley, & Edwards, 2003; Vance et al., 2007; Wadley et al., 2006).

While many of the cognitive intervention studies to date have looked at the effect of training on a variety of functional abilities, only a few have looked directly at the impact on driving abilities with older adults. One such study was based on the UFOV® screening test described earlier. Specifically, Ball and Owsley (2000) sampled 77 older drivers who had performed below threshold on the UFOV®, and randomised them into training on either a speed of processing training program, or classroom based sessions. Participants in the speed group were trained to a criterion level of improvement on the UFOV® and performed fewer dangerous manoeuvres in an on-road test than did the classroom group. In contrast, the classroom training group were better at signalling, turning and stopping in an appropriate position. A follow-up evaluation at 18 months found a persistent reduction on dangerous driving manoeuvres for the speed of processing versus the classroom training groups, although by this stage, all improvement on the UFOV® test itself had disappeared (Roenker et al., 2003).

Given the possibility of improvement or maintenance of abilities and functioning across a broad set of domains (Ball, Edwards, & Ross, 2007), cognitive training programs show perhaps the most promise for interventions with older drivers at the individual level. Importantly, these programs are becoming increasingly sophisticated, using high-tech hardware, sophisticated software algorithms, and in some cases, internet-based distribution (Wadley et al., 2006) to deliver individualised programs that provide maximum training efficiency. The software for the UFOV® training procedure used by Ball and colleagues enjoys patent protection (Ball et al., 2002) and has been successfully commercialised, with penetration into a range of markets through industry partners. Further research, evaluating the benefits of improving older drivers' visual processing efficiency using adaptive software algorithms and sophisticated interface hardware to present optimal targets or training stimuli at optimal locations and speeds will likely demonstrate the potential for long-term benefits at the capacity side for older adults in activities such as driving.

TRANSPORT INFRASTRUCTURE

The second component of the safe systems framework is that of transport infrastructure. Transport infrastructure in this context refers broadly to roadway design, traffic management systems and traffic regulation. Research and understanding of the safety impacts of transport infrastructure have increased dramatically over the past two decades. In relation to older drivers, several recent reports and studies have examined the effects of road signage and speed limits (Wang & Carr, 2004), lighting (Wood & Owens, 2005), and intersection design (Lord et al., 2007; Oxley et al., 2006). Most of the findings and recommendations from such reports and studies focus on issues and solutions relating to engineering rather than technological factors, and given the practicalities of infrastructure design and construction, the widespread implementation of safe system principles will take many years. Over the same time period however, and in conjunction with engineering developments, it is likely that we will see the beginnings of widespread incorporation of technology into transport infrastructure in the form of infrastructure based ITS. All advanced ITS technologies currently on the marketplace operate at the level of the vehicle, however work on integrated infrastructure ITS that incorporate an exchange of information between the vehicle and the environment are in the development pipeline, and will be touched upon briefly here. First, however, a short summary of current, non-technological infrastructure initiatives targeting older drivers is presented.

Safe Road Systems for Older Drivers

Many jurisdictions are now adopting a safe systems approach to transport infrastructure and design (Langford & Oxley, 2006). The goal of such systems is generally twofold, attempting to "make the road transport system more forgiving of human error", and to "minimise the level of unsafe road user behaviour" (Australian Transport Council, 2008, p. 2). For younger drivers, a prominent feature of safe systems, addressing the second of these priorities, is the development and appropriate enforcement of traffic regulations (Evans, 1991). As discussed earlier, however, older drivers rarely intentionally break the law, meaning that such approaches are unlikely to result in safer driving for this group. Instead, infrastructure systems that encourage safer driving through engineering solutions, known as self-explanatory road systems (Peden et al., 2004) are likely to be more useful. Self-explanatory road systems include such features as slow points, roundabouts, and clear and obvious signage that make appropriate driving behaviour both obvious to, and easy for the driver.

Other non-technological infrastructure systems that have attracted recent focus include safer roadsides (i.e., minimising poles or trees that might be impacted when a vehicle leaves the carriageway), safer road surfaces (using new materials to produce faster stopping in conjunction with ABS braking systems; Peden et al., 2004), and safer intersection design, with specific reference to roundabouts. Roundabouts, which differ from traffic circles or rotaries in requiring entering traffic to give way, and requiring relatively slow speeds for negotiation, are common in Europe, the UK, Australia and several other developed nations, but are less often seen in America. However, several studies have demonstrated significant safety benefits of roundabouts, particularly for older drivers (Lord et al., 2007; Persaud, Retting, Garder, & Lord, 2000). For example, Persaud and colleagues found that the number of serious accidents decreased by an estimated 90% following installation of a roundabout, and that this reduction was the same for both younger and older drivers.

There is a significant body of research on similar non-technological aspects of road infrastructure design in addition to the studies mentioned above. Interested readers are referred to an excellent review and design recommendations by Staplin, Lococo, Byington and Harkey (2001).

Current Transport Infrastructure Technologies

Current infrastructure-based ITS can be divided into three categories. The first focusses on enforcement with speed and red-light cameras the most prominent examples. The second includes systems that allow short-term variation of signage, speed limits or directional regulation or lane markings to maximise the efficiency of traffic flows at different times of day or in different weather or lighting conditions. The third category involves systems for traffic information display, such as centrally controlled digital road signage.

Of these, only the first category – enforcement measures – has received much research attention in relation to road safety outcomes and few, if any studies have evaluated the impact of such technologies on older drivers. Several however have looked at the safety implications more generally of such systems, and the findings of these have been mixed. For example, enforcement technologies such as speed and red-light cameras, designed primarily to increase adherence to regulation and thus improve road safety, have in some cases been found to have a questionable impact. A recent meta-analysis of 21 studies on traffic accidents at intersections with red-light cameras found that while some accident types such as right-hand turn crashes decreased, others, such as rear-end collisions, significantly increased (Erke, in press). Further, while most of these studies found an overall reduction in the number of accidents with red-light cameras, those that controlled for a statistical artefact known as regression to the mean found an increase. The authors of this review conclude that red-light cameras may not significantly improve traffic safety.

Future Smart Roadway Designs

Looking finally at the future of infrastructure based ITS, there has been significant research and development over the past decade, particularly on the side of communication technology (see for example the suggestions for further reading at the end of this chapter). One of the major research and development programs currently underway in the US is a public-private collaboration funded by US state and federal Departments of Transportation and several major auto companies. This project, called IntelliDrive^{SM}, aims to develop, test, and commercialise integrated vehicle-to-vehicle (V2V) and vehicle-to-infrastructure (V2I) systems that will provide first the driver, and eventually, automated vehicle control systems with enhanced safety and traffic information. The main focus of IntelliDrive^{SM} at present is wireless communications, and it uses a dedicated short range communications (DSRC) band that has been set aside for future ITS applications. A report on a pilot of the system in 2008 showed that the technology could support the data and communication requirements of multiple information systems, both safety focussed, and commercial (Row, Schagrin, & Briggs, 2008). These authors concluded that within the next 5-10 years, such systems are likely to be deployed on large scales, with an initial focus on high-risk locations in busy urban transport environments. These results are promising and indicate that a critical component of future safe transport systems, machine-environment communication, is certainly feasible. The issue of human interaction with such technology however is yet to be addressed, and the question of how such systems will apply to, and be utilised by older drivers remains to be seen.

VEHICLE

The final component of the safe systems approach involves the vehicle, and it is at this level where most work on ITS technologies has taken place. Vehicle based ITS includes a range of current technologies such as cruise control, power steering, a range of convenience technologies (e.g., entertainment and climate control systems), and advanced safety technologies such as systems for collision avoidance, vision enhancement and hazard alerting that are just beginning to appear in top-end vehicles. This section will outline the limited research that has looked at advanced safety technologies in relation older drivers. First however, a brief overview of vehicle design considerations relevant to those marketing to, or making policy for older drivers is presented.

Vehicle Design

A famous adage in the auto industry states: "You can sell a young man's car to an old man, but you cannot sell an old man's car to a young man" (Setright, 2002). This principle, accredited to Semon Knudsen, head of Pontiac in the 1950s and 60s, has had a profound influence on automobile design and marketing that continues today. Despite the fact that a majority of those purchasing new vehicles are aged over 40 (Eby et al., 2009), marketing strategies continue to promote features useful primarily to young drivers (Mueller, 2003). Furthermore, the majority of vehicle and ITS designers are young or mid-life adults for whom the physical or sensory declines associated with age may be difficult to imagine (although it is interesting to note that during the 1990s Ford's ergonomics department developed a 'Third Age Suit' for their designers that decreased strength and flexibility, and impeded the senses; Coughlin, 2005). Evidence of this problem comes from studies that suggest that standard design features such as seatbelts and airbags that are intended to protect, may actually cause significant injury to some frail older adults (Smith & Hall, 2005). This is not to say that drivers would be better off without seatbelts or airbags, but simply that systems designed with older adults in mind may provide better safety outcomes.

Some commentators have also speculated that with the demographic changes that will occur over the coming decades, the market for the less stylish but more functional 'old man's car' will become increasingly prominent, particularly given the fact that the primary purchasers of vehicles in the older age groups are, in fact, women (Eby et al., 2009). Today however, most vehicles are not designed with the older driver in mind, and only a few have features more relevant to the older driver such as easy access doors and seats, and larger knobs and controls on instrumentation (Molnar, Eby, St. Louis, & Neumeyer, 2007).

To compensate for these failings of existing vehicle design, numerous programs have appeared which help older adults adjust their vehicles to increase their mobility and safety. One of the largest of these is the CarFit program (www.carfit.org), which aims to provide expert advice to older drivers on simple ways in which they can adjust their vehicles, for example, by repositioning mirrors, seatbelts, and seat position (distance, tilt and height where available). CarFit involves a free 20-30 minute consultation (generally at a travelling drive-in centre), and although no permanent modifications are made to vehicles, the assessors do discuss options and make recommendations. Importantly, although these adjustments are at the very simplest end of what could be considered vehicle technologies for the elderly, they have been shown to be highly effective. A pilot study across 12 US cities showed that a majority of those who participated in CarFit made at least one beneficial adjustment to their vehicles, and follow-up interviews showed that most had changed their behaviours and were more likely to use safety devices such as seatbelts (Finn, 2006). In addition, older drivers who had participated in the program were also more likely to talk to their friends and relatives about their driving future, a critical issue in the broader field of mobility and aging (e.g.; Windsor & Anstey, 2006).

Vehicle design for older drivers at the technological level will become increasingly important as ITS technologies become more integrated into vehicles in the future. At present however, all of the research on vehicle design and the implications for older drivers has focussed on non-technological aspects such as those discussed above. Interested readers are recommended an excellent review by Shaheen and Neimeier (2001).

Current Vehicle Technologies

Non-mechanical safety technologies have been incorporated into vehicles for some time. Features such as automatic transmission, power steering, cruise control, anti-lock brakes, and electronic traction and stability control have been in higher end cars since the 1980s, and studies have demonstrated that many of these systems are effective in increasing driver safety (see, for example, Ferguson, 2007; Poindexter, 2003). The remainder of this section will focus on advanced technologies that have only recently appeared in top-end vehicles, and which are likely to have a significant impact on older driver safety in the future.

Advanced Technologies

There are a number of advanced ITS technologies that have entered the market since the early 2000s, and many more that are at various points along the development pathway. Current and near future advanced technologies that will be discussed include GPS and route guidance systems; vision enhancement systems; hazard alerting and warning systems; and adaptive cruise control and collision avoidance systems. Importantly, while all of these technologies hold the promise of increased safety, convenience and reliability, few have been evaluated with older drivers, and fewer still designed specifically to meet their particular needs (Caird, 1999; Coughlin, 2005). As such, little is known about the safety implications of advanced ITS for older drivers despite a long history of research documenting the fact that older adults have different skills and abilities, as well as different requirements for, attitudes towards, and ways of interacting with technology. Before reviewing the research that has looked specifically at advanced ITS technologies in relation to older drivers, a brief outline of the relevant human factors and acceptability considerations.

Usability, Reliability and Acceptability of Advanced ITS for Older Drivers

The design and implementation of ITS technologies for older drivers requires a human factors approach which recognises not only that the abilities and requirements of this group are different to those of younger adults, but also that there is enormous heterogeneity in skills, abilities, knowledge, and experience within the population of older drivers themselves (Fisk, Rogers, Charness, Czaja, & Sharit, 2004). This second factor is more complex than the former, however ITS technologies that incorporate computer learning methodologies and can adapt to some extent to meet the needs of individual users do hold promise for satisfying this requirement (Sussman, 2005).

Usability

Any ITS technology designed for use by older drivers must first be usable, and general principles of universal design apply (Story, 1998). Primarily, this means that technologies should be simple and intuitive to use (for all age groups), require low physical effort, and have an inherent tolerance for human error (Fisk et al., 2004). If these conditions are not met, then the technology, for all its potential, is likely to be either underutilised, or distracting to the point of impairing rather than enhancing driver safety (Bayly et al., 2009). It is considered far safer, for example, to navigate with the assistance of an auditory turn-by-turn GPS navigation system than to drive whilst reading a map. However, a device involving a complex interface is likely either to be ignored by the driver, or demand more of their attention than the paper map it is intending to replace. Usability considerations are particularly relevant for older adults, who in general have lower levels of familiarity with technology, and who often have greater difficulty with systems that require fine motor control such as small buttons and menus (Fisk et al., 2004).

Reliability

In order to reduce the cognitive and attentional load on the driver and improve their safety, ITS technologies must be reliable. If the user perceives a systems to be unreliable, it is likely either to be distracting (requiring greater attention to determine if an alert, for example, is valid), or simply ignored. Reliability is also critically important given the possibility of drivers becoming over-reliant on ITS. News outlets occasionally carry reports of drivers who have doggedly followed the voice instructions of their GPS into a river or lake which was not included in the device's map data (Menon, 2008). In addition, simulator studies have found that collision alerting systems result in higher speeds and closer following distances when drivers perceive them to be reliable (Maltz, Sun, Wu, & Mourant, 2007; Yamada & Kuchar, 2006). Reliance on technology in safety systems is not a bad thing of course, as long as the systems are essentially fail-safe. In many ways such systems can make the driving task significantly safer for drivers of all ages. However, there is a need to ensure that systems do not reduce the driver's attention to, and/or ability to react to events that require rapid decision making and manual vehicle control for safety (Stanton & Young, 1998).

Acceptability

Another critical factor in considering ITS applications, and a topic that is covered elsewhere in this book, is that of acceptability. One of the few studies to examine the acceptability of vehicle-based ITS for older drivers was a series of focus groups conducted by Sixsmith in the late 1980s (Sixsmith, 1990). Technologies discussed were systems for route-guidance, collision avoidance, hazard alerting, breakdown detection, and information delivery. Noting that at the time, all of these technologies were at very early stages of development and not available to consumers, participants expressed mixed feelings. In general, these older drivers were enthusiastic about breakdown alerting and information delivery systems, but more wary of collision avoidance or hazard alerting technologies, both of which were felt might unreliably take away control of the vehicle, or prove distracting. In general, women were also more hesitant than men about the benefits or usefulness of vehicle-based ITS, and many participants expressed a belief that such technologies would be more useful to younger drivers.

Guidance Systems

Vehicle based GPS navigation systems are becoming commonplace in modern cars, either as portable after-market accessories, or as integrated systems built into the dashboard. Of all the advanced technologies discussed here, most research relating to older drivers has focussed on this area (May, Ross, & Osman, 2005; Pohlman & Traenkel, 1994). One study that is particularly noteworthy evaluated usage of an early GPS navigation system (TravTek®) by younger, middle-aged, and older drivers, first in an instrumented car with an experimenter present, and secondly using data collected from a fleet of rental cars equipped with the devices (Dingus et al., 1997). These authors found numerous age differences in a range of outcome measures relating to driving performance and interactions with the devices. Specifically, older drivers spent significantly longer looking at the device per glance, and made more inappropriately long glances (more than 2.5 seconds) than did younger drivers. They also had more variability in speed and were less adept at maintaining lane position while looking at the device than the younger group, although their acceleration variance was lower overall, possibly as a result of slower and more cautious driving styles. In relation to route planning using the system, older drivers took longer than younger, however there were no differences in navigational errors. Older drivers also expressed a strong preference for synthesised turn-by-turn voice instructions over other interface options (including electronic map only, turn-by-turn instructions on-screen, and route-map with voice instructions). Most importantly however, Dingus and colleagues (1997) found that over an extended period using the device, drivers of all ages improved on these outcomes. They concluded that GPS route guidance devices could potentially increase safety for all drivers, but that systems imposing increased attentional demands may be particularly detrimental for older drivers.

A more recent study investigated a method of reducing the potential visual monitoring requirement of GPS route guidance devices by modifying the auditory instructions from distance based (e.g., 'turn right in 150m'), to landmark based (e.g., 'turn right after the petrol station'; Maltz et al., 2007, p. 646). Results showed that using landmark instead of distance information reduced the number and duration of glances to the navigation device by around 40%, reduced the number of navigational errors, and increased navigational confidence. Although this study incorporated a young-old design (younger drivers aged 21-40, and older aged 55+), the benefits were consistent across both groups, with no significant age-differences found.

Finally, a recent focus-group study looked at the degree of navigational collaboration between older drivers and their passengers (Vrkljan & Polgar, 2007). This study found that for many participants, driving, particularly in unfamiliar areas, was a shared experience, and that the use of a navigational device could increase the level of this collaborative effort, potentially increasing driving safety in certain situations.

Despite the relative wealth of studies looking at the safety implications of route guidance for older adults, it is important to note that most were conducted in the 1990s. In the same way and in the same timeframe as mobile phones have gone from brick-size analogue devices to high-tech digital computers, the satellite navigation systems of today – Garmin®, TomTom®, and integrated proprietary systems – are very different from those of the 1990s, using different interfaces, software, hardware, and technology. Similarly, most older adults have become more familiar with technology in general over the past decade, and as they might interact differently with such devices now than then, further research on older drivers' interaction with GPS route guidance devices, and the safety implications thereof is required.

Night Vision Enhancement Systems

Night vision enhancement (NVE) systems are intended to increase the visual information available to drivers in low-visibility conditions (Eby et al., 2009; Rumar, 2002). This is particularly relevant to older drivers, for whom low-beam lighting generally does not provide nearly enough illumination for safe travel at normal speeds (Plainis, Murray, & Pallikaris, 2006). The NVE systems currently being developed use near or far infrared sensors in combination with infrared emitting headlights to present low-visibility roadway objects and hazards to the driver in either a head-down (i.e., dash-mounted) or head-up (windscreen projected) display (Rumar, 2002). As of 2009, such systems are just beginning to emerge as standard or additional features in top end luxury vehicles of manufacturers such as Mercedes and BMW.

Several recent studies have evaluated different NVE systems. Mahlke and colleagues (2007) tested 6 different prototype systems with a small sample of 15 drivers aged 40-65. Interestingly, they found that there were no significant differences in hazard recognition rates between the control and instrumented groups (in fact, the control group, without an NVE system detected more pedestrians than any of those using NVE technology). However NVE systems did result in a significant improvement in detection time, with those using conformal near-infrared systems (which produce sharp images directly mapped onto the road environment), and non-conformal LED alerting systems (which indicate the presence but not location of a hazard via an illuminated diode) performing best (Mahlke et al., 2007). A further study, this time with 24 younger and 24 older participants, presented conformal and nonconformal NVE information in a high-fidelity driving simulator (Caird, Horrey, & Edwards, 2001). Potential hazards outlined by the conformal system produced faster reaction times than the nonconformal system, although there were no differences between younger and older participants, and also no control condition. Importantly, several other studies on NVE systems have found relatively low levels of acceptability amongst older drivers, with most saying they would not use the devices often (Caird et al., 2001; Gish & Staplin, 1995). However, as with guidance systems, these studies were conducted on early versions of the technology, and it is therefore uncertain to what extent such findings would apply to the commercially available systems of today.

Hazard Warning Systems

Hazard warning systems are designed to provide a warning (visual, auditory, tactile, or a combination) to the driver to alert them to a potential hazard (Eby et al., 2009). One type of hazard warning system that is beginning to enter the luxury car market is a class of blind-spot information system. These systems use a camera and/or laser or radar distance sensor to detect vehicles in the driver's blind spot, and use a light (sometimes adjacent to the relevant side-mirror), to alert the driver to the potential hazard. No studies to date have examined the safety implications of such systems with older drivers; however it is likely, given the reduced neck and shoulder flexibility of many older drivers, that systems to assist with blind-spot monitoring may be particularly useful.

The other common type of hazard warning systems are Headway Detection and Alerting (HDA) devices, that monitor the following distance to a vehicle ahead, and alert the driver when either the distance, or more usefully, the time headway (i.e., absolute time gap), decrease beyond a specified level (Eby et al., 2009). One study that evaluated such a system in a high-fidelity driving simulator compared the time headway of older and younger drivers with and without an auditory HDA warning system in operation (Maltz et al., 2007). They found that drivers maintained a safer time headway (>2 seconds) with than without the device, and that decreasing the reliability of the warnings with false alarms increased the headway time. There were no differences between age groups in this study; however, they did report high levels of confusion amongst the older group with the auditory stimuli, suggesting that multi-modal ITS applications may not be appropriate for older drivers, at least without significant training.

A further consideration in the design of hazard warning systems is the types of alerts to use. Spence and Ho (2008) address this issue, reviewing research that has examined responses to stimuli in peri-personal (i.e., near self, inside the vehicle) as opposed to extra-personal space. They found that proximal peri-personal stimuli demanded far greater, automatic attention than stimuli more distant from the body. These authors also reported differences based on the type of stimulus, auditory cues resulting in faster reactions when presented from behind than in front of the head for example. Based on their review, Spence and Ho (2008) recommended alerting systems that combine a range of modalities (auditory, tactile, and visual), at a range of locations within the vehicle to make driving hazards more behaviourally relevant to the driver and to elicit automatic, safe responses. This field is still in its infancy and will require much more research to determine optimal parameters for safety.

Finally, more sophisticated alerting systems are being developed that use computer vision methods to recognise and alert the driver to specific classes of potential hazards (e.g., pedestrians or side-entering vehicles; McCarthy, Barnes, Anstey, & Horswill, 2008). Future technology may combine such techniques with eye monitoring systems to provide alerts to drivers only when they have not registered a saccade (rapid eye movement) to a potential hazard within a specific timeframe (when looking at a mirror, or vehicle instrumentation for example). Development and evaluation of such technologies is however some way off.

Adaptive Cruise Control and Collision Avoidance Systems

Like NVE systems, adaptive cruise control and collision avoidance systems are gradually entering the market in top-end luxury cars. The 2008 model Volvo XC70 for example incorporates a technology called 'Collision Warning with Brake Support' (www.volvocars.com) that combines headway monitoring and alerting with adaptive cruise control to provide warning of an imminent collision in the first instance, and then if required, to assume throttle and brake control. These systems do not at present take over full control of the vehicle, although the technology is certainly available to do so. Instead, they significantly reduce impact speed in order to increase safety. In some cases, such systems also pre-tension seatbelts, and prime airbags for faster deployment on impact (Eby et al., 2009).

While there are no published studies directly evaluating collision avoidance systems, there are several which have looked at younger and older drivers' use of automatic cruise control (ACC). ACC systems work in a similar way to collision avoidance systems, monitoring headway and automatically adjusting speed, but are designed to maintain headway with slight accelerations and decelerations, rather than to avoid impact per se (Hoedemaeker & Brookhuis, 1998). One of the primary concerns with ACC systems is that the automation of the driving task may decrease attention and result in slower responses to unpredictable driving hazards. Rudin-Brown and Parker (2004) demonstrated such an effect, requiring a sample of younger drivers, all of whom had experience using conventional cruise control, to follow a lead vehicle around a test-track for 2 hours. They found that with longer headway settings, participants relied more heavily on the ACC system to maintain safe following distance. They performed better on a secondary task (i.e., diverting more attention away from driving), and reacted more slowly to simulated ACC system failure. A similar study using simulators looked at driver workload and locus-of-control for participants aged 18-73 (Stanton & Young, 2005). Data showed a reduced workload under ACC conditions, but contrary to the author's predictions, no reduction in locus-of-control. They reported that in high-traffic conditions the reduced workload appeared beneficial but speculated that for highway driving, the lower attention levels may lead to problems, particularly for older drivers.

Finally, ACC systems are designed to increase driver safety by reducing the distraction associated with monitoring headway, speed, and manipulating throttle and braking controls (Koppel, Charlton, & Fildes, 2009). However as with most advanced ITS technologies, the systems themselves have controls that need periodic manipulation (in the case of ACC, setting headway, maximum speed etc). One recent simulator study varied the placement of these controls – in one condition on the steering wheel, and the other on the dashboard – while measuring the frequency and duration of glances away from the road (Thompson, Tonnis, & Lange, 2006). They found that manipulation of dashboard controls required significantly longer and more frequent glances than did controls on the wheel. Reducing the visual monitoring requirements of control manipulation with efficient interface design and placement may be particularly important for older drivers, who generally require longer to locate, and manipulate vehicle controls (Koppel et al., 2009), resulting in less time looking at the road, and consequently, reduced driving safety.

FUTURE TECHNOLOGIES

The preceding sections have discussed current and future ITS systems at three different levels: the individual, the transport infrastructure, and the vehicle. On the vehicle side, driverless cars – perhaps the ultimate future technology – have actually been in operation for many years. In the mid-1990s, a German research team equipped a Mercedes S-Class with automatic guidance and control systems and drove it from Munich to Copenhagen and back in traffic and at highway speeds with minimal human intervention (at one stage, completing a 157km stretch under full machine control; Behringer & Muller, 1998). More recently, a team from Carnegie Mellon University won the 2008 Defence Advanced Research Projects Agency Urban Challenge, their autonomous Chevy Tahoe completing a 153km course in just over 4 hours, obeying all road rules, and interacting naturalistically with other traffic and staged obstacles and driving hazards (DARPA, 2008). However, system wide automation requires the development of ITS technologies that interact seamlessly between the infrastructure and the vehicle, a prospect of decades rather than years due to the early stage of development of such systems, and the time and resource requirements for implementation of large infrastructure projects on nationwide scales.

As mentioned at the outset, the next 20-30 years will likely see as significant an advance in transportation as the century before. This will undoubtedly produce many dilemmas and problems to be overcome. For example, in the same way that many vehicles on the roads today were manufactured 20 years ago, it is likely that many of the vehicles produced today will be in service on the roads of 2030. The challenge then will be to design system-wide intelligent transportation systems that are backwards compatible with preceding technology, or at least amenable to wide-spread retrofitting programs.

RECOMMENDATIONS FOR CONSUMERS, RESEARCHERS AND POLICY MAKERS

This chapter has discussed issues and reviewed research on older drivers and technology using a systems framework that incorporates the road user, the transport infrastructure, and the vehicle. While the evidence for an 'older driver problem' remains ambiguous, it has been repeatedly demonstrated that older drivers are more likely to be injured or killed in accidents than those aged under 65. Furthermore, demographic changes and shifts in transportation patterns mean that the number of older drivers in developed countries is increasing faster than any other segment of the driving population, and importantly, that these individuals have different capabilities, expectations and attitudes than older drivers in the past in regard to both their driving and mobility, and to their interactions with technology.

This final section will briefly summarise the current state of ITS technology at each of the three levels, with key recommendations for both consumers, and researchers and policy makers.

Road User

ITS at the level of the road user is currently restricted to technologies for screening, and emerging techniques for cognitive intervention.

Consumers

- The most important factor is to be aware of any declining abilities and adjust driving behaviour and exposure to suit (limiting night-time, wet-weather or peak hour driving for example).
- There are a number of vehicle-based technologies that can help to overcome some of these declines in abilities (see below).
- Validated technologies that can be used for self-screening are available. Visit www.visualawareness.com, or http://www.aaaseniors.com for more information. Those with concerns for themselves or others are encouraged to speak to a healthcare provider or visit a specialist driving instructor or assessor.
- Improvement is possible. There are a range of consumer oriented 'brain-training' games and activities, and those that focus on visual speed and hand-eye coordination activities are most likely to be of benefit for improving alertness and reaction times behind the wheel.
- Formal instruction with a driving instructor for a refresher on road rules and safe driving techniques is also likely to be of significant benefit.

Researchers and Policy Makers

- Technology driven screening tests have come a long way in the past two decades, but still require further development and validation before they will be suitable for wide-scale deployment.
- Technological interventions are less developed, but show significant promise. Methods that use adaptive algorithms to adjust difficulty or delivery to target individual weaknesses appear to offer the possibility of the most significant benefit.

Transport Infrastructure

Infrastructure based ITS is less developed than technology at the individual or vehicle level, and as such there are no applications as yet for consumers. As the technology develops, however, it is important that researchers and policy makers engage in efforts to ensure that the technologies are appropriate for older drivers, particularly as this group of road users will, by then, constitute a significant proportion of the road user population.

Vehicle

ITS technologies at the level of the vehicle have the longest history of research and development, and consequently, the largest presence at the consumer level. Many of these technologies promise better safety outcomes for older drivers; however, there are also important factors that need to be considered.

Consumers

- Older drivers are not necessarily less safe than other drivers, but are more likely to be injured or killed if involved in an accident. The newest vehicles are generally the safest, and it is therefore recommended that older drivers use the newest vehicles they can afford.
- At the same time, when purchasing a new vehicle, drivers should look for features such as adjustability and simple controls that are easy to use. Visit www.aaaseniors.com for advice and recommendations.
- Seeking advice on appropriate adjustment of a vehicle in terms of seating, control, and mirror position is highly recommended. Programs such as CarFit (www.car-fit.org) provide helpful advice and ideas.
- Vehicle based ITS systems have the potential to increase safety either directly (in the case of hazard warning or collision avoidance systems), or by reducing the attentional requirements of secondary tasks such as navigation or monitoring of speed. Such systems are recommended to older drivers; however it is very important to undergo appropriate familiarisation or training in order that these systems do not become an additional driving distraction.

Researchers and Policy Makers

- Development of vehicle-based ITS is largely industry driven, but this R&D effort in most cases does not seek to cater specifically to older drivers. There remains a need for research to continually address the needs, acceptability and usability of advanced, vehicle-based ITS technologies for older drivers.
- Further research on the ways in which older drivers interact with vehicle based ITS will help to improve the safety, acceptability and usability of this technology.

CONCLUSION

In summary, technology has the potential to dramatically increase road safety for drivers of all ages, but particularly for older drivers. At the level of the road user, new computerised screening tests and cognitive training programs hold the promise of identifying individuals for whom the capacity to drive safely in complex traffic environments is starting to decline, and more importantly, to assist such individuals to maintain, or in some cases improve these capacities to extend their driving longevity. Intelligent Transportation Systems at the infrastructure level are much less developed, although eventually these will allow for system wide coordination of traffic flows and vehicle-to-vehicle, and vehicle-to-infrastructure exchanges of digital information to enhance the safety and efficiency of traffic and road users. On the vehicle side, ITS technologies have a much longer history of development and commercial implementation, and as such are more sophisticated and advanced than technologies elsewhere within this framework. A significant research literature demonstrates the utility of numerous technologies such as satellite navigation systems, vision enhancement, and collision warning and avoidance systems for older drivers, although it is important that such technologies are developed and tested with universal design and human factors considerations in mind. It is also vital that technology designers, researchers and policy makers keep in mind the principles of usability, reliability and acceptability, as deficits in any of these domains will potentially nullify or reverse the potential safety benefits available from the technologies. Finally, it is important to note that most of the relevant studies on vehicle-based ITS were conducted during the development stage of these technologies, and may therefore not strictly apply to the polished, mass-produced consumer versions that appear in the following years. Further research evaluating the implications of consumer ITS technologies for older drivers is required.

It may be the case that the next two to three decades will see ITS develop to the point where land-based transport is largely or completely automated, and the safety implications addressed throughout this chapter will no longer apply. However given the very complex and multi-factorial nature of the driving task, of transportation networks and infrastructure development, along with the broad variability in vehicle types and road user abilities, interests and aptitudes, it is likely that this future is still a long way off. In any case, between now and then there remain innumerable technological, logistical and very likely psychological and political issues to be overcome. This chapter addresses some of the key issues, priorities and considerations as they apply to older drivers in the hope that they will be relevant to those engaged in solving these problems and improving road safety and mobility for all.

REFERENCES

Anstey, K. J., Wood, J., Lord, S., & Walker, J. G. (2005). Cognitive, sensory and physical factors enabling driving safety in older adults. *Clinical Psychology Review*, *25*(1), 45–65. doi:10.1016/j.cpr.2004.07.008

Arentze, T., Timmermans, H., Jorritsma, P., Olde-Kalter, M.-J., & Schoemakers, A. (2008). More gray hair—but for whom? Scenario-based simulations of elderly activity travel patterns in 2020. *Transportation*, *35*(5), 613–627. doi:10.1007/s11116-008-9170-z

Australian Transport Council. (2008). *National Road Safety Action Plan: 2009 and 2010.*

Austroads. (2004). *Model licence re-assessment procedure for older drivers: Stage 2 research.* Sydney: Austroads Incorporated.

Ball, K. K., Beard, B. L., Miller, R. L., & Roenker, D. L. (1987). Mapping the useful field of view as a function of age. *Gerontologist, 27*(A), 166-167.

Ball, K. K., Beard, B. L., Roenker, D. L., Miller, R. L., & Griggs, D. S. (1988). Age and visual search: Expanding the useful field of view. *Journal of the Ophthalmological Society of America, Series A*, *5*(12), 2210–2219.

Ball, K. K., Berch, D. B., Helmers, K. F., Jobe, J. B., Leveck, M. D., & Marsiske, M. (2002). Effects of cognitive training interventions with older adults: A randomized controlled trial. *Journal of the American Medical Association*, *288*(18), 2271–2281. doi:10.1001/jama.288.18.2271

Ball, K. K., Edwards, J. D., & Ross, L. A. (2007). The impact of speed of processing training on cognitive and everyday functions. *The Journals of Gerontology. Series B, Psychological Sciences and Social Sciences*, *62*(S1), 19–31.

Ball, K. K., & Owsley, C. (2000). Increasing mobility and reducing accidents of older drivers. In Schaie, K. W., & Pietrucha, M. (Eds.), *Mobility and transportation in the elderly*. New York: Springer Publishing Company, Inc.

Ball, K. K., Owsley, C., Sloane, M. E., Roenker, D. L., & Bruni, J. R. (1993). Visual attention problems as a predictor of vehicle crashes in older drivers. *Investigative Ophthalmology & Visual Science*, *34*(11), 3110–3121.

Ball, K. K., Owsley, C., Stalvey, B., Roenker, D. L., Sloane, M. E., & Graves, M. (1998). Driving avoidance and functional impairment in older drivers. *Accident; Analysis and Prevention*, *30*(3), 313–322. doi:10.1016/S0001-4575(97)00102-4

Ball, K. K., Roenker, D. L., & Bruni, J. R. (1990). Developmental changes in attention and visual search throughout adulthood. In Enns, J. T. (Ed.), *The development of attention: Research and theory*. Amsterdam: Elsevier Science Publishers B. V. doi:10.1016/S0166-4115(08)60472-0

Ball, K. K., Roenker, D. L., Wadley, V. G., Edwards, J. D., Roth, D. L., & McGwin, G. (2006). Can high-risk older drivers be identified through performance-based measures in a Department of Motor Vehicles setting? *Journal of the American Geriatrics Society*, *54*(1), 77–84. doi:10.1111/j.1532-5415.2005.00568.x

Bayly, M., Young, K. L., & Regen, M. A. (2009). Sources of distraction inside the vehicle and their effects on driving performance. In Regen, M. A., Lee, J. D., & Young, K. L. (Eds.), *Driver Distraction: Theory, Effects, and Mitigation*. Boca Raton, Florida: CRC Press.

Behringer, R., & Muller, N. (1998). Autonomous road vehicle guidance from autobahnen to narrow curves. *IEEE Transactions on Robotics and Automation*, *14*(5), 810–815. doi:10.1109/70.720356

Berger, M. L. (2001). *The automobile in American history and culture: A reference guide*. Westport, Connecticut: Greenwood Publishing Group.

Birren, J. E., Schaie, K. W., Gatz, M., & Salthouse, T. A. (Eds.). (2006). *Handbook of the Psychology of Aging* (6th ed.). Amsterdam, The Netherlands: Elsevier.

Blows, S., Ivers, R. Q., Woodward, M., Connor, J., Ameratunga, S., & Norton, R. (2003). Vehicle year and the risk of car crash injury. *Injury Prevention*, *9*(4), 353–356. doi:10.1136/ip.9.4.353

Brabyn, J. A., Shchneck, M. E., Lott, L. A., & Haegerstrom-Portnoy, G. (2005). Night driving self-restriction: Visual function and gender differences. *Optometry and Vision Science*, *82*(8), 755–764. doi:10.1097/01.opx.0000174723.64798.2b

Braitman, K. A., Kirley, B. B., Ferguson, S., & Chaudhary, N. K. (2007). Factors leading to older drivers' intersection crashes. *Traffic Injury Prevention*, *8*, 267–274. doi:10.1080/15389580701272346

Brown, L. B. (2004). Driving and dementia: A review of the literature. *Journal of Geriatric Psychiatry and Neurology*, *17*(4), 232–240. doi:10.1177/0891988704269825

Caird, J. (1999). *In-vehicle intelligent transportation systems: Safety and mobility of older drivers.* Paper presented at the Conference on Transportation in an Aging Society: A Decade of Experience, Bethesda, Maryland.

Caird, J., Horrey, W. J., & Edwards, C. J. (2001). Effects of conformal and nonconformal vision enhancement systems on older-driver performance. *Transportation Research Record*, *1759*, 38–45. doi:10.3141/1759-05

Chimpan, M. L., Payne, J., & McDonough, P. (1998). To drive or not to drive: The influence of social factors on the decisions of elderly drivers. *Accident; Analysis and Prevention*, *30*(3), 299–304. doi:10.1016/S0001-4575(97)00107-3

Choo, S., & Mokhtarian, P. L. (2004). What type of vehicle do people drive? The role of attitude and lifestyle in influencing vehicle type choice. *Transportation Research Part A, Policy and Practice*, *38*(3), 201–222. doi:10.1016/j.tra.2003.10.005

Colcombe, S. J., Kramer, A. F., Erickson, K. I., Scalf, P., McAuley, E., & Cohen, N. J. (2004). Cardiovascular fitness, cortical plasticity, and aging. *Proceedings of the National Academy of Sciences of the United States of America*, *101*(9), 3316–3321. doi:10.1073/pnas.0400266101

Cole, B. L. (2002). Who's responsible for safe vision on the roads? [Editorial]. *Clinical & Experimental Optometry*, *85*(4), 207–209. doi:10.1111/j.1444-0938.2002.tb03038.x

Coughlin, J. F. (2005). Not your father's auto industry? Aging, the automobile, and the drive for product innovation. *Generations (San Francisco, Calif.)*, *28*(4), 38–44.

Cutler, S. J., & Coward, R. T. (1992). Availability of personal transportation in households of elders: Age, gender, and residence differences. *The Gerontologist*, *32*(1), 77–81.

DARPA. (2008). DARPA Urban Challenge. Retrieved 10.02.09, from http://www.darpa.mil/grandchallenge/index.asp.

DeSilva, H. (1938). Age and highway accidents. *Scientific Monthly, New York*, *47*, 536–545.

Dingus, T. A., Hulse, M. C., Mollenhauer, M. A., Fleischman, R. N., McGehee, D. V., & Manakkal, N. (1997). Effects of age, system experience, and navigation technique on driving with an Advanced Traveller Information System. *Human Factors*, *39*(2), 177–199. doi:10.1518/001872097778543804

Eby, D. W., Molnar, L. J., & Kartje, P. S. (2009). *Maintaining Safe Mobility in an Aging Society*. Boca Raton, Florida: CRC Press.

Edwards, J. D., Leonard, K. M., Lunsman, M., Dodson, J., Bradley, S., & Myers, C. A. (2008). Acceptability and validity of older driver screening with the Driving Health Reg. Inventory. *Accident; Analysis and Prevention*, *40*(3), 1157–1163. doi:10.1016/j.aap.2007.12.008

Edwards, J. D., Vance, D. E., Wadley, V. G., Cissell, G. M., Roenker, D. L., & Ball, K. K. (2005). Reliability and validity of useful field of view test scores as administered by personal computer. *Journal of Clinical and Experimental Neuropsychology*, *27*, 529–543. doi:10.1080/13803390490515432

Edwards, J. D., Wadley, V. G., Vance, D. E., Wood, K., Roenker, D. L., & Ball, K. K. (2005). The impact of speed of processing training on cognitive and everyday performance. *Aging & Mental Health*, *9*, 262–271. doi:10.1080/13607860412331336788

Erke, A. (in press). Red light for red-light cameras? A meta-analysis of the effects of red-light cameras on crashes. [Corrected Proof]. *Accident; Analysis and Prevention*.

Evans, L. (1991). *Traffic safety and the driver*. New York: Van Nostrand Reinhold.

Federal Highway Administration. (1997). *Highway Statistics 1997: Section VIII Nationwide Personal Transportation Survey*: Office of Highway Information Management.

Ferguson, S. A. (2007). The effectiveness of electronic stability control in reducing real-world crashes: A literature review. *Traffic Injury Prevention*, *8*(4), 329–338. doi:10.1080/15389580701588949

Finn, J. (2006, June). Fitting cars to their older drivers. *Healthword: Putting Health promotion Back in Motion*.

Fisk, A. D., Rogers, W. A., Charness, N., Czaja, S. J., & Sharit, J. (2004). *Designing for Older Adults: Principles and Creative Human Factors Approaches*. Boca Raton, Florida: CRC Press.

Gish, K., & Staplin, L. (1995). *Human factors aspects of using head up displays in automobiles: A review of the literature (No. DOT HS 808320)*. Washington, D. C.: U.S. Department of Transportation.

Graham, D. P., Kunick, M. E., Doody, R., & Snow, A. L. (2005). Self-reported awareness of performance in dementia. *Brain Research. Cognitive Brain Research*, *25*(1), 144–152. doi:10.1016/j.cogbrainres.2005.05.001

Hakamies-Blomqvist, L. (1999). *Safety of older persons in traffic.* Paper presented at the Conference on Transportation in an Aging Society: A Decade of Experience, Bethesda, Maryland.

Hakamies-Blomqvist, L. (2006). Are there safe and unsafe drivers? *Transportation Research Part F: Traffic Psychology and Behaviour*, *9*(5), 347–352. doi:10.1016/j.trf.2006.06.004

Hakamies-Blomqvist, L., & Henriksson, P. (1999). Cohort effects in older drivers' accident type distribution: Are older drivers as old as they used to be? *Transportation Research Part F: Traffic Psychology and Behaviour*, *2*(3), 131–138. doi:10.1016/S1369-8478(99)00009-1

Hakamies-Blomqvist, L., Raitanen, T., & O'Neill, D. (2002). Driver ageing does not cause higher accident rates per km. *Transportation Research Part F: Traffic Psychology and Behaviour*, *5*, 271–274. doi:10.1016/S1369-8478(03)00005-6

Hakamies-Blomqvist, L., & Siren, A. (2003). Deconstructing a gender difference: Driving cessation and personal driving history of older women. *Journal of Safety Research*, *34*(4), 383–388. doi:10.1016/j.jsr.2003.09.008

Hakamies-Blomqvist, L., & Wahlstrom, B. (1998). Why do older drivers give up driving? *Accident; Analysis and Prevention*, *30*(3), 305–312. doi:10.1016/S0001-4575(97)00106-1

Hatherly, C., & Anstey, K. J. (2008). *Extending the Useful Field of View paradigm for screening older drivers*. Paper presented at the ACRS/Qld Travelsafe Committee Joint Conference.

Haworth, N., & Bowland, L. (2000). *Serious injury single vehicle crashes (No. 175)*. Monash University Accident Research Centre.

Hills, B. L. (1980). Vision, visibility and perception in driving. *Perception*, *3*, 434–467.

Hoedemaeker, M., & Brookhuis, K. A. (1998). Behavioural adaptations to driving with an adaptive cruise control (ACC). *Transportation Research Part F: Traffic Psychology and Behaviour*, *1*, 95–106. doi:10.1016/S1369-8478(98)00008-4

Hole, G. (2007). *The psychology of driving*. Mahwah, New Jersey: Lawrence Erlbaum Associates.

Horswill, M. S., Marrington, S. A., McCullough, C. M., Wood, J., Pachana, N. A., & McWilliam, J. (2008). The hazard perception ability of older drivers. *The Journals of Gerontology. Series B, Psychological Sciences and Social Sciences*, *63*(4), 212–218.

Janke, M. K. (1991). Accidents, mileage, and the exaggeration of risk. *Accident; Analysis and Prevention*, *23*(2-3), 183–188. doi:10.1016/0001-4575(91)90048-A

Johnson, C. A., & Keltner, J. L. (1983). Incidence of visual field loss in 20,000 eyes and its relationship to driving performance. *Archives of Ophthalmology*, *101*(3), 371–375.

Johnson, H. (1946). The detection and treatment of accident-prone drivers. *Psychological Bulletin*, *43*(6), 489–532. doi:10.1037/h0061866

Klein, R. (1991). Age-related eye disease, visual impairment, and driving in the elderly. *Human Factors: The Journal of the Human Factors and Ergonomics Society*, *33*, 521–525.

Koppel, S., Charlton, J. L., & Fildes, B. (2009). Distraction and the older driver. In Regen, M. A., Lee, J. D., & Young, K. L. (Eds.), *Driver distraction: Theory, effects, and mitigation*. Boca Raton: Taylor & Francis Group.

Kosnik, W. D., Sekuler, R., & Kline, D. W. (1990). Self-reported visual problems of older drivers. *Human Factors: The Journal of the Human Factors and Ergonomics Society*, *32*, 597–608.

Langford, J., & Koppel, S. (2006). Epidemiology of older driver crashes - Identifying older driver risk factors and exposure patterns. *Transportation Research Part F: Traffic Psychology and Behaviour*, *9*(5), 309–321. doi:10.1016/j.trf.2006.03.005

Langford, J., Koppel, S., McCarthy, D., & Srinivasan, S. (2008). In defence of the 'low-mileage bias'. *Accident; Analysis and Prevention*, *40*, 1996–1999. doi:10.1016/j.aap.2008.08.027

Langford, J., Methorst, R., & Hakamies-Blomqvist, L. (2006). Older drivers do not have a high crash risk--A replication of low mileage bias. *Accident; Analysis and Prevention*, *38*(3), 574–578. doi:10.1016/j.aap.2005.12.002

Langford, J., & Oxley, J. (2006). Using the safe system approach to keep older drivers safely mobile. *IATSS Research*, *30*(2), 97–109.

Leduff, C. (2004, 5 November). Elderly driver to stand trial in deaths of 10. *The New York Times*. Retrieved 19 February, 2009, from http://query.nytimes.com/gst/fullpage.html?res=9B06E7D9143CF936A35752C1A9629C8B63&sec=&spon=&pagewanted=all.

Li, G., Braver, E. R., & Chen, C.-L. (2003). Fragility versus excessive crash involvement as determinants of high death rates per vehicle-mile of travel among older drivers. *Accident; Analysis and Prevention*, *35*, 227–235. doi:10.1016/S0001-4575(01)00107-5

Liu, C., Utter, D., & Chen, C.-L. (2007). *Characteristics of crash injuries among young, middle-aged, and older drivers*. National Highway Traffic Safety Administration.

Lord, D., van Schalkwyk, I., Chrysler, S., & Staplin, L. (2007). A strategy to reduce older driver injuries at intersections using more accommodating roundabout design practices. *Accident; Analysis and Prevention*, *39*(3), 427–432. doi:10.1016/j.aap.2006.09.011

Lutz, R. (2004). Detroit's Mr. Car Guy says driving is dead. *Fortune*, *149*(12), 68.

Lyman, S., Ferguson, S. A., Braver, E. R., & Williams, A. F. (2002). Older driver involvements in police reported and fatal crashes: Trends and projections. *Injury Prevention*, *8*, 116–120. doi:10.1136/ip.8.2.116

Mahlke, S., Roesler, D., Seifert, K., Krems, J. F., & Thuering, M. (2007). Evaluation of six night vision enhancement systems: Qualitative and quantitative support for intelligent image processing. *Human Factors: The Journal of the Human Factors and Ergonomics Society*, *49*, 518–531. doi:10.1518/001872007X200148

Maltz, M., Sun, H., Wu, Q., & Mourant, R. (2007). In-vehicle alerting system for older and younger drivers: Does experience count? *Transportation Research Record*, *1899*, 64–70. doi:10.3141/1899-08

Marottoli, R. A., H., V. P., Araujo, K. L. B., Iannone, L. P., Acampora, D., Charpentier, P., et al. (2007). A randomized trial of an education program to enhance older driver performance. *Journals of Gerontology: Series A: Medical Sciences*, *62*(10), 1113–1119.

Marottoli, R. A., & Richardson, E. D. (1998). Confidence in, and self-rating of, driving ability among older drivers. *Accident; Analysis and Prevention*, *30*(3), 331–336. doi:10.1016/S0001-4575(97)00100-0

May, A., Ross, T., & Osman, Z. (2005). The design of next generation in-vehicle navigation systems for the older driver. *Interacting with Computers*, *17*(6), 643–659. doi:10.1016/j.intcom.2005.09.004

McCarthy, C., Barnes, N., Anstey, K. J., & Horswill, M. S. (2008). *Towards a hazard perception assistance system using visual motion*. Paper presented at the 10th European Conference on Computer Vision.

McCurry, J. (2006). Video games for the elderly: an answer to dementia or a marketing tool? *The Guardian*. Retrieved 8 February, 2009, from http://www.guardian.co.uk/technology/2006/mar/07/nintendods.games.

McFarland, R., Tune, G., & Welford, A. (1964). On the driving of automobiles by older people. *Journal of Gerontology*, *19*, 190–197.

Menon, V. (2008, 28 October). Scary when GPS voice has it wrong. *Toronto Star*.

Meuleners, L. B., Harding, A., Lee, A. H., & Legge, M. (2006). Fragility and crash over-representation among older drivers in Western Australia. *Accident; Analysis and Prevention*, *38*(5), 1006–1010. doi:10.1016/j.aap.2006.04.005

Molnar, L. J., & Eby, D. W. (2008). Getting around: Meeting the boomers' mobility needs. In R. Houston (Ed.), *Boomer or Bust? The New Political Economy of Aging*. Westport, Connecticut: Praeger Publishing.

Molnar, L. J., Eby, D. W., St. Louis, R. M., & Neumeyer, A. L. (2007). *Promising Approaches for Promoting Lifelong Community Mobility*. Washington, D.C.: AARP.

Mueller, J. (2003). Universal products in the U.S. In Clarkson, J., Coleman, R., Keates, S., & Lebbon, C. (Eds.), *Inclusive Design: Design for the Whole Population*. New York: Springer.

Nasvardi, G. E., & Vavrik, J. (2007). Crash risk of older drivers after attending a mature driver education program. *Accident; Analysis and Prevention*, *39*, 1073–1079. doi:10.1016/j.aap.2007.02.005

NHTSA. (2006). *Traffic Safety Facts 2006: Older Population*. National Highway Traffic Safety Administration.

Nutley, S., & Thomas, C. (1995). Spatial mobility and social change: The mobile and the immobile. *Sociologia Ruralis*, *35*(1), 24–39. doi:10.1111/j.1467-9523.1995.tb00824.x

OECD. (2001). *Ageing and transport: Mobility needs and safety issues*. Paris, France: Organisation for Economic Co-operation and Development.

Owsley, C., Ball, K. K., McGwin, G., Sloane, M. E., Roenker, D. L., & White, M. F. (1998). Visual processing impairment and risk of motor vehicle crash among older adults. *Journal of the American Medical Association*, *279*(14), 1083–1088. doi:10.1001/jama.279.14.1083

Owsley, C., Ball, K. K., Sloane, M. E., Roenker, D. L., & Bruni, J. R. (1991). Visual/cognitive correlates of vehicle accidents in older drivers. *Psychology and Aging*, *6*(3), 403–415. doi:10.1037/0882-7974.6.3.403

Owsley, C., McGwin, G., Phillips, J. M., McNeal, S., & Stalvey, B. T. (2004). Impact of an educational program on the safety of high-risk, visually impaired, older drivers. *American Journal of Preventive Medicine*, *26*, 222–229. doi:10.1016/j.amepre.2003.12.005

Oxley, J., Fildes, B., Corben, B., & Langford, J. (2006). Intersection design for older drivers. *Transportation Research Part F: Traffic Psychology and Behaviour*, *9*(5), 335–346. doi:10.1016/j.trf.2006.06.005

Pachana, N. A., & Petriwskyj, A. M. (2006). Assessment of insight and self-awareness in older drivers. *Clinical Gerontologist*, *30*(1), 23–38. doi:10.1300/J018v30n01_03

Peden, M., Scurfield, R., Sleet, D., Mohan, D., Hyder, A. A., & Jarawan, E. (Eds.). (2004). *World Report on Road Traffic Injury Prevention*. Geneva, Switzerland: World Health Organization.

Persaud, B. N., Retting, R. A., Garder, P. E., & Lord, D. (2000). *Crash reductions following installation of roundabouts in the United States*. Arlington, VA: Insurance Institute for Highway Safety.

Plainis, S., Murray, I. J., & Pallikaris, I. G. (2006). Road traffic casualties: Understanding the night-time death toll. *Injury Prevention*, *12*(2), 125–138. doi:10.1136/ip.2005.011056

Pohlman, S., & Traenkel, U. (1994). Orientation in road traffic: Age-related differences using an in-vehicle navigation system and a conventional map. *Accident; Analysis and Prevention*, *26*(6), 689–702. doi:10.1016/0001-4575(94)90048-5

Poindexter, K. N. (2003). *Passenger vehicle crash involvement rates by vehicle model year*. Washington, DC: U.S. Department of Transportation.

Preusser, D. F., Williams, A. F., Ferguson, S. A., Ulmer, R. G., & Weinstein, H. B. (1998). Fatal crash risk for older drivers at intersections. *Accident; Analysis and Prevention*, *30*(2), 151–159. doi:10.1016/S0001-4575(97)00090-0

Roenker, D. L., Cissell, G. M., Ball, K. K., Wadley, V. G., & Edwards, J. D. (2003). Speed-of-processing and driving simulator training result in improved driving performance. *Human Factors*, *45*(2), 218–233. doi:10.1518/hfes.45.2.218.27241

Rogè, J., Pèbayle, T., Aurèlie, C., & Muzet, A. (2005). Useful visual field reduction as a function of age and risk of accident in simulated car driving. *Investigative Ophthalmology & Visual Science*, *46*(5), 1774–1779. doi:10.1167/iovs.04-0540

Rosel, N. (2003). Aging in place: Knowing where you are. *International Journal of Aging & Human Development*, *57*(1), 77–90. doi:10.2190/AMUD-8XVX-9FPK-MR8G

Row, S., Schagrin, M., & Briggs, V. (2008). [*ITS International, August.*]. *Future*, VII.

Rubin, G. S., Ng, E. S. W., Bandeen-Roche, K., Keyl, P. M., Freeman, E. E., & West, S. K. (2007). A prospective, population-based study of the role of visual impairment in motor vehicle crashes among older drivers: The SEE study. *Investigative Ophthalmology & Visual Science*, *48*(4), 1483–1491. doi:10.1167/iovs.06-0474

Rudin-Brown, C. M., & Parker, H. A. (2004). Behavioural adaptation to adaptive cruise control (ACC): implications for preventive strategies. *Transportation Research Part F: Traffic Psychology and Behaviour*, *7*(2), 59–76. doi:10.1016/j.trf.2004.02.001

Rumar, K. (2002). *Night vision enhancement systems: What should they do and what more do we need to know? University of Michigan*. Ann Arbor: Transportation Research Institute.

Ryan, G., Legge, M., & Rosman, D. (1998). Age related changes in drivers' crash risk and crash type. *Accident; Analysis and Prevention*, *30*(3), 379–387. doi:10.1016/S0001-4575(97)00098-5

Sekuler, R., & Ball, K. K. (1986). Visual localization: Age and practice. *Journal of the Ophthalmological Society of America, Series A*, *3*(6), 864–867.

Setright, L. K. J. (2002). *Drive on!: A social history of the motor car*. London: Palawan Press.

Shaheen, S. A., & Neimeier, D. A. (2001). Integrating vehicle design and human factors: Minimizing elderly driving constraints. *Transportation Research Part C, Emerging Technologies*, *9*, 155–174. doi:10.1016/S0968-090X(99)00027-3

Sims, R. V., McGwin, G. Jr, Allman, R. M., Ball, K., & Owsley, C. (2000). Exploratory study of incident vehicle crashes among older drivers. *The Journals of Gerontology. Series A, Biological Sciences and Medical Sciences*, *55A*(1), 22–27.

Sixsmith, J. (1990). *Driving experiences and new technology: Evaluations and expectations of older drivers*. London: Occasional Paper 31. Department of Geography, King's College.

Smiley, A. (1999). *Adaptive strategies of older drivers*. Paper presented at the Conference on Transportation in an Aging Society: A Decade of Experience, Bethesda, Maryland.

Smith, J. E., & Hall, M. J. (2005). Injuries caused by seatbelts. *Trauma*, *7*(4), 211–215. doi:10.1191/1460408605ta348oa

Spence, C., & Ho, C. (2008). Multisensory warning signals for event perception and safe driving. *Theoretical Issues in Ergonomics Science*, *9*(6), 523–554. doi:10.1080/14639220701816765

Stanton, N. A., & Young, M. S. (1998). Vehicle automation and driving performance. *Ergonomics*, *41*(7), 1014–1028. doi:10.1080/001401398186568

Stanton, N. A., & Young, M. S. (2005). Driver behaviour with adaptive cruise control. *Ergonomics*, *48*, 1294–1313. doi:10.1080/00140130500252990

Staplin, L., Lococo, K., Byington, S., & Harkey, D. (2001). *Highway Design Handbook for Older Drivers and Pedestrians*. McLean, VA: U.S Department of Transportation, Federal Highway Administration.

Story, M. F. (1998). Maximizing usability: the principles of universal design. *Assistive Technology*, *10*(1), 4–12.

Subzwari, S., Desapriya, E., Babul-Wellar, S., Pike, I., Turcotte, K., & Rajabali, F. (2009). *Vision screening of older drivers for preventing road traffic injuries and fatalities*. Chichester, UK: John Wiley & Sons, Ltd.

Sussman, J. M. (2005). *Perspectives on Intelligent Transportation Systems (ITS)*. New York: Springer.

Thompson, L. K., Tonnis, M., & Lange, C. (2006). *Using glance behaviour to evaluate ACC driver controls in a driving simulator*. Paper presented at the Human Factors and Ergonomics Society 50th Annual Meeting.

Ulfarsson, G., Kim, S., & Lentz, E. (2006). Factors affecting common vehicle-to-vehicle collision types: Road safety priorities in an aging society. *Transportation Research Record: Journal of the Transportation Research Board*, *1980*(1), 70–78. doi:10.3141/1980-12

Ulleberg, P., & Rundmo, T. (2003). Personality, attitudes and risk perception as predictors of risky driving behaviour among young drivers. *Safety Science*, *41*(5), 427–443. doi:10.1016/S0925-7535(01)00077-7

Utz, R. L., Carr, D. B., Nesse, R., & Wortman, C. B. (2002). The effect of widowhood on older adults' social participation: An evaluation of activity, disengagement, and continuity theories. *The Gerontologist*, *42*(4), 522–533.

Van Mierlo, J., Maggetto, G., & Lataire, P. (2006). Which energy source for road transport in the future? A comparison of battery, hybrid and fuel cell vehicles. *Energy Conversion and Management*, *47*(17), 2748–2760. doi:10.1016/j.enconman.2006.02.004

Vance, D., Dawson, J., Wadley, V., Edwards, J., Roenker, D., & Rizzo, M. (2007). The accelerate study: The longitudinal effect of speed of processing training on cognitive performance of older adults. *Rehabilitation Psychology*, *52*(1), 89–96. doi:10.1037/0090-5550.52.1.89

Vrkljan, B. H., & Polgar, J. M. (2007). Driving, navigation, and vehicular technology: experiences of older drivers and their co-pilots. *Traffic Injury Prevention*, *8*(4), 403–410. doi:10.1080/15389580701576423

Wadley, V. G., Benz, R. L., Ball, K. K., Roenker, D. L., Edwards, J. D., & Vance, D. E. (2006). Development and evaluation of home-based speed-of-processing training for older adults. *Archives of Physical Medicine and Rehabilitation*, *87*(6), 757–763. doi:10.1016/j.apmr.2006.02.027

Wang, C. C., & Carr, D. B. (2004). Older driver safety: A report from the older drivers project. *Journal of the American Geriatrics Society*, *52*(1), 143–149. doi:10.1111/j.1532-5415.2004.52025.x

Windsor, T. D., & Anstey, K. J. (2006). Interventions to reduce the adverse psychosocial impact of driving cessation in older adults. *Clinical Interventions in Aging*, *1*(3), 205–211. doi:10.2147/ciia.2006.1.3.205

Witkowski, J. M., & Buick, T. R. (1985). Travel behavior of residents of retirement communities. *Transportation Research Record*, *1018*, 13–22.

Wood, J. M., Anstey, K. J., Kerr, G. K., Lacherez, P. F., & Lord, S. (2008). A multidomain approach for predicting older driver safety under in-traffic road conditions. *Journal of the American Geriatrics Society*, *56*(6), 986–993. doi:10.1111/j.1532-5415.2008.01709.x

Wood, J. M., & Owens, A. D. (2005). Standard measures of visual acuity do not predict drivers' recognition performance under day or night conditions. *Optometry and Vision Science*, *82*(8), 698–705. doi:10.1097/01.opx.0000175562.27101.51

Yagil, D. (1998). Instrumental and normative motives for compliance with traffic laws among young and older drivers. *Accident; Analysis and Prevention*, *40*(4), 417–424.

Yamada, K., & Kuchar, J. K. (2006). Preliminary study of behavioural and safety effects of driver dependence on a warning system in a driving simulator. *IEEE Transactions on Systems, Man, and Cybernetics. Part A, Systems and Humans*, *36*(3), 602–610. doi:10.1109/TSMCA.2006.871646

ADDITIONAL READING

Books and Journals

Eby, D. W., Molnar, L. J., & Kartje, P. S. (2009). *Maintaining Safe Mobility in an Aging Society*. Boca Raton, Florida: CRC Press.

IEEE Transactions on Intelligent Transportation Systems.

Regan, M. A., Lee, J. D., & Young, K. L. (Eds.). (2009). *Driver Distraction: Theory, Effects and Mitigation*. Boca Raton, Florida: CRC Press.

Schaie, K. W., & Pietrucha, M. (Eds.). (2000). *Mobility and Transport in the Elderly*. New York: Springer.

Sussman, J. M. (2005). *Perspectives on Intelligent Transportation Systems*. New York: Springer.

US Department of Transportation ITS Initiative: http://www.rita.dot.gov/; http://www.its.dot.gov/library.htm

Websites

www.aaaseniors.com

www.car-fit.org

www.visualawareness.com

http://www.itsinternational.com/

IntelliDrive[SM]: http://www.intellidriveusa.org/

Intelligent Transportation Society of America. http://www.itsa.org/

Chapter 12
Low Usage of Intelligent Technologies by the Aged:
New Initiatives to Bridge the Digital Divide

John Heng
Nanyang Technological University, Singapore

Subhasis Banerji
Nanyang Technological University, Singapore

ABSTRACT

Contrary to expectations, assistive technology (AT) usage by the elderly has not increased in proportion to availability and ease of access. This is despite a belief that technology can contribute significantly towards improving their quality-of-life. Our Rehabilitation Mechatronics research group at NTU Singapore is developing a "unified neuro-physio platform", taking a cue from Eastern philosophies which emphasize that the "internal environment" of the users strongly affects how they interact with the "external environment." This chapter highlights the need to bridge these two environments meaningfully through "sensitive" technologies which address the mindsets and learning mechanisms of users. The technology platform we propose helps the elderly to understand and enhance their internal environment in order to interact at various levels with AT in their external environment. It provides a fresh approach to understanding and minimizing the persistent "digital divide" between the elderly and high technology.

INTRODUCTION

The Internal Environment and its Relation to Health

Human beings exist simultaneously in two environments, internal and external. The internal environment relates to perceptions, self image, emotions and motivation levels. The external environment is the physical body and the world around it. These two environments constantly interact with and affect each other. The development of assistive technology (AT) has focused primarily on helping the elderly to cope with physical tasks, activities of daily living, accessing entertainment and using communication tools to exchange information. Hence the approach has so far been to enable interaction with what we refer to as the "external environment". In spite of impressive advances in technology, the usage

DOI: 10.4018/978-1-61520-825-8.ch012

of such devices among the elderly has not shown the rise that may have been expected. Studies show that in general, those using simple devices feel more self-sufficient and are less likely to use formal care, whereas those using complex devices are more likely to feel the need for formal care (Agree & Freedman, 2000). Does this mean that elderly populations are more comfortable and confident using a technology which is simple and usable, even though the device may have a low level of intelligence? If so, one wonders how high technology can meaningfully contribute to raising their quality of life.

One of the potential ways for increasing AT uptake would be to successfully tap the "internal environment" of the user, and link it to the user's external environment. The brain interacts within itself far more than it interacts with the external world (Harris, 1998; Taylor, 2009). The neuronal connections are constantly being reinforced or reworked, even when we sleep. This enables the development and maintenance of memory, motor function, audio sensitivity, cognition, mobility, and so on. Research in medicine, neuroscience and physiology has shown that it is possible, at least partially, to recover or maintain these faculties in the elderly, which may have deteriorated due to disuse or damage. (Clark & Stump, 1998; Hofgren, Bjorkdahl, Esbjornsson & Stibrant-Sunnerhagen, 2007; Williams, Ramaswamy & Oulhaji, 2006). The internal environment also includes the perceptions, self-image and motivation levels of the person. We know from the self-determination theory that humans who are naturally motivated tend to incorporate an internal regulation strategy for all important activities (Deci, Eghrari, Patrick & Leone, 1994). Several studies have also shown that attention, motivation and repetitive task practice are essential factors in the reorganization of the brain (Bach-y-Rita, 2001; Berthoz, 1996; Robertson & Murre, 1999) and this reorganization can take place well into old age.

The major factors affecting this recovery or maintenance depend on the high level of engagement of the individual with the task at hand. Studies in psychology and accelerated learning demonstrate that such high levels of engagement occur when there is an "emotional connect" for the individual to the task and when all sensory pathways - visual, auditory and kinesthetic - are brought into play. This can happen in an active, collaborative environment (Loureiro, Johnson & Harwin, 2006). A notable example of the effectiveness of engaging the internal environment can be seen with the success of pet therapy for elders in Japan using artificial pets such as "Paro the seal" (Inoue, Wada & Ito, 2008). This highlights the importance of managing both the external and the internal environments. Perhaps it makes sense to develop technologies that help maintain abilities in the internal environment as an important complement to devices which help the elderly in everyday physical tasks.

BACKGROUND

The Traditional Approach to AT

The "raison d'être" of AT is the improvement of quality of life (QoL). Technologists have believed so far that a better QoL means an easier way of executing activities of daily living (ADLs) and certain other tasks related to personal physical comfort, transport, communication and health monitoring.

Traditionally, AT started as devices to help accomplish simple tasks. Hence early devices such as walking aids and spectacles were strictly functional. A simple device such as a remote was created to establish control over a reasonably smart device such as a television set. Although the remote controls a wide array of features, most of them are not regularly accessed by the elderly. They still use the remote for the basic functions: to switch on/off, surf channels, and adjust volume. The same cannot be said, though, for mobile phones. Some features such as text messaging and

Figure 1. Traditional approach to AT design (adapted from Freedman, Agree & Cornman, 2005)

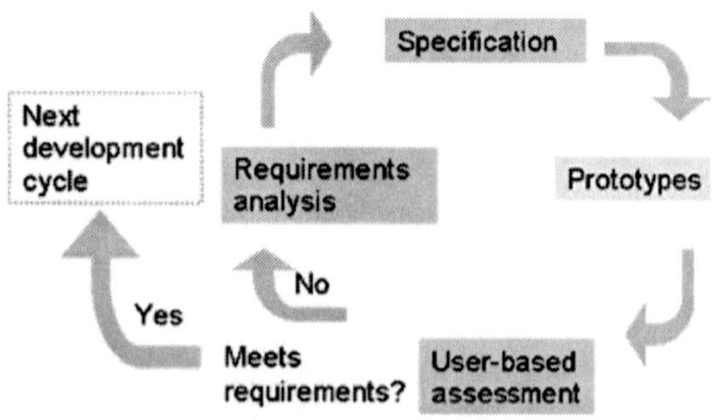

sharing photographs have succeeded in making mobile phones a more widely used tool than was achieved by mere basic telephone features. This brought into focus the importance of "valued activities" over and above the "basic activities".

Figure 1 illustrates the traditional approach to AT design over the past few decades (Freedman, Agree & Cornman, 2005).

The starting point in drawing up the specifications in this model is an assessment of the person's functional capabilities at the physical, sensory and cognitive levels. Next, the activities that the device is meant to help with are identified. The types of accommodations are then established for the effective execution of these activities. Technological intervention is generally deployed for the following:

1. Augmenting the person's capabilities by enabling better mobility, stability, positioning ability, force generation, control and so on (Refer box "Person's Capabilities" in Figure 1).
2. Providing external accommodations by engineering the environment or device such that the task in question is easier to execute (Refer box "External Accommodations" in Figure 1).

The early approach to focus largely on basic tasks has persisted, resulting in an emphasis on activities of daily living, communication, mobility and accessing entertainment. To illustrate this, Figure 1 shows the "Basic Activities" block is much bigger than the "Valued Activities" block.

Access, Affordability, Awareness and Usage

Socio-economic developmental disparities within and between countries is a major impediment to easier access and higher usage of AT. This has contributed significantly to what we call the digital divide (Milner, 2006). While several countries and organizations are working towards closing this gap ("Ushering in the second digital revolution" n.d.), affordability of several key AT products is an important issue.

The disabled population is particularly disadvantaged in this respect. As one example, over 70% of blind and low vision citizens in the United States are reported unemployed (Findings about the awareness and use of accessible technology, n.d.). A screen reader that enables blind people to use their computers costs more than $1000, which effectively places this valuable example of AT out of reach of the majority of vision impaired Americans. People with other severe disabilities have similar adverse employment statistics and are likewise unable to afford appropriate AT (Findings about the awareness and use of accessible technology, n.d.). The affordability problem is amplified in developing countries.

For the issues of awareness and usage, let us next consider the scenario in the computer industry which has been one of the pioneers in the propagation of accessibility features and assistive technologies for its users. Although most accessible technology was originally intended and designed for individuals with severe difficulties/ impairments, it is widely used by computer users of all abilities today. The technology includes accessibility options built into products (such as the option that changes font size and colors,) and assistive technology products (specialty hardware and software products such as a screen reader or voice recognition products).

Microsoft (2004) found that the majority of computer users (54%) were aware of some form of accessible technology but few were using it ("Findings about the awareness and use of accessible technology" n.d.). AT product usage was higher among products that were more widely used by the general population and lower among specialty products that were designed for specific difficulties/impairments. The Microsoft study also showed another interesting result. Individuals with and without difficulties/impairments were turning to accessibility options/utilities to improve their "overall computing experience". Participants who used assistive technology were asked to report if their use of such technology was due to an ongoing health issue, a health issue they had recovered from, avoiding a health issue, or assisting someone in their household with an ongoing health issue. The majority, 65%, of users did not report any of these health issues as reasons for using assistive technology products. However, the study showed that the second most likely reason users report using assistive technology products was to avoid a health issue. The overall usage percentage of such products among computer users ranged from 1-9%, with only 24% of users with severe difficulties or impairments using such products.

This low usage of AT may be related to the fact that users do not find that current AT features enhance their overall computing experience (79-83% of the population in the Microsoft study). This may indicate that such subjective perceptions as "computing experience" play a larger role in usage than acknowledged earlier when compared to cost, accessibility and the amelioration of disabilities.

A CLOSER LOOK AT PERCEPTIONS

Perceptions of Dependency and Independent Living

When the decrements associated with ageing begin to set in, the elderly find it harder to remain functional. Motor and cognitive impairments become the new reality. The ageing person may perceive himself/herself as a dependant and an increasing burden on family and society. This gives rise to new independence and relation needs (Goldberg, 1984; Maclean & Pound, 2000). If hit by a sudden disability, individuals above 65 years of age may also lose interest in independent living and believe they will never improve (Lewis, 1984). On the other hand, in traditional joint family societies, elders do not mind being physically and materially dependent if they are seen as contributing members of the family (Gupta, 2000). They may help the family in an advisory capacity and look after the values education of the grandchildren. These and other contributions are tangible and economically valuable, particularly in those families with "double-income" parents.

The question that arises now is should we design AT devices to focus on merely independent living or to focus more on "dignified and useful living"? In the emerging scenario, the lower functionalities such as ADLs may be best left to low intelligence devices which are safe, cheap and easily adopted. The smart devices may make sense to the elderly only if they can enable higher living goals that justify the purchase cost and the time taken to understand the technology. In short, the devices offer a richer life experience. These higher goals would logically seem to include greater social participation and a more useful role to play in society. Activities related to these higher goals would typically fall into the category of "Valued Activities" in Figure 1.

Emerging Perceptions about Health in Old Age

The emerging research on brain plasticity is changing the way in which we perceive the ageing process. For example, recent studies have proven that mental imagery activities result in improvement of motor and cognition recovery after stroke (Pfurtschellar & Neuper, 2001). For centuries, both yoga and martial arts have used mental imagery and visualization to enhance levels of co-ordination, balance, speed and power. This combination of physical activity, heightened awareness and visio-audio-kinesthetic (VAK) sensory feedback seems to generate an enhanced sense of psychological and emotional well-being, resulting in a richer life experience well into old age.

These traditional practices of healthy living emphasize two modes of practice - individual and collaborative. In solitary individual practice, one gets in touch with one's internal environment more intimately. In collaborative practice, one establishes one's position with respect to the external environment and one's peers. Long time practitioners seem to become adept at quickly adapting to changes in both environments, even with advancing age. Several studies have shown that even those who start after the onset of disabilities due to osteoarthritis or stroke benefit from yoga and martial arts practice, gaining a new awareness and control over their daily activities (Bastille & Gill-Body, 2004; Song, Lee, Lam & Bae, 2003). A shining example from Singapore is Ms. Teresa Hsu who was born in China in 1898 and set up Heart To Heart, Singapore ("Sister Teresa-Never too old to care for others", n.d.). Already past 112 years, she cheerfully and tirelessly works for the care of the old and disabled, practicing yoga every day.

In Chinese literature, "Xin" can be translated as mind and "Yi" as a sense of intention. When used together, the two words represent "the desire to do something specific". "Qi" is the intrinsic energy which arises out of this desire, triggering the physiological functions that prepare the physical body for action and movement. Eastern philosophies emphasize the interdependence of "Xin-Yi-Qi" (Yang, 1996) or "Thought-purpose-energy-action" and its cyclic nature. This is illustrated in Figure 2.

Figure 2. Movement in the user's inner world manifesting as action and effect in the outer world. This in turn affects the thought process, hence feedback and acknowledgement of small successes are important

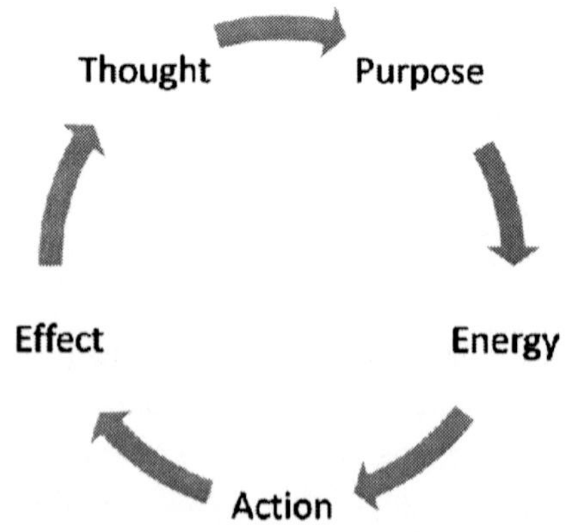

Both Yoga and Chinese medicine treat the mind and the body as a whole unit. They emphasize the benefits of an increase in inner awareness, sensitivity, self confidence and modification in perceptions of self and society. These factors have been shown to directly inhibit not only progressive degeneration due to ageing but also sudden acute events such as stroke (Bastille & Gill-Body, 2004; Kolasinski, Garfinkel, Tsai, Matz, Van Dyke & Schumacher, 2005; Song, Lee, Lam & Bae, 2003). Today, we see increasing scientific evidence that thought, energy and action are intimately connected. Motivation or purpose plays a significant part in the performance and re-learning of both basic and valued activities (Vallerand, & O'Connor, 1989). Certain developments in modalities such as biofeedback and collaborative therapy have shown very promising results (Hayashi, 2002; Martinez, Bakardjian & Cichocki, 2007; Wallace, Wagner, Wagner & McDeavitt,

Figure 3. The user's capabilities form the interface between the inner and outer worlds and reflect the quality of the integration of these two aspects. These allow for "inner accommodations"

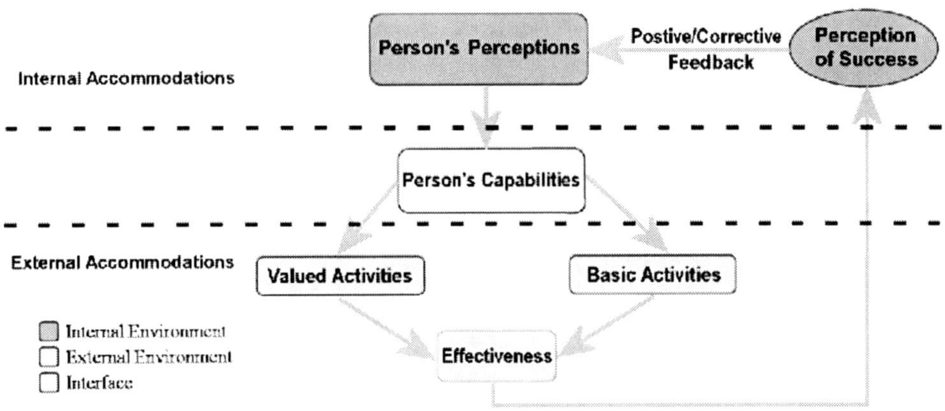

2001). However, these aspects have somehow been largely neglected in the design of AT products in the past few decades because mechanical task performance has received the maximum attention. The new scientific evidence supporting these age-old theories demands that we take a fresh look at how we have approached the design of AT so far.

A Wider Perception of AT

What are the factors that could influence the perception that high technology AT is usable, value-for-money and empowering?

Humans do not use their bodies, minds and sensory faculties in isolation. The activity of going about life in a fulfilling manner involves the integration of these abilities. People with motor impairments use their unique motor abilities to operate assistive technology devices to facilitate their work, recreation and daily living tasks. AT devices are at their most effective when users deploy their own unique motor abilities instead of trying to move in a manner that is considered "normal" (Bain & Leger, 1996). People who are aware of their residual strengths adapt fastest and lead productive lives. Being essentially multi-tasking in nature, they are best served by a system which allows them some facility to do so.

Hence, there is a need to highlight new initiatives being taken in various studies and experiments to develop technology platforms and interfaces that train the integration of human faculties in a measurable and assistive manner. They may facilitate the engagement of the users with their inner and outer worlds as well as the interaction with the AT device at multiple levels. This will make it possible for the elderly to re-connect with their residual capabilities at the physical, sensory, cognitive and adaptive levels. As the elderly user improves or deteriorates over a period of time, such devices can "sense" and respond with appropriate levels of assistance.

Figure 3 illustrates the aspects of the internal environment which are shaping the use of assistive technology today.

In the new scheme, the person's perceptions and understanding play a large role in the design of the AT system. In Figure 3, the perception (i.e. the box labeled "Person's Perceptions) may typically include,

- Self image (Phillips, 1957),
- Benefits of doing a given task,

- Perceived degree of difficulty,
- Perception of progress/recovery/success in task/activity,
- Role in society (Brubaker & Powers, 1976)
- Cost and utility of AT devices

These issues would directly impact the person's capabilities (in the box labeled "Person's Capabilities" in Figure 3), which now would have to include certain new parameters, such as

- Physical, cognitive, sensory abilities
- Level of training on the technology platform
- Levels of motivation, confidence/anxiety based on perceptions listed above

The earlier definition of "Effectiveness" was centered on the successful completion of a given task. The new approach acknowledges that the capabilities undergo changes at levels other than, but closely related to, physical, cognitive and sensory faculties. The "internal accommodations" level in Figure 3 indicates the user's changing inner belief about his/her capabilities and the life decisions that lead to a change in mindset. In the new approach, therefore, "Effectiveness" is extended to include the ability to generate and receive appropriate feedback through existing sensory channels and an ability to interpret this feedback for the user's benefit.

We have seen in the previous sections that it is not necessary that people's choice of technologies is dictated by their levels and type of disability. What they are looking for is a "richer experience". The example given earlier was the rise in use of mobile phones for messaging and sharing by the elderly, who traditionally are regarded as technology averse. This suggests the need for a closer look at what we, as designers, perceive as "Valued Activities". Rather than just work and leisure then, Valued Activities also need to incorporate:

- Social engagement
- Self-expression, self growth
- Social contribution.

This new way of looking at "Effectiveness" and "Valued Activities" is more sensitive to users and represents the new, more sensitive and inclusive approach to AT.

DESIGN APPROACH TO "SENSITIVE" AT

In its simplest form, an assistive device such as a walking stick provides support along with some form of tactile feedback about load distribution and imbalance. Anybody who uses crutches for the first time knows that it takes several days to learn how to use them to walk, sit, get up and climb stairs. The care giver may give verbal instruction and physical assistance during the learning process, but the most over-riding form of feedback is visual and kinesthetic. In this manner, a low intelligence technology such as a crutch becomes a 'sensitive" device, allowing the user to utilize his or her residual intelligence and capability.

Newell (1995) has suggested that researchers should focus on the relationship between the functionality of users and the environment in which they may operate. This concept has been fully exploited by the "Jaipur foot", a prosthetic device tailored to the user and the environment in India. It is probably the world's cheapest (basic versions cost less than USD 50) and highest selling prosthetic leg, allowing thousands of users to lead their rural lifestyle - walking barefoot, squatting on the floor, and even climbing trees. ("What is our special technology?" n.d.). In devices of higher intelligence, if portability and functionality is required, the user interface is limited in its bandwidth of channels as in the case of mobile phones with alpha-numeric input requirements. This limited bandwidth then becomes the limiting factor in the human-machine system (Angelo,

2000). That is why the Human Activity Assistive Technology Model (HAAT) encompasses four parts (Nielsen, 1993):

- The human-technology interface
- The processor
- The activity output
- The environmental interface

This model acknowledges that the activity enabled by AT takes place not only in the physical context but also in the social and cultural context. "User centered design" developers formerly focused on the interface of the user and his external environment (Helander, Landauer & Prabhu, 1997; Nielsen, 1993). "User sensitive design" is now exploring how best to present information to the disabled user in various modalities, such as visio-audio-kinesthetic (VAK) cues and biofeedback.

With regard to usability, the principles of Universal Design (Story, 1998) indicate that assistive technology should be usable by all categories of people - impaired and otherwise. Apart from encouraging social inclusion, this is useful in the hitherto unheralded context of familiarizing people early with technology that may be useful for future rehabilitation needs. If a person has already used a technology when he/she was unimpaired earlier in life, the chances are that they will be less resistant to using such technology if impairment due to ageing eventually sets in. Biofeedback, entrainment, HMHI and the other approaches to AT design explained in the following sections can be gainfully used to enhance physical and mental ability even when there is no impairment, and can also be instrumental in bridging the internal and external environments.

VAK and Bio-Feedback Approach

Concepts being developed for children with disabilities also show great promise for the ageing. The "Siftables" is a new interface which involves VAK cues and feedback at every stage, in the process of solving problems by understanding spatial relationships. These are building blocks which are intelligent and capable of guiding the user intuitively (Merrill, Kalanithi & Maes, 2007). While the blocks exercise no control over what the user does, they provide both visual and audio cues and feedback for creating various combinations, whether they are used to create an image or create music. Since the blocks engage the motor function, we see a high level of "engagement" of users with their internal and external environments.

Progress in the field of acquiring, processing and using biofeedback in a simple, portable format is gaining momentum all over the world. EEG systems such as Emotiv (http://www.emotiv.com) and new communication protocols (Paulson, 2008) are demonstrating that one need no longer be hampered by high cost and long set-up times. While Emotiv is planning to use brain signals for gaming, other companies are developing special data acquisition electrodes and wireless systems. It is now possible for the user to "see" and "measure" the events occurring in the internal environment, and use it to carry out "internal accommodations" or adjustments in perceptions about oneself and the environment (See Figure 3).

Neurofeedback can identify the onset of many states such as high stress, low attention, and hemispheric asymmetry and allow people to train their brain waves to help slow the deterioration of their faculties. Neurofeedback is a direct method of intensive attention training. During training, the brain's activity is controlled consciously and unconsciously by the direction of attention. As clients become aware of how they can control and maintain the feedback signal by staying calm, alert and generating the right brain patterns, they can choose to stay in this state for up to 40 minutes. The brain gradually tunes in on the feedback signal intuitively. Similarly surface electromyographic (SEMG) feedback has been shown to be very useful in the retraining of the kinetic chain and functional movements after surgery or injury in old age, helping the person to recover a substantial percentage of motor capability and co-ordinated movement. These new skills are internalized during the training and automatically transferred to the persons' daily activities.

Training with attention seems to stimulate and promote neurological coherence, growth and maturation processes in the brain. This occurs because the neurons are stimulated to create new synaptic connections improving brain functions in the concerned areas. There is evidence that brain wave training increases blood flow to the brain (Madsen, Hasselbalch, Hagemann, Olsen & Bulow, 1995). Brain scientists found a negative correlation between delta/theta (lower frequency brain waves) activity and blood flow, and a positive correlation between alpha activity (8-13 Hz brain waves that lie in the middle of the brain waves frequency band) and blood flow to the brain. In other words, when a user succeeds in maintaining a high alpha state for some time, his/her brain receives more blood and therefore more oxygen and nutrition. This also stimulates impaired neurons to regenerate and improve their conduction of electric signals.

Thus, biofeedback is an important tool for "seeing" and measuring engagement of the user in a task. This modality can be interfaced with many high technology products for both old and young, including video gaming platforms such as Playstation and Xbox (www.smartbraintech.com). This can serve as a preventive intervention against normal degeneration due to ageing. If the person is already familiar with such a technology, it will be easier to return to using biofeedback as one ages or recovers from disease or trauma. Affordable systems marketed by companies such as Somatic Vision Inc. and others combine gaming and biofeedback to induce beneficial states and moods in persons ("How do skin conductance…" n.d.). These beneficial moods in the user encourage the prolonged engagement with assistive and rehabilitative technology.

Brain Entrainment Approach

With the discovery of brainwaves came the discovery that electrical activity in the brain will change depending on what the person is doing. For instance, the brainwaves of a sleeping person are vastly different than the brainwaves of someone wide awake. Over the years, more sensitive equipment has brought us closer to figuring out exactly what brainwaves represent and with that, what they mean about a person's health and state of mind. For example, anxious people tend to produce an overabundance of certain (high beta) waves while people with very low attention tend to produce very low amplitude alpha and beta waves (Prichep et al., 1994). Researchers have found that not only are brainwaves representative of mental state, but they can be externally stimulated to *change* a person's mental state, and even help treat a variety of mental disorders (Huang & Charyton, 2008).

"Brain entrainment" refers to the brain's electrical response to rhythmic sensory stimulation, such as pulses of sound or light. When the brain is given a stimulus through the ears, eyes or other senses, it emits an electrical charge in response, called a Cortical Evoked Response (Figure 4).

When the brain is presented with a rhythmic stimulus such as a drum beat, the rhythm is reflected in the brain waves. If the rhythm becomes fast and consistent enough, it can start to resemble the natural internal rhythms of the brain, as seen in the EEG. When this happens, the brain responds by synchronizing its own electric cycles to the same rhythm. For example, a 4 Hz brainwave is associated with sleep, so a 4 Hz sound pattern would help reproduce the sleep state in your brain. The same concept can be applied to nearly all mental states, including attention, frustration, stress and many others. As the therapy session progresses, the frequency rate of these pulses is changed slowly, thereby gradually changing one's brainwave patterns and guiding the mind to various useful mental states.

Figure 4. Reflection of external pulse in the EEG as an evoked potential

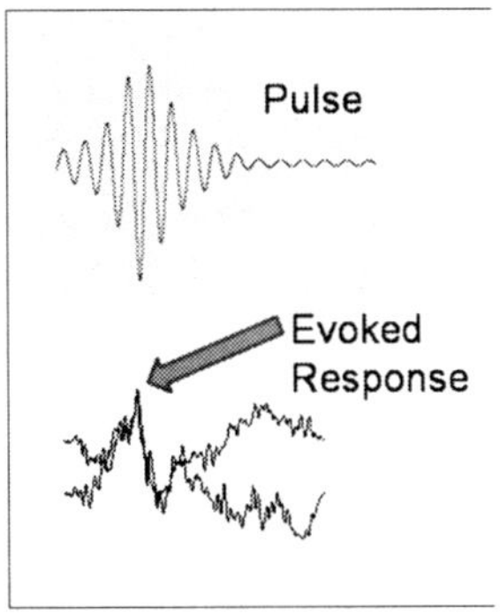

Brainwave Entrainment has been shown to have beneficial effects on the elderly disabled, especially in inducing 10Hz alpha waves which enhance short term memory and relaxed wakefulness (Williams, Ramaswamy & Oulhaji, 2006). The pulses are usually audio or visual stimuli.

Human-Machine-Human Interaction (HMHI) Approach

Senior citizens feel motivated to come together in groups for recreation, socializing and traveling (Nawate, Kaneko, Hanaoka & Okamura, 2007). Community rehabilitation projects in some countries like Japan and Turkey have demonstrated several advantages. Thus it seems that socializing is important for the elderly. However, in most clinics, there is little scope for socializing. While new patients get the major part of the attention from the overworked and outnumbered clinicians and therapists, the older patients have to struggle through their routines largely on their own. Some studies have shown that de-motivation is one of the major reasons for patients stopping rehabilitation prematurely. Two acknowledged de-motivating factors are progressively decreasing therapist contact and steadily decreasing rate of improvement (Damush, Plue, Bakas, Schmid & Williams, 2007; Johnson et al., 2006; Johnson, 2007). This scenario is in sharp focus now with a dramatically increasing disabled population. In 2007, the US population of those disabled by stroke, TBI and hip fracture grew by almost 2 million people. The number of people with significant disability in the US alone now totals more than 10 million. The disparity between the number of health professionals and number of patients grows daily.

This disparity suggests that it may be beneficial to design robotic rehabilitation and assistive devices to be multi-station systems instead of single station systems. In these devices two or more patients could play against each other, motivating themselves or even physically sharing strength and mobility resources to assist each other in exercise and functional movement. It is possible that this would go a long way to addressing current problems of de-motivation and high cost. For example, a well tested rehabilitation system such as the MIT Hand Guide (Krebs et al., 2004) or the Gentle/s System (Loureiro, Johnson & Harwin, 2006) can be reconfigured so that one patient can assist the other to complete the movement correctly. The performance of each may be recorded for future reference, analysis and assessment. We believe the ability to help a fellow patient would be a considerable boost to self esteem and motivation for a patient who has struggled with therapy for many months (Maritz, 2007). To the clinic it will mean less therapist load and cost. For the user, it would be more economical in terms of time and money, and more fun to boot.

The authors' general observations at clinics in Singapore and India and subsequent discussions with therapists and special education professionals seem to suggest that children with special needs and elderly people struggling with disability may have common challenges as follows:

1. In both cases, given the right conditions, neuroplasticity can occur and the brain can rewire itself.
2. Both suffer from low self-image and low social interaction.

3. Both have reduced attention spans and may have difficulties with motor function
4. Motivation to improve is generally low.

People from any age group may be struggling with one or more of the above conditions. This highlights the importance of "Collaborative therapy" where two persons play with each other or with their care givers or friends. Importantly, it may help re-introduce the patient (who has felt isolated so far as an invalid) into the social milieu. Using universal design principles in the design of "Collaborative Play Devices" will enable the patient to interact with whosoever he or she pleases, be it an infant or an elderly friend, able bodied or physically/ mentally challenged (Banerji & Heng, 2009). So far, the case of interactive play has been seriously addressed only by Virtual Reality, where a patient is able to respond to / elicit response from a virtual object or person. But the experience of interacting with a real person is far richer and more stimulating to the various senses. It also brings into play more hand movements and upper extremity manipulations rather than being restricted to a mouse or a joy stick, and a computer screen.

Studies show that collaboration between users has a positive effect on prolonged usage. This prolonged engagement in the activity is the first step for brain plasticity to occur and restore some of the impaired functions in part or full (Meinzer et al., 2004).

Multi-Level Interaction Approach

Apart from the need to communicate, people with disabilities also need to be as active as possible with whatever muscles are at their command to prevent further muscle wastage. If a television remote is hooked up with a bio-signal electrode to switch every time there is a muscle contraction (on the forearm or thigh for example), it will reduce overuse of the finger and distribute muscle load more appropriately. A television set can be rigged to run for 60 seconds for every 15 seconds of pedaling on a stationary bicycle for those who need lower limb exercise and mobility. This is very easily done with today's wireless technology and microelectronics. Gadgets such as these can be used by everyone in the house to enhance health. It is also preventive in function. Such technology platforms can also enable simultaneous selection of more than one trigger, thus speeding up a person's functions and enabling some level of multi-tasking. One such system which can use EEG or facial muscle activity is explained in the following section.

Rehabilitation is likely to be effective if those muscles which clinically need the most exercise are targeted to operate the device. We feel that the human-machine interface literature should emphasize this aspect more strongly. Keeping safety in mind, the device must enable the patient to improve the health of various muscles and joints instead of solely making the task easier. The Unified Platform Project explained below allows a person to exercise not just body, but also the mind. It has the capability to incorporate one or all of the other key approaches mentioned above, namely biofeedback, entrainment and HMHI. The concept behind the Unified Platform was first presented by the authors as part of a study on motor function recovery of the upper limb (Banerji, Heng & Kangdra, 2008).

EXPERIMENTS WITH THE UNIFIED PLATFORM PROJECT

Developing awareness about what is constant and what is changing inside our bodies at the deepest levels is one of the benefits of practices such as yoga and martial arts. This takes many years of dedicated practice and study. Biosignals such as EEG and EMG are a window to our internal environment. These signals open up a whole new world which we always knew existed but could not see, measure and experience easily. The

Figure 5. Schematic representation of a plug-n-play system which engages the internal and external environments of the user

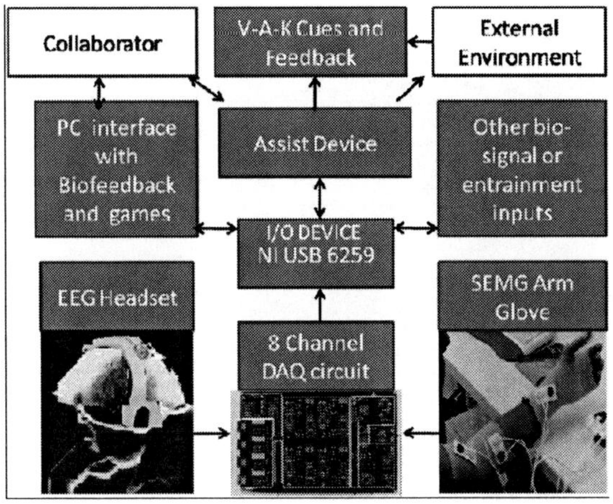

effects of meditation, hypnosis, and relaxation (Banquet, 1973; Lixin, Yunfa, Kanichi & Shigeo, 2007; Yunfa, Kanichi, Lixin & Komei, 2003) can now be seen and relatively measured using these biosignals. Results of some of the SEMG and EEG experiments by the authors were reported in 2009 (Heng & Banerji, 2009). The unified EEG/SEMG platform is sensitive to changes in SEMG and EEG differences and these changes can be used to trigger a motor or some other actuator in an assist device, in a collaborative or individual manner. A pictorial representation of the Unified Platform concept is shown in Figure 5.

Recording the SEMG provides the immediate activity triggers while the quantitative EEG analysis periodically updates and illustrates the brain states (Raichur, Wihardjo, Banerji & Heng, 2009). The virtual game or device for individual and collaborative use can be operated by voluntarily altering the muscle and brain waves towards more optimum values. The twin purposes of training the mind-body internal environment and operating functional or play/work devices in the external environment are thus both met.

The use of muscle contractions in the real time operation of switches and motors was tested in several formats. One of these was the combining of SEMG from muscle contractions of two persons jointly to achieve a simple task. Figure 6(A) shows the difference in contraction strength of two healthy young adults each using the same muscle. A strong muscle contraction of one of the participants was programmed to pull the pointer of the scale shown in Fig. 6(A) to one side. If the other person's muscle contraction was stronger, the scale would get pulled to the opposite side. Based on such a system, a range of competitive and collaborative games can encourage training and rehabilitation in a fun, collaborative, inclusive environment. It makes each "player" also aware of the imbalances in muscle co-ordination, timing and strength. It allows the therapist to evaluate important parameters such as force, compensatory muscle use and fatigue.

The algorithm was further modified so that it could generate real-time statistical triggers even with small twitches of intrinsic forearm muscles like finger flexors and extensors, showing sensitivity even with dry electrodes which can be implanted in an easy-to-wear glove. These triggers can serve as switches for different devices of daily use, and this is currently under investigation. A range of virtual games which mimic co-ordinated movements and functional tasks have also been created for testing with stroke patients in Singapore.

Although qualitative EEG signal acquisition and display is not noise-free at present, we find it is possible to tap into some EEG signals which are repeatable enough to act as triggers for certain functions. Fig 6(B) shows the difference in the alpha wave in the brain, as seen in the occipital lobe in the rear of the head due to eyes blinking. It has been found to be reliable, repeatable and suitable for use in real time, especially for those who cannot use their hands anymore. In the development of an "Active" assist device for which the sub-system is being designed, the use of quantitative EEG (QEEG) analysis is significant for detecting certain triggers and mind states of

Figure 6. A. LabView front panel showing simultaneous processing of signals from two persons. B. Alpha wave increase detected during eyes closure

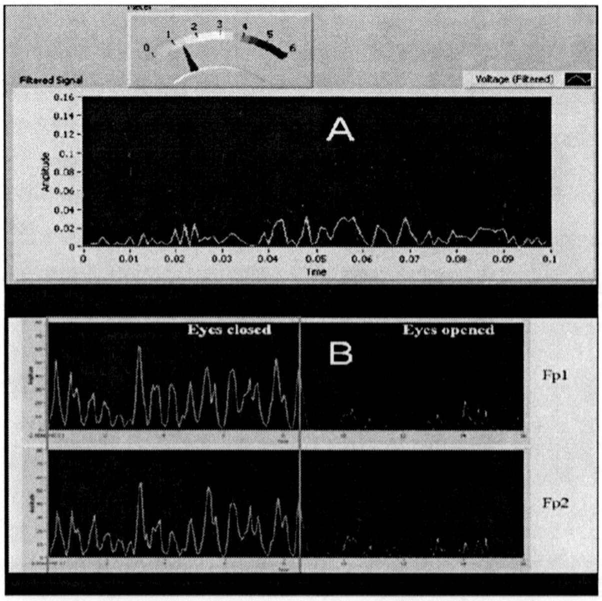

the patient (Clarke, Johnstone, Magee & Rushby, 2007; Van Putten & Tavy, 2004). Clinical studies of using such SEMG and EEG triggers and EEG power spectrums are currently being undertaken at a major rehabilitation clinic in Singapore.

The unified "neuro-physio" platform has the analog and digital ports to communicate with any automated assist device. At present, the person controls muscle and brain signals, using bio-feedback in solitary play and strength and timing feedback in collaborative play. At a later stage, it may facilitate the ability to play and train with another person freely, as well as set personalized game parameters. The data acquisition system can also accept other inputs such as electrocardiogram, skin conductance, force and motion. Ultimately, the ability to combine inputs from multiple sources such as SEMG, EEG, pressure transducers, goniometers and motion sensors, among others, will enable a level of multi tasking not seen in assistive technology so far. The hardware and software development for such a system in a wireless format will be a useful pursuit for the future. Some preliminary work in developing a mobile, home-use workstation with the unified platform and the real-time data transfer of performance and health parameters from such a device to a central server is underway at Nanyang Technological University, Singapore.

Such a multi-level interface which is robust, easy to set-up, versatile, adaptable and of low complexity increases the possibility of having a portable, miniaturized system with several interaction levels,

Level 1 - direct physical input e.g. keyboard, mouse, joystick.
Level 2 - secondary input e.g. head tracking, eye tracking, force feedback.
Level 3 - neuro and muscle input e.g. EEG, SEMG.
Level 4 - involuntary bio-signal input e.g. heart rate, respiratory rate, skin conductance, blood oxygen saturation.

This proposed interface will effectively bridge the users' internal and external environments when it is used simultaneously for operating various devices and self-training through the VAK feedback loop.

CONCLUSION

In the course of the next decade, it seems likely that an improved cochlear implant (McDermott & Looi, 2004) will emerge which will enable people to hear better than normal by being sensitive to a wider frequency range. Similarly, an artificial eye may someday not only enable the visually impaired to recognize faces, but also allow them to see in the ultraviolet and infrared range. Emerging knowledge in neuroscience and artificial intelligence suggests that it may be possible to augment the capacities of the body and mind artificially. However, Louise-Bender Pape (2002) concluded from experiments that successful integration of assistive technology into daily lives requires potential device users to explore the meanings they assign to devices and to understand that disability is one, but not the defining, feature of one's identity.

Moving the user away from "Isolation" to a more "Relational" environment where he or she is able to interact with oneself and others at various levels, HMHI will allow the user several options including:

1. Sharing of resources such as strength, mobility and motivation between two or more elderly users or between a physically impaired person and a healthy person.
2. Using the system for a wider range of impairments as well as facilitating more variety in activity.
3. Interacting with the system at multiple levels with their residual functions, so that they can adapt, communicate and respond faster.
4. Providing a tool to see and measure incremental improvements at mind, body and functional levels.

Such technology should be usable for both the young and elderly populations. Greater familiarity with modalities such as entrainment and biofeedback earlier in life could result in people managing some of the decrements that accompany advancing age. As a result, acceptance and usage of such technology after onset of disability may increase because of expertise developed earlier. If a device reinforces the elderly persons' inner resources (e.g. improves self image, confidence, encourages social inclusion) in all probability it will provide incentive for them to use the device.

This new approach to AT design can be the springboard for a new generation of simple, universally-used assistive devices. The acid test of the effectiveness of such technologies will be to restore in the ageing and impaired users the desire to continue living a productive and happy life, even after injury or disease. The role of AT must be widened to include this goal, if we wish to see higher usage and a substantial reduction in the grey digital divide.

REFERENCES

Agree, E. M., & Freedman, V. A. (2000). Incorporating assistive devices into community-based long term care. *Journal of Aging and Health, 12*(3), 426–450. doi:10.1177/089826430001200307

Angelo, J. (2000). Factors affecting the use of a single switch with assistive technology devices. *Journal of Rehabilitation Research and Development, 37*(5), 591–598.

Bach-y-Rita, P. (2001). Theoretical and practical considerations in the restoration of functions following stroke. *Topics in Stroke Rehabilitation, 8*(3), 1–15. doi:10.1310/8T1T-ETXU-8PDF-9X7F

Bain, B. K., & Leger, D. (1996). Environmental controls and robotics. In Hammel, J. (Ed.), *Assistive technology and occupational therapy: A link to function*. Bethesda, MD: American Occupational Therapy Association.

Banerji, S., & Heng, J. (2009). A unified, neurophysio platform to facilitate collaborative play in children with learning disabilities. In *Proceedings of the 2009 IEEE 11th International Conference on Rehabilitation Robotics*, 23-26 June 2009, Kyoto, Japan (pp. 912-917).

Banerji, S., Heng, J., & Kangdra, W. (2008). New directions in the creation of upper extremity robotic rehabilitation devices for stroke patients. In *Proceedings of the 2nd International Conference on Assistive Technology and Rehabilitation Engineering iCREATe 2008*, Bangkok, Thailand.

Banquet, J. P. (1973). Spectral analysis of EEG in meditation. *Electroencephalography and Clinical Neurophysiology*, *35*, 143–151. doi:10.1016/0013-4694(73)90170-3

Barry, R. J., Clarke, A. R., Johnstone, S. J., Magee, C. A., & Rushby, J. A. (2007). EEG differences between eyes-closed and eyes-open resting conditions. *Clinical Neurophysiology*, *118*, 2765–2773. doi:10.1016/j.clinph.2007.07.028

Bastille, J. V., & Gill-Body, K. M. (2004). A yoga-based exercise program for people with chronic poststroke hemiparesis. *Physical Therapy*, *84*(1), 33–48.

Berthoz, A. (1996). Neural basis of decision in perception and control of movement. *Neurobiology in Decision Making*, 83-100.

Brubaker, T. H., & Powers, E. A. (1976). The stereotype of 'old': a review and alternative approach. *Journal of Gerontology*, *31*(4), 441–447.

Clark, D. O., & Stump, D. E. (1998). Predictors of onset of and recovery from mobility difficulty among adults aged 51-61 years. *American Journal of Epidemiology*, *148*(1), 63–71.

Damush, T.M., Plue, L., Bakas, T., Schmid, A., & Williams, L.S. (2007). Barriers and facilitators to exercise among stroke survivors. *Rehabilitation Nursing, 32*(6), 253-260+262.

Deci, E. L., Eghrari, H., Patrick, B. C., & Leone, D. R. (1994). Facilitating internalization: the self determination theory perspective. *Journal of Personality*, *62*(1). doi:10.1111/j.1467-6494.1994.tb00797.x

Emotiv Systems Inc. (n.d.). Retrieved January 25, 2009 from http://emotiv.com/corporate/3_0/3_1.htm

Findings About the Awareness and Use of Accessible Technology. (n.d.). Retrieved February 10, 2009 from http://www.microsoft.com/enable/research/acctechnology.aspx.

Freedman, V. A., Agree, E. M., & Cornman, J. C. (2005). Development of an assistive technology and environmental assessment instrument for national surveys: Final report. Retrieved February 10, 2009 from http://aspe.hhs.gov/daltcp/reports/ATEAdevI.htm

Goldberg, R. (1984). Psychosocial aspects of stroke. In Kruger, D. W., & Collins, L. B. (Eds.), *Rehabilitation psychology*. Rockville: Aspen Publication.

Gupta, R. (2000). A path model of elder caregiver burden in Indian/Pakistani families in the United States. *International Journal of Aging & Human Development*, *51*(4), 295–313. doi:10.2190/J9XY-V3E0-NP1B-UNA5

Harris, J. E. (1998). *How the brain talks to itself.* USA: The Howarth Press Inc.

Hayashi, K. (2002). Striving for the greatest enjoyment through Collaborative Therapy: The role of the speech therapist in collaborative therapy treatment of patients with communication disorders. *Japanese Journal of Communication Disorders*, *19*(3), 236–241.

Helander, M., Landauer, T. K., & Prabhu, P. (Eds.). (1997). *Handbook of Human-Computer Interaction* (pp. 813–824). Elsevier Science BV.

Heng, J., & Banerji, S. (2010). A step towards multi-level human interface devices: A system that responds to EEG/SEMG triggers. *International Journal of Biorobotics and Biomechatronics, special issue on Rehabilitation Robotics, 1*(2), 93-98.

Hofgren, C., Bjorkdahl, A., Esbjornsson, E., & Stibrant-Sunnerhagen, K. (2007). Recovery after stroke: cognition, ADL function and return to work. *Acta Neurologica Scandinavica*, *115*(2), 73–80. doi:10.1111/j.1600-0404.2006.00768.x

How do skin conductance and heart rate rhythms measure stress? (n.d.). Retrieved February 15, 2009 from http://somaticvision.com/measurements.php.

Huang, T. L., & Charyton, C. (2008). A comprehensive review of the psychological effects of brainwave entrainment. *Alternative Therapies in Health and Medicine*, *14*(5), 38–50.

Inoue, K., Wada, K., & Ito, Y. (2008). Effective application of Paro: Seal type robots for disabled people in According to Ideas of Occupational Therapists. *Computers Helping People with Special Needs, Springer Berlin/Hiedelberg. 5105*, 1321-1324.

Johnson, M. J. (2007). Potential for a suite of robot/computer assisted motivating systems for personalized home based, stroke rehabilitation. *Journal of Neuroengineering and Rehabilitation*, *4*(6).

Johnson, M. J., Feng, X., Johnson, L. M., Ramachandran, B., Winters, J. M., & Kosasih, J. B. (2006). Robotic systems that rehabilitate as well as motivate: Three strategies for motivating impaired arm use. In *Proceedings IEEE / RASEMBS Int. Conf. on Biomedical robotics and Biomechatronics*, BioRob 2006, art.no.1639095 (pp. 254-259).

Kolasinski, S. L., Garfinkel, M., Tsai, A. G., Matz, W., Van Dyke, A., & Schumacher, H. R. (2005). Iyengar yoga for treating symptoms of osteoarthritis of the knees: A Pilot Study. *Journal of Alternative and Complementary Medicine (New York, N.Y.)*, *11*(4), 689–693..doi:10.1089/acm.2005.11.689

Krebs, H. I., Ferraro, M., Buerger, S. P., Newbery, M. J., Makiyama, A., & Sandmann, M. (2004). Rehabilitation Robotics- A pilot trial for spatial extension of MIT Manus. *Journal of Neuroengineering and Rehabilitation*, *1*(5). doi:. doi:10.1186/1743-0003-1-5

Lewis, C. B. (1984). Rehabilitation of an older person: a psychosocial focus. *Physical Therapy*, *64*(4), 517–522.

Lixin, W., Yunfa, L., Kanichi, M., & Shigeo, F. (2007). The psycho-physiological effects of "Taiji sense" in taijiquan exercise. *Japan Journal of Physical Fitness and Sports Medicine*, *56*, 131–140.

Louise-Bender Pape, T., Kim, J., & Weiner, B. (2002). The shaping of individual meanings assigned to assistive technology: A review of personal factors. *Disability and Rehabilitation*, *24*(1-3), 5–30. doi:10.1080/09638280110066235

Loureiro, R. C. V., Johnson, M. J., & Harwin, W. S. (2006). Collaborative tele-rehabilitation: a strategy for increasing engagement. In *Proceedings of the 1st IEEE Int. Conference on Biomedical Robotics and Biomechatronics,* art. 1639198 (pp. 859-864).

Maclean, N., & Pound, P. (2000). A critical review of the concept of patient motivation in the literature on physical rehabilitation. *British Medical Journal*, *50*(4), 495–506.

Madsen, P. L., Hasselbalch, S. G., Hagemann, L. P., Olsen, K. S., & Bulow, J. (1995). Persistent resetting of cerebral oxygen/glucose uptake ratio by brain activation: evidence obtained by Kety-Schmidt technique. *Journal of Cerebral Blood Flow and Metabolism*, *15*, 485–491.

Maritz, C. A. (2007). Using a model of reciprocal mentorship to develop, implement and sustain a group based exercise program for the frail elderly. *Physical & Occupational Therapy in Geriatrics*, *26*(3), 41–56.

Martinez, P., Bakardjian, H., & Cichocki, A. (2007). Fully online multicommand brain-computer interface with visual neurofeedback using SSVEP paradigm. *Computational Intelligence and Neuroscience*, 2007: 94561, PubMed Central. doi: 10.1155/2007/94561.

McDermott, H. J., & Looi, V. (2004). Perception of complex signals, including musical sounds, with cochlear implants. International Congress Series, Cochlear Implants. In *Proceedings of the VIII International Cochlear Implant Conference, 1273* (pp. 201-204).

Meinzer, M., Elbert, T., Wienbruch, C., Djundja, D., Barthel, G., & Rockstroh, B. (2004). Intensive language training enhances brain plasticity in chronic aphasia. *BMC Biology*, *2*, 20.. doi:10.1186/1741-7007-2-20

Merrill, D., Kalanithi, J., & Maes, P. (2007). Siftables: towards sensor network user interfaces. In *Proceedings of the 1st international conference on Tangible and embedded interaction* (pp. 75–78).

Milner, H. V. (2006). The digital divide: The role of political institutions in technology diffusion. *Comparative Political Studies*, *39*(2), 176–199. doi:10.1177/0010414005282983

Nawate, Y., Kaneko, F., Hanaoka, H., & Okamura, H. (2007). Efficacy of a group reminiscence therapy for elderly dementia patients residing at home. *Physical & Occupational Therapy in Geriatrics*, *26*(3), 57–68.

Newell, A. F. (1995). Extraordinary human computer operation. In Edwards, A. D. N. (Ed.), *Extraordinary human-computer interactions*. Cambridge University Press.

Nielsen, J. (1993). *Usability Engineering*. London: Academic Press.

Paulson, L. D. (2008). A New Wi-Fi for Peer-to-Peer Communications. *Computer*, *41*(6), 19–21. doi:10.1109/MC.2008.171

Pfurtschellar, G., & Neuper, C. (2001). Motor imagery and direct brain-computer communication. *Proceedings of the IEEE*, *89*(7), 1123–1134. doi:10.1109/5.939829

Phillips, B. S. (1957). *A Role Theory Approach to Adjustment in Old Age*. American Sociological Review.

Prichep, L., John, E., Ferris, S., Reisberg, B., Almas, M., Alper, K., & Cancro, R. (1994). Quantitative EEG correlates of cognitive deterioration in the elderly. *Neurobiology of Aging*, *15*(1), 85–90. doi:10.1016/0197-4580(94)90147-3

Raichur, A., Wihardo, G., Banerji, S., & Heng, J. (2009). A step towards home-based robotic rehabilitation: An interface circuit for EEG/SEMG actuated orthosis. In *Proceedings of the 2009 IEEE/ASME International Conference on Advanced Intelligent Mechatronics*, Singapore, 1998-2003.

Robertson, I. H., & Murre, J. M. J. (1999). Rehabilitation of brain damage: Brain plasticity and principles of guided recovery. *Psychological Bulletin*, *125*(5), 544–547. doi:10.1037/0033-2909.125.5.544

Sister Theresa-Never too old to help others, (n.d.). Retrieved September 18, 2009 from http://www.hearttoheartservice.org/AboutFounder.htm

Song, R., Lee, E., Lam, P., & Bae, S. C. (2003). Effects of tai chi exercise on pain, balance, muscle strength, and perceived difficulties in physical functioning in older women with osteoarthritis: A randomized clinical trial. *The Journal of Rheumatology*, *30*(9), 2039–2044.

Story, M.F. (1998). Maximising usability: The principles of universal design. *Assistive Technology-The official journal of RESNA, 10*(1), 4-12.

Taylor, J. B. (2009). *My stroke of insight* (pp. 147–158). UK: Hodder & Stoughton.

Ushering in the second digital revolution, (n.d.). Retrieved February 19, 2009 from http://www.digitaldivide.org/dd/index.html

Vallerand, R. J., & O'Connor, B. P. (1989). Motivation in the elderly: A theoretical framework and some interesting findings. *Canadian Psychology*, *30*(3). doi:10.1037/h0079828

Van Putten, M. J. A. M., & Tavy, D. L. J. (2004). Continuous quantitative EEG monitoring in hemispheric stroke patients using the brain symmetry index. *Stroke*, *35*, 2489–2492. doi:10.1161/01.STR.0000144649.49861.1d

Wallace, B. E., Wagner, A. K., Wagner, E. P., & McDeavitt, J. T. (2001). A history and review of quantitative electroencephalography in traumatic brain injury. *The Journal of Head Trauma Rehabilitation*, *16*(2), 165–190. doi:10.1097/00001199-200104000-00006

What is our special technology? (n.d.). Retrieved February 2, 2009 from http://www.jaipurfoot.org/03_Technology_ourspecialtech.asp

Williams, J., Ramaswamy, D., & Oulhaji, A. (2006). 10Hz flicker improves recognition memory in older people. *BMC Neuroscience,* 7(21), 1471-2202/7/21.

Yang, J. W. (1996). *Tai chi theory and martial power* (pp. 27–32). Boston: YMAA Publications.

Yunfa, L., Kanichi, M., Lixin, W., & Komei, I. (2003). Physiological benefits of 24-style taijiquan exercise in middle-aged women. *Journal of Physiological Anthropology and Applied Human Science*, *22*, 219–225. doi:10.2114/jpa.22.219

ADDITIONAL READING

Arena, J. G., Hannah, S. L., Bruno, G. M., & Meador, K. J. (1991). Electromyographic biofeedback training for tension headache in the elderly: a prospective study. *Biofeedback and Self-Regulation*, *16*(4), 379–390. doi:10.1007/BF00999991

Bernstein, N.A. (1957). Some emergent problems of the regulation of Motor Acts. *Questions of Psychology* No.6.

Berthoz, A. (1997). *The brain's sense of movement* (pp. 137–153). Harvard University Press.

Carmel, S. (2001). The will to live: gender differences among elderly persons. *Social Science & Medicine*, *52*(6), 949–958. doi:10.1016/S0277-9536(00)00198-2

Collura, T. F. (2002). Application of Repetitive Visual Stimulation to EEG Neurofeedback Protocols. *Journal of Neurotherapy*, *6*(2), 47–70. doi:10.1300/J184v06n02_07

Coulter, D. (2001). *Anatomy of Hatha Yoga: A manual for students, teachers and practitioners*. India: Motilal Banarsidas Publishers.

Doidge, N. (2007). *The brain that changes itself.* Penguin.

Galante, L. (1981). *Tai chi: The supreme ultimate*. USA: Weisner.

Hawkins, J., & Blakeslee, S. (2005). *On intelligence*. Times Books.

Kerr, K. (2000). Relaxation techniques: A critical review. *Critical Reviews in Physical and Rehabilitation Medicine*, *12*(1), 40.

Mannarino, M. (1991). The present and future role of biofeedback in successful ageing. *Applied Psychophysiology and Biofeedback*, *16*(4), 391–397.

Mikalsen, M. & Walderhaug, S. (2007). Empowering the elderly and cognitively disabled. *IEEE Pervasive Magazine, 6*(1).

Townsend, R. E., Lubin, A., & Naitoh, P. (1975). Stabilisation of alpha frequency by sinusoidal modulated light. *Electroencephalography and Clinical Neurophysiology*, *39*, 515–518. doi:10.1016/0013-4694(75)90053-X

Wisocki, P. A. (1991). *Handbook of Clinical Behaviour Therapy with the Elderly Client*. Plenum Press.

Chapter 13
Building a Mutual Assistance Community for Elderly People

Hong Sun
University of Antwerp, Belgium & Interdisciplinary Institute for Broadband Technology (IBBT), Belgium

Vincenzo De Florio
University of Antwerp, Belgium & Interdisciplinary Institute for Broadband Technology (IBBT), Belgium

Ning Gui
University of Antwerp, Belgium & Interdisciplinary Institute for Broadband Technology (IBBT), Belgium

Chris Blondia
University of Antwerp, Belgium & Interdisciplinary Institute for Broadband Technology (IBBT), Belgium

ABSTRACT

Efficient and cost-effective solutions are needed to meet the demands for services required by an ever increasing number of users. We discuss the characteristics of Ambient Assisted Living (AAL) as a new approach that promises to address the needs of elderly people. We propose combining social aspects with technology to build a community of mutual care which, among other things, can serve as a platform to effectively organize the social resources, promote social connection, and introduce intergenerational activities. Our research analyzes the characteristics of a mutual assistance community to help elderly people age well. The needed technologies are investigated, challenges of building such a community are reviewed, and the design of some prototypic solutions and preliminary research on organizing services inside the community are discussed.

DOI: 10.4018/978-1-61520-825-8.ch013

INTRODUCTION

A well known trend and a dominant characteristic of most of our societies is the rapid increase in the elderly population. Several statistical reports have revealed that the proportion of elderly people has kept increasing since the end of last century. For example, EUROSTAT (2004) indicated that "the share of the total European population (EU 15) older than 65 is set to increase from 16.3% in 2000 to 22% by 2025 and 27.5% by 2050." The European overview report of Ambient Assisted Living (AAL) also investigated this trend (Steg et al., 2006). Several research programmes that focus on AAL have been started, such as the Ambient Assisted Living Joint Programme launched by the European Union in 2008, which aims to find an efficient solution to help elderly people live independently.

Supporting independent living is a key goal of AAL services. Research indicates that elderly people would prefer to live in their own homes rather than in nursing homes but they need support to remain independent in their homes (Counsel and Care, 2005). Research has also shown that remote clinical therapy at home will not negatively affect the therapy process (Deutsch, Lewis & Burdea, 2007). However, one significant characteristic of the elderly and people with disabilities is reduced mobility and social contact. Reduced mobility can make simple tasks such as feeding a pet or mowing the lawn difficult. To improve the quality of life for the elderly, it is important to provide timely assistance in home settings.

AAL aims at extending the time that elderly people can live in their home environment by increasing their autonomy and assisting them in carrying out daily activities through the use of intelligent products and the provision of remote services including care services. Most efforts towards building ambient assisted living systems are based on developing pervasive devices and using Ambient Intelligence to integrate these devices in a safe environment. Ambient Intelligence refers to electronic systems that provide services in a sensitive and responsive way to the presence of people, and are unobtrusively integrated into our daily environment (Aarts, Harwig & Schuurmans, 2001). Living assistance systems and assistive devices are being developed to facilitate daily living and show promise in helping elderly people to live independently and in comfort. However, these systems and devices do not fully express the power of people or the importance of social connections and social activities. Although such efforts aspire to assist elderly people to live independently by transferring dependence from the human side to assistive devices, we observe how such transfers often reduce the social connections of those assisted in this way.

Home assistance systems developed using Ambient Intelligence can produce a safer environment for elderly people. Currently available solutions appear to overemphasize the technology and inadequately address the human element. This is evident in the low level of adoption of the technology. We suggest combining the mechanical power of assistive devices and the human power from "social computing"—seamlessly integrated— to provide timely, needed services and effective utilization of social resources. This means focusing not only on keeping elderly people physically healthy, but also on taking other daily requirements into consideration to improve their quality of life.

In the next sections, we introduce a prototype of a mutual assistance community.

RELATED WORK

Much research has been carried out on building intelligent environments around people such as Aware Home (Aware Home 2007) and I-Living (I-Living 2007). These studies found that "smart houses" improved the independence of elderly people, and reduced manual work. Devices such as RFID (Radio Frequency Identification), and motion detectors assist elderly people in the activities of daily living. The Aware Home project included a living laboratory where user acceptance of technology was tested, and a bridging framework for universal device interoperability in pervasive systems was built. The project also assessed devices for pervasive computing environments, medical monitoring, and human computer interaction interfaces. The mission of I-Living is similar to that of Aware Home: that is in developing an assisted-living, supportive software infrastructure that allows disparate technologies, software components, and wireless devices to work together. Tasks provided in I-Living included activity-reminding, health monitoring, and location detection.

These projects set out to provide assistive services in pervasive technology environments and offered people better lives by assisting with daily activities and keeping them safe by monitoring aspects of their health status. The Amigo project (Amigo, 2007), though not specifically designed for assisting elderly people, investigated ambient intelligence for the networked home environment to provide attractive services and improve end-user usability. Pervasive devices are managed in the Amigo project in an adaptive, context-aware and autonomous way. The system combines research in home automation, consumer electronics, mobile communications and PC (Personal Computer) technology to deliver services in a user-centric way. The scenarios of this project demonstrated that this system is able to provide users with customized services. The applications are not restricted to the home environment but extend to connecting the work environment through mobile devices, as well as connecting family members.

The Amigo project is a huge step towards general introduction of the networked home and towards Ambient Intelligence by increasing the usability of a networked home system. The achievements made in the Amigo project could be applied in Ambient Assisted Living for the elderly to provide services through advanced ICT (Information and Communications Technology).

The AAL country report for Finland noted that the (assistive) devices are not useful if not combined with services and formal or informal support and help (AAL Fin, 2005). Informal care from relatives, friends and neighbors is indispensable when constructing timely and cost-effective services in addition to formal care support arrangements. The use of assistive devices helps transfer dependence from the human side to the mechanical side and enhances the degree of independence. However, dependence on assistive devices can potentially reduce social connections and can mean that people are merely surviving safely, but not actively living. The cartoon in Figure 1 shows a humorous depiction of the possible side-effect of over-using technology. Although the effect is exaggerated, the picture reminds us that we should be cautious of over-reliance on assistive devices, and that we should never overlook human and social aspects.

Much effort is also being made around communication between people. One such project is COPLINTHO (COPLINTHO 2008), which built an eHomeCare system to link the patient's family, friends and the overall care team. This was focused on the recovery progress of a patient, thus on exchanging patient medical data rather than more generalized application.

Advanced Ambient Intelligence technology is able to construct safe environments, provide customized services, and improve quality of life. Greater participation of people could help fully harness the potential of smart devices, and maintain the social awareness of the elderly; the usage of advanced ICT could connect elderly people more effectively and help to organize community activities. In the following section, we propose a possible approach to constructing such a system.

Figure 1. Side effect of over-using assistive devices (Karlsson, 1996) (© 1996, Helsingin Sanomate. Used with permission.)

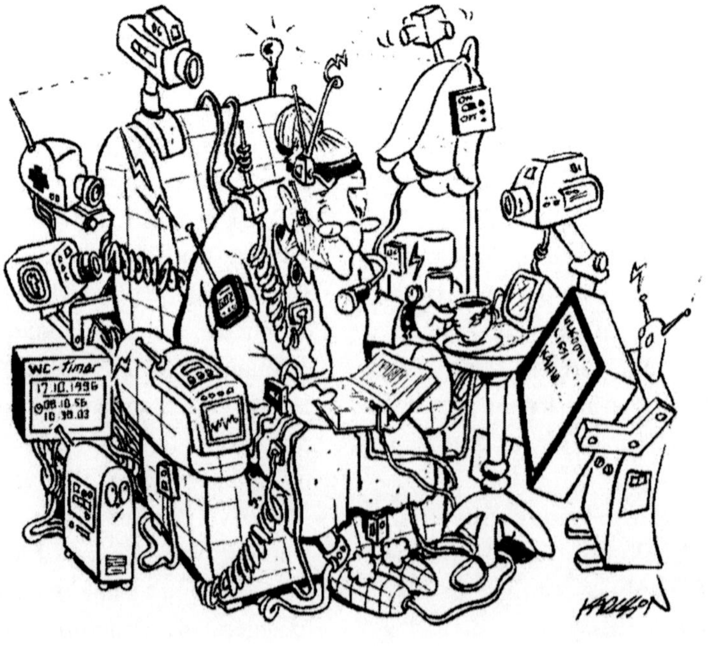

MUTUAL ASSISTANCE COMMUNITY

Rather than focusing solely on technology to solve the problem of assisting aging people, we propose combining relevant advances in technology and sociology. We propose building a mutual assistance community where dwellers may help each other when they are able to, supported by assistive devices which also contribute to a smart environment. Participants are able to make contributions to the health of the community. The technology and social forces are more seamlessly combined, providing the best services to people.

The architecture of our proposal for a mutual assistance community is shown in Figure 2. This combines assistive and ICT technologies and social interaction. Assistive devices are deployed to construct a smart house environment around the assisted people. These assistive devices will be developed as OSGi (Open Systems Gateway initiative) bundles and managed by a local OSGi gateway (OSGi 2007).

The mutual assistance community brings together technologies and people. People who are able to provide services are encouraged to act as informal caregivers for those requesting assistance. Elderly people are also encouraged to participate in group activities, which not only help to maintain their physical and psychological health but also reduce the requests for professional medical resources. Professional caregivers are included in the community to provide emergency and professional care services.

Aware Home (2008) points out that technology should support networks of formal and informal caregivers. The link between informal caregivers and the elderly can be quite static. Our proposed community can flexibly connect the needed help and available informal caregiver services through web service publication, matching and binding. The elderly can also use this approach to initiate and join group activities. Inter-generational activities can also be supported.

Figure 2. Organization of a mutual assistance community

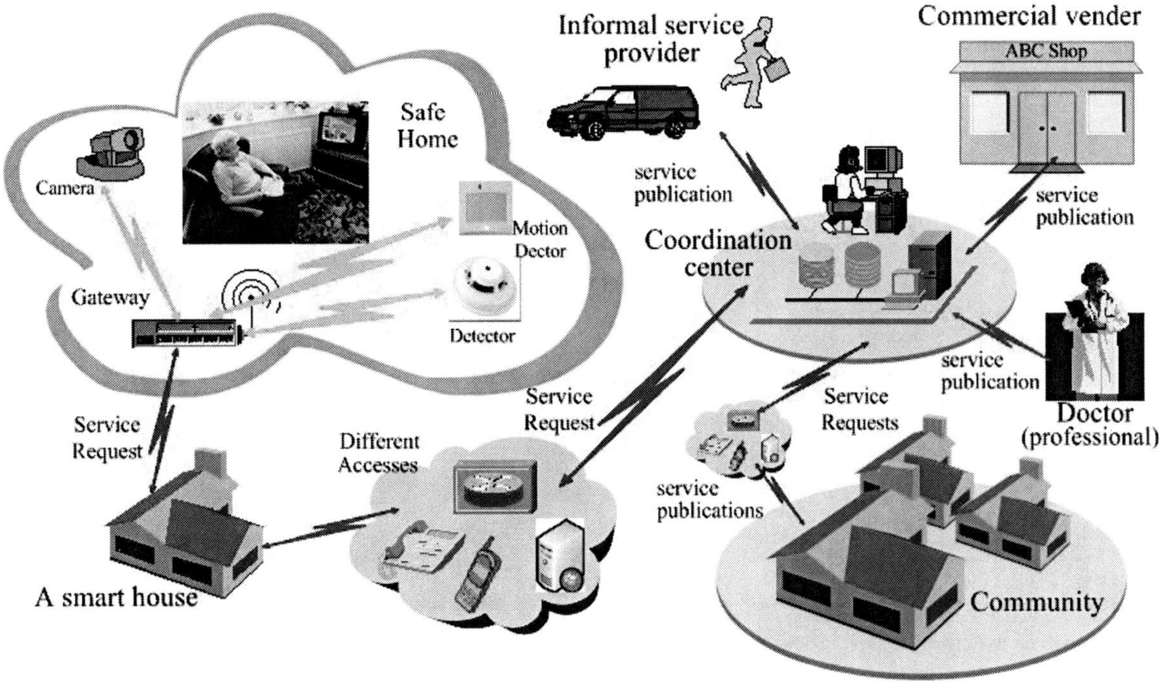

The interaction between assistive devices, human services, and end users, under the coordination of a service oriented management layer, are shown in Figure 3. Assistive devices and human services would interact to provide integrated services to people in need. Both assistive devices and human services would indicate their availability through a service oriented management framework. Requested and available services would be rationalized in the framework, and matched available services would be invoked. End users would interact with the framework through a user-friendly technology interface. In the proposed mutual assistance community, a user could be registered as both a service consumer and a service provider at the same time, based on the type of services they need and could provide. For instance, an elderly person could request physically challenging services, while providing knowledge/experience-based advisory/consulting services to others.

Figure 3. Service integration

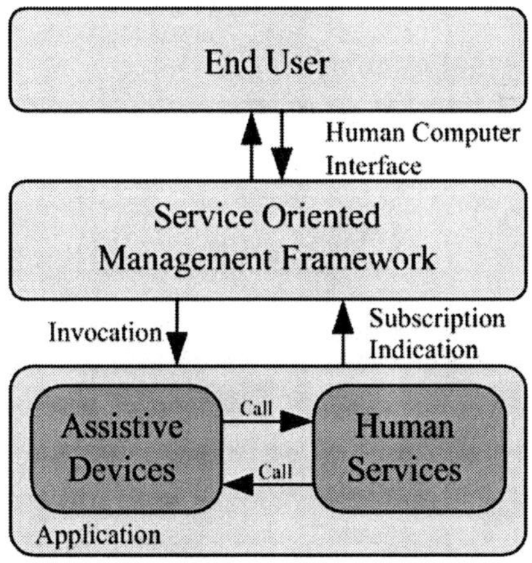

In preliminary research, we carried out simulations which included the participation of informal caregivers. Our simulation results indicate that the presence of informal caregivers helps to reduce the dependence on social resources and provides timely daily assistance (Sun et al., 2006). We also proposed a participant model to encour-

Figure 4. Technologies to construct a mutual assistance community

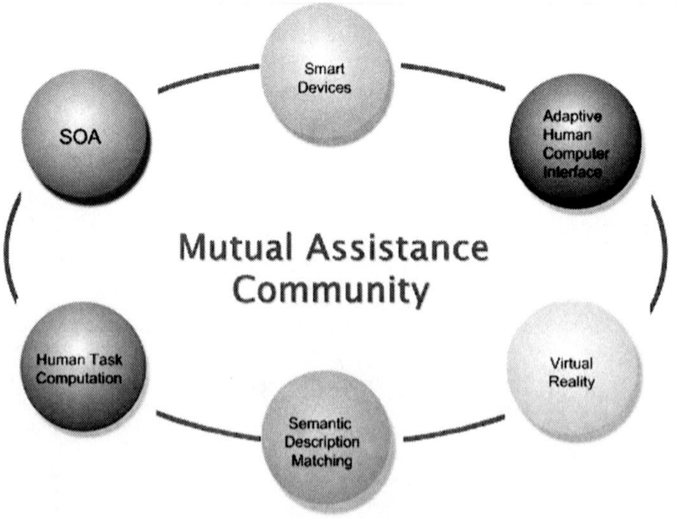

age elderly people to be active in group activities. As a result of introducing this model, the dependence on social resources is further reduced, while social connections are retained and even strengthened (Sun et al., 2007a).

CONSTRUCTING THE COMMUNITY AND ENCOURAGING PARTICIPATION

Figure 4 illustrates some important components for constructing a mutual assistance community. Smart assistive devices are important in building safe environments for people; however, in our proposed mutual assistance community, the most significant contribution is to integrate the services from the human side and the applications from assistive technologies. Challenges include managing the dynamic aspect of human services and integrating them with technology.

Generally, these challenges could be met through a service oriented approach. Service Oriented Architecture (SOA) is a flexible, standardized architecture that supports the connection of various services, and is an ideal tool to tackle the dynamic nature of the problem. The application of SOA, such as the OSGi (Open Systems Gateway initiative) platform, can also help establish a framework where various smart devices could be integrated and automatically called, started or stopped. Research using OSGi to build safe home environments is reported in Aiello and Dustdar (2008).

With the rising awareness of the importance of human roles in service-oriented organizations, much effort has been directed towards integrating people activities into service frameworks. This culminated in two specifications launched in the summer of 2007: WS-BPEL Extension for People (BPEL4People 2007) and Web Services Human Task (WS-HumanTask 2007). The WS-HumanTask targets the integration of humans in service-oriented applications. It provides a notation, state diagram and API (Application Programming Interface) for human tasks, as well as a coordination protocol that allows interaction with human tasks in a service-oriented fashion and, at the same time, controls the tasks' autonomy. A human-based activity (service) could be described as human tasks in the WS-HumanTask specification. The BPEL4People specification supports a broad range of scenarios that involve people within business processes, using human tasks defined in the WS-HumanTask specification. These two specifications could help meet the challenges of integrating human services in the SOA framework of the proposed mutual assistance community.

When the availability of services from the human side and device side are heterogeneously represented in service oriented architectures, the remaining challenge is how to automatically and semantically map the requested and available services. The foundation for service mapping is service description. A Semantic Knowledge Base is required to describe the advertised services precisely; certain ontology libraries describing the domain knowledge of the home-care environment should be developed. With such domain knowledge, a conceptual model for semantic service matching could be applied. OWL-S (OWL-S, 2002) is currently the most used technology in this domain; it is able to provide a framework for semantically describing web services from several perspectives such as service inquiry, invocation, or composition.

There are some service matching tools developed for matching OWL-S services, such as OWL-S Matcher (Tang & Liebetruth, 2006), OWL-S UDDI/Matchmaker (Srinivasan, 2004), and OWLS-MX Matchmaker (Klusch et al., 2005). The drawback of the first two is that the matching process takes a large amount of time, while the drawback of the latter one lies in its being memory intensive (Georgantas et al., 2006). These tools serve as good starting points to investigate web service matching while we believe more elegant and efficient matching engines should be developed. We have made some preliminary tests of service matching in home-care service matching (see Sun et al., 2007b).

The proposed mutual assistance community could be implemented in many different forms, but in any case, technologies of virtual reality and adaptive human computer interface could help to build up a user-friendly application. One way is to build an online virtual community (Sun et al., 2008a), where people may use their avatars to communicate more easily with each other. Daily activities and instruments (such as sensors, cameras, and the like) of physical life may be translated into their virtual community equivalents, and activities happening in the virtual world may trigger corresponding actions in the real world, so that inter-reality may be obtained through this virtual community.

Group activities can be enhanced through a virtual community. Communication between elderly persons may also be increased. Some websites have been constructed to provide an online space for elderly people to communicate as a community, such as U3A Online (www.u3aonline.org.au) and others. We envisage that an online community could better connect people and assist them to hold group activities. The online virtual community could also provide an easier way to implement intergenerational mutual assistance.

By combining services such as Google Earth and YouTube, the online community may also provide a greater sense of connectivity with the outside world. Due to health conditions, some requests by elderly people are difficult to realize due to physical constraints– such as visiting places for which they retain nostalgic memories from youth, or to places they always dreamed to go to but never had the chance. These requests may also be realized in the virtual community by taking a virtual tour. The virtual community could deliver services in the virtual world to elderly people such as entertainment. Physical limitations are less important in virtual environments.

RAISING USER ACCEPTANCE

As people enter old age, they need to contend with the likelihood of physical and cognitive decline. In addition there may be psychological issues. They may become passive consumers of societal services rather than active creators. In so doing, their self-esteem may suffer. There is a risk that some AAL systems for elderly people may consider their users as people who are weak and need to be passively assisted by others. The technology needs to be designed and implemented to recognize that elderly can still make their contributions to society and have a wealth of valuable experience to share. Our proposed mutual assistance community could help encourage elderly people to participate actively in group activities as peer participants, and possibly even to use their experiences to help the younger generations solve issues, for example, work and school problems (Sun et al., 2008b). Such possibilities will be discussed in more detail in the following section. Such activities provide elderly people with the chance to live creatively and with greater self-esteem.

Overcoming Technical Barriers

Elderly people may have more difficulties getting accustomed to the application of new technology than younger people (for example, see the chapter *Promoting Active Ageing through Technology Training in Korea* in this book). In order to help them get used to the ambient assistive devices and "bridge the grey digital divide," we must construct user friendly interfaces, and also provide appropriate training for users. Developing adaptive, straightforward, and multimodal human computer interfaces is a challenge in terms of the design of user interfaces to assisted living technologies (Kleinberger et al., 2007). The issue of improving the ICT knowledge of the elderly people so as to include them in the information society is receiving more and more attention from governments, and appropriate courses are provided to the elderly people in many countries. It is proposed that people should be involved in training on how to use assistive devices before they really need it (Floeck & Litz, 2007).

Technical barriers can be bridged when people have a strong drive to do so. Social connectivity is one such drive. Andreessen, former CEO of Netscape, recalled how people broke the technical barrier to surf online when Netscape first came to the public:

There was no shortage of skeptics at the time, who said that none of this would work because it was all too complicated. 'You had to go out and get a PC and a dial-up modem. The skeptics all said, 'It takes people a long time to change their habits and learn a new technology.' [But] people did it very quickly, and ten years later there were eight hundred million people on the Internet. People will change their habits quickly when they have a strong reason to do so, and people have an innate urge to connect with other people. (Friedman, 2005, pp. 62-63)

In a mutual assistance community, elderly people not only benefit from keeping connected with other people, but also are provided with chances to make contributions to society, to feel that they are still useful, and to live in an active way with increased self-esteem. Such benefits could provide our elderly people with further stimuli to break the grey digital divide.

A PARTICIPANT MODEL FOR GROUP ACTIVITIES

The concept of participant (Sun et al., 2007a) comes from the fact that many activities in which elderly people want to engage, require the involvement of others. Examples include playing chess and conversing. Instead of asking for nurses or informal caregivers to meet these requests, the participant model would encourage the people to participate in or initiate group activities in order to meet such needs autonomously, whenever this is possible and safe. When elderly people want to initiate or join a group activity, they could send a request to participate. The request will be parsed by a service center. If such a group activity is ongoing, the requester could join this activity directly; otherwise, based on the time constraint of the requester, the system will either initiate

Figure 5. Comparison between traditional model and participant model

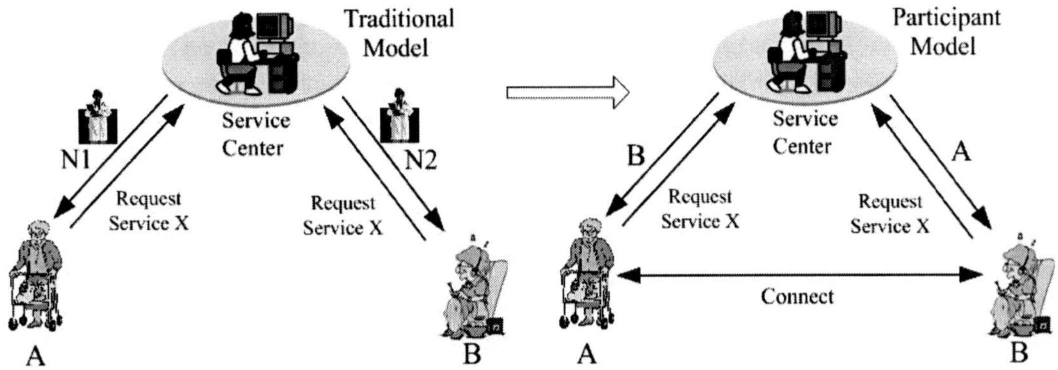

a new joint activity or try to find service from informal or professional caregivers to fulfill the user's requirement.

Figure 5 compares the participant model with the traditional one. A and B represent elderly people; N1 and N2 represent care-givers. In the participant model, when A and B want to participate in the same event, the service center will try to establish a link between them rather than requesting help as in the traditional model. Additional services and costs are thereby reduced, social networks are increased and self-esteem is also possibly increased because the participants have a greater sense of control over the process. Moreover, the peer-to-peer nature of the participant model does not classify the participants into caregivers and caretakers, which also helps preserve the dignity of elderly people.

Intergenerational Mutual Assistance

Intergenerational mutual assistance refers to activities between the older and younger generations, each participant using their special knowledge and capabilities to help the other. When people grow older, their mobility can be reduced, and they may become physically weaker. In intergenerational mutual assistance the younger generation could help the older one in physically demanding tasks. Older people have accumulated valuable experiences and knowledge during their lives. They may use such knowledge to assist the younger generation solve their problems in work and studies. During this process, not only the younger generation gets assistance but the older generation also finds a means to contribute to society.

SCENARIO

To better illustrate the functions of our proposed mutual assistance community, we will use a scenario to explain how the community organizes group activities.

Scenario: Participation in Group Activities

Mary is 70 years old and lives alone in Antwerp, Belgium. In the afternoon of a sunny day, Mary wants to take a walk in Middelheim Park, which is close to her home. She wants to have somebody accompany her during her walk. Mary decides to use the mutual assistance community to find someone who also wants to walk in the park. She switches on the TV, which is the graphical interface of the mutual assistance community. She navigates the service menu, which is built as an ontology tree, and selects the "Group Activity". A few photos will be presented to her, representing group activities such as chatting, exercising together, to name two. Mary chooses the symbol for walking and types in the location where she wants to hold this event as "Middelheim Park". For the service organization, Mary chooses to receive service from peer "participants", specifies the deadline as "today, 8pm", and forwards the service request to "relatives" in case no such service is found by the deadline.

After these inputs, the service matching engine will start searching for the appropriate services. The service matching engine is located in the service matching center. Available services are advertised in the service matching center which then produces a list of available services, and ranks them by their relevance to the users' requirements. The settings for the search, translated from Mary are as follows:

Required Service: Walk with someone.
Location: Middelheim Park, Antwerp.
Deadline: 8pm, 1st, August, 2007.
Service Form: Participant of Group Activities.
Action if no match found: Forward to "relatives"

Unfortunately, the service matching engine could not find a matched or similar service for Mary, so it will notify Mary that no matched services/requests are found. Nevertheless, the request from Mary is still kept in the service center until the deadline arrives.

Luckily, some minutes later, Kate submitted a similar request, which is also displayed in Figure 6. This time the system found that Kate's request is similar to the one from Mary. The degrees of match on different criteria are shown in Table 1.

The screen in Mary's interactive TV will notify her that it is now possible to meet her request: "*Kate* initiated a *walking* activity in *some park (includes Middelheim Park)* by *7pm today*; if you agree to take this *group activity* with *Kate*, press the **confirm** button and we will forward *Kate* your contact information."

Mary agrees to join this activity and she presses "confirm", while Kate also confirms the participation of Mary, agreeing on Middelheim Park as an acceptable venue. Their contact information is then displayed on their TV screens respectively, they call each other to confirm the time and place to meet, and have an enjoyable time walking in the park later.

In this scenario, Mary and Kate take the group activity – walking in the park – together. No additional help is required to meet their requests, so that social resources are effectively saved, and they also avoid the possible frustration of having to be taken care of by others. Figure 6 illustrates the actions taken in this scenario; the numbers displayed indicate the steps of the indicated action, the indicator "NA" means "not available". For technical details about service matching, readers may refer to our previous paper (Sun et al., 2007b).

CONCLUSION

This chapter discussed what we consider as being some crucial issues in building AAL systems. We proposed to solve those issues by building a mutual assistance community to effectively provide services for elderly people. Current research efforts at building pervasive home-care environments are also discussed in this chapter. Much work is focused on building pervasive home-care environments with advanced Ambient Intelligence. However, such approaches also face a concrete threat, namely possible social isolation due to the over-use of technology and lack of the communication between the assisted people and the outside community. Solutions to assist elderly people living independently and actively should leverage the efforts from both the technical and social sides.

In this chapter, we also introduced a prototypic implementation of a mutual assistance community, where people are mutually assisting each other, and human services and device applications are

Figure 6. A Scenario of Organizing a "Participant Activity"

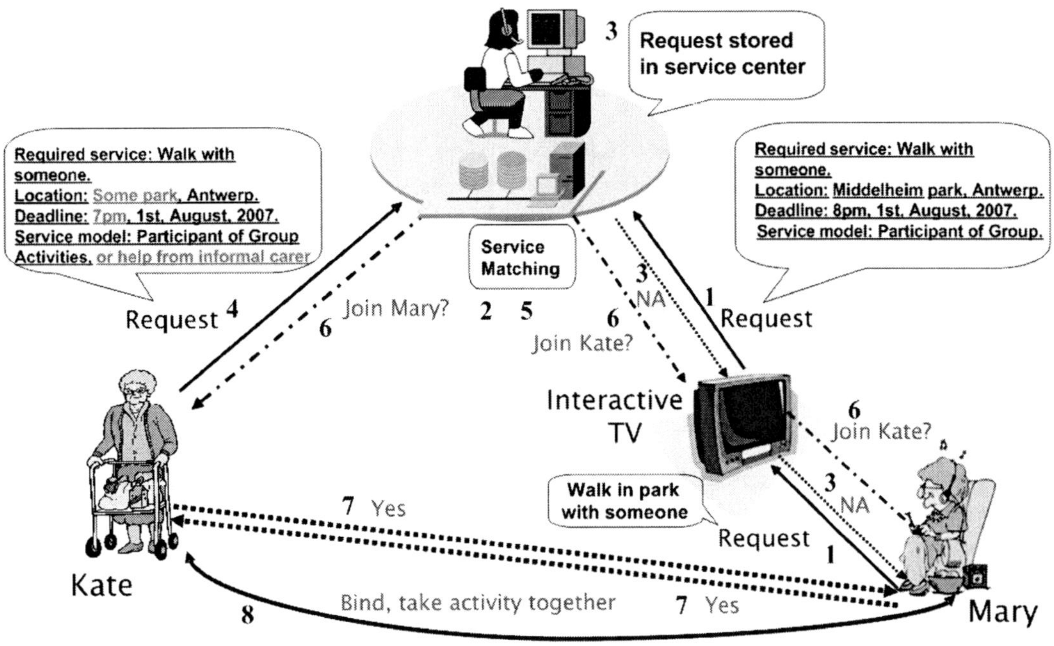

Table 1. Service Matching

Criteria	Mary	Match Degree	Kate
Required Service:	Walk with someone.	Match	Walk with someone.
Location:	Middelheim Park, Antwerp.	Sub_class of	Some Park, Antwerp.
Deadline:	8pm, 1st, August 2007	Parent_class of	7pm, 1st, August, 2007.
Service Form:	Participant of Group Activities.	Sub_class of	Participant of Group Activities, or Informal Caregiver

heterogeneously integrated. Smart devices can still be used in such a community to guarantee the safety of elderly people. Informal caregivers and professional caregivers are also actively involved.

The active roles of the elderly people envisaged in our mutual assistance community were also presented. The elderly could organize group activities according to a 'participant model', where people may participate as peers rather than receiving help from others. Societal resources may be saved as additional services are reduced. Intergenerational mutual assistance activities are also better enabled where the younger and the older generations mutually help each other. Elderly people may also find themselves better able to make contributions to society, thus raising their self-esteem. The mutual assistance community presented in this chapter is a vision of how to assist people to age well.

REFERENCES

Aarts, E., Harwig, R., & Schuurmans, M. (2001). Ambient intelligence. In *The invisible future: The seamless integration of technology into everyday life*. McGraw-Hill.

Aiello, M., & Dustdar, S. (2008). Are our homes ready for services? A domotic infrastructure based on the Web service stack. *Pervasive and Mobile Computing, 4*(4). doi:10.1016/j.pmcj.2008.01.002

Amigo (2007). Amigo: Ambient intelligence for the networked home environment. Retrieved August 24, 2009, from http://www.hitech-projects.com/euprojects/amigo/.

Aware Home. (2008). Aware Home Research Initiative Project, Georgia Institute of Technology. Retrieved August 24, 2009 from http://awarehome.imtc.gatech.edu/.

BPEL4People (2007) Specification: WS-BPEL Extension for People, (BPEL4People). Retrieved August 24, 2009, from https://www.sdn.sap.com/irj/sdn/go/portal/prtroot/docs/library/uuid/30c6f5b5-ef02-2a10-c8b5-cc1147f4d58c.

COPLINTHO. (2008). COPLINTHO Project, IBBT. Retrieved August 24, 2009, from https://projects.ibbt.be/coplintho/.

Counsel and Care (2005). *Community care assessment and services.*

Deutsch, J., Lewis, J., & Burdea, G. (2007). Technical and patient performance with a virtual reality-integrated telerehabilitation system. *IEEE Transactions on Neural Systems and Rehabilitation Engineering, 15*(1), 30–35. doi:10.1109/TNSRE.2007.891384

EUROSTAT. (2004.). Retrieved from www.eurostat.com.

Finland, A. A. L. (2005). *Ambient assisted living.* Country report, Finland.

Floeck, M., & Litz, L. (2007). Aging in place: Supporting senior citizens' independence with ambient assistive living technology. *mst / news.*

Friedman, T. L. (2005). *The world is flat – A brief history of the twenty-first century.* US: Farrar, Straus and Giroux.

Georgantas, N. (2006). Amigo middleware core: Prototype implementation & documentation. *IST Amigo Project Deliverable D3.2.*

Gui, N., Sun, H., De Florio, V., & Blondia, C. (2007). A service oriented infrastructure approach for mutual assistance communities. In *Proceedings of the First IEEE WoWMoM Workshop on Adaptive and DependAble Mission- and bUsiness-critical mobile Systems (ADAMUS 2007), Helsinki, Finland.*

I-living. (2007). I Assisted Living Project. Retrieved August 24, 2009, from http://lion.cs.uiuc.edu/assistedliving/.

Karlsson, R. (1996). Cartoon printed in *Helsingin Sanoma, October 18.*

Kleinberger, T., Becker, M., Ras, E., Holzinger, A., & Muller, P. (2007). *Ambient Intelligence in Assisted Living: Enable Elderly People to Handle Future Interfaces. Universal Access in Human-Computer Interaction. Ambient Interaction, Part II.* HCII.

Klusch, M. (2005). Retrieved August 24, 2009, from OWL-MX Matcher. Retrieved from http://projects.semwebcentral.org/frs/?group_id=90.

OSGi. (2007). OSGi Service Platform Release 4. Retrieved August 24, 2009, from http://www.osgi.org/Release4/Download.

OWL-S. (2002). OWL-S Technical Committee (T.C), Web Ontology Language for Web Services (OWL-S), http://www.w3.org/Submission/OWL-S/.

Srinivasan, N. OWL-S UDDI Matchmaker (2004). Retrieved August 24, 2009, from http://projects.semwebcentral.org/projects/owl-s-uddi-mm.

Steg, H. Strese. H., Loroff, C., Hull, J., & Schmidt, S. (2006). Europe is facing a demographic challenge: Ambient assisted living offers solutions. *Ambient Assisted Living – European overview report. VDI/VDE/IT,* Berlin, Germany.

Sun, H., De Florio, V., & Blondia, C. (2006). A design tool to reason about ambient assisted living systems. In *Proceedings of the International Conference on Intelligent Systems Design and Applications* (ISDA06), IEEE Computer Society, Jinan, China.

Sun, H., De Florio, V., Gui, N., & Blondia, C. (2007.a). *Participant: A new concept for optimally assisting the elder people.* In *Proceedings of the 20th IEEE International Symposium on Computer-Based Medical Systems* (CBMS-2007), Maribor, Slovenia.

Sun, H., De Florio, V., Gui, N., & Blondia, C. (2007.b). Service matching in online community for mutual assisted living. In *Proceedings of The Third International Conference on Signal-Image Technology & Internet Based Systems* (SITIS' 2007). IEEE Computer Society. Shanghai, China.

Sun, H., De Florio, V., Gui, N., & Blondia, C. (2008a). Towards building virtual community for ambient assisted living. In *Proceedings of 16th Euromicro International Conference on Parallel, Distributed and network-based Processing* (PDP2008). IEEE Computer Society. Toulouse, France.

Sun, H., De Florio, V., Gui, N., & Blondia, C. (2008b). Towards longer, better, and more active lives: Building mutual assisted living community for elder people. In the *Proceedings of the 47th European FITCE Congress*, FITCE, London.

Tang, S., & Liebetruth, C. (2006.). *The TUB OWL-S Matcher*. Retrieved August 24, 2009 from http://owlsm.projects.semwebcentral.org.

WS-HumanTask. (2007). *Specification: Web Services for Human Task (WS-HumanTask), version 1.0.* Retrieved August 24, 2009 from https://www.sdn.sap.com/irj/sdn/go/portal/prtroot/docs/library/uuid/a0c9ce4c-ee02-2a10-4b96-cb205464aa02

Chapter 14
Preventative Healthcare:
A Proposed Holistic Assistive Technology Model Based on Industry Practice

James Barrientos
LifeTec Queensland, Australia

Michele Barry
LifeTec Queensland, Australia

ABSTRACT

Australia's ageing population has escalated the demand for current health services and the trend could compound to unsustainable levels under the current health system. This chapter proposes a preventative healthcare model based on assistive technology to strengthen wellbeing at the individual and community level. The proposed model could minimise premature and inappropriate admission of Australians to care facilities while enhancing their independence and self care. It could also present a cost effective approach for policy makers by helping to alleviate the escalating costs of the health system. Importantly, this program offers an effective and sustainable alternative for delivering future health services.

INTRODUCTION

LifeTec Queensland is a not-for-profit consultative organisation that delivers professional advisory and educational services on the appropriate application of assistive technology (http://www.lifetec.org.au). LifeTec health professionals who include occupational therapists and speech pathologists provide state-wide information, consultation and education services to assist people to choose assistive technology which meets their needs and improves their independence and quality of life.

DOI: 10.4018/978-1-61520-825-8.ch014

Because LifeTec is a not-for-profit organisation, it can work in close partnership with suppliers of assistive technology without entering into commercial arrangements. This independent approach helps define LifeTec as a valuable provider of quality advice on assistive technology to its clients.

Assistive technology intervention is a strategy which can facilitate the independence and wellbeing of people and contribute to preventative health models (McCreadie & Tinker, 2005). Assistive technology refers to devices or systems that provide people with practical solutions to everyday life activities. It includes a wide range of devices, systems or designs that also allow a

Figure 1. Some common assistive technology that can assist people of all ages, including (a) large screen clock and large number dial phone; (b) adaptable tap turner; (c) computer access joystick, trackball and mouse configurations; (d) speech generating devices; (e) battery operated one handed jar opener; (f) mobility equipment

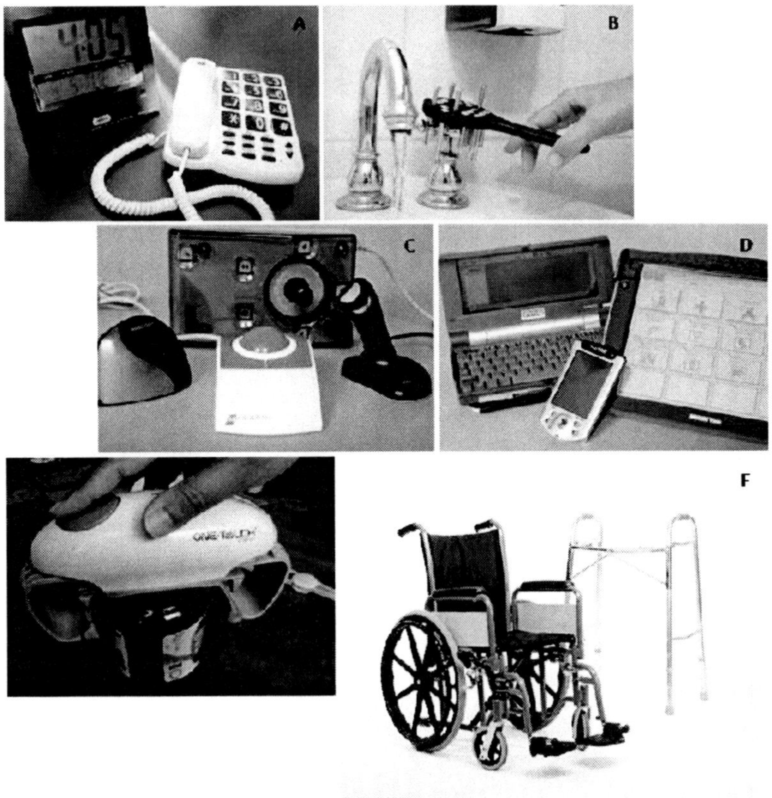

person to perform a task they would otherwise not do, or increase the ease and safety of performing a task. Assistive technology covers an array of both high and low technology solutions. These include mobility equipment, jar openers and tap turners, computer access hardware and software, bathroom and hygiene equipment, communication devices, home modification and accessible building design, eating equipment, personal alarm systems, and recreational aids. A small selection of low technology assistive devices is illustrated in Figure 1.

Although many devices appear to meet the desired needs of people, high levels of assistive technology abandonment are well documented (Wessels, 2003; Scherer, 2002). Inappropriate selection of assistive technology and social reasons are behind these high levels of abandonment. Many social and practical reasons induce people to purchase 'off the shelf' assistive devices without seeking clinical advice to inform their selection. For some, a reluctance to seek advice is part of a denial of disability (Livneh, 2009). This is especially the case for those people who may suffer from chronic conditions.

The goal for assistive technology professionals should not be to merely reach people with a disability, but to reach everyone who can benefit from technology. Traditionally, assistive technology has been marketed to those with disabilities; however, a larger group has emerged who do not necessarily identify as having a disability. This group often needs assistive technology to manage chronic health conditions or the effects of ageing.

The public stigma that is associated with disability can create adverse perceptions of assistive technology devices in general, and of the organisations that supply these devices (Parette & Scherer, 2004). These adverse perceptions have been observed by LifeTec staff following frequent interactions with potential users around Queensland. Staff have reported instances where people have heard of LifeTec services but have identified it as a 'disability' organisation and therefore largely irrelevant to their own specific needs. Ironically, our increasing success with improving the quality of life of many Queenslanders goes hand in hand with negative perceptions of LifeTec services by the public at large.

LifeTec was established in 1981 as the Independent Living Centre. Today it provides services to over 20,000 Queenslanders annually. The organisation's major challenge every year is to meet the needs of a population that is decentralised, growing, and, of course, ageing. As a state-wide service, LifeTec health professionals regularly travel throughout Queensland on a schedule that includes some of Australia's most remote communities, especially in Cape York and the Torres Strait Islands in the far north-east of Australia. By 2006, the organisation had become aware that its clientele was composed of people of essentially the same population profile as people who had been using the service in 1981: that is, people connected to disability services and who identified with disability culture. Both management and staff of LifeTec had become aware that wider demographic changes evident in the community were not reflected in this client data and that the service was not matching emerging trends. In particular, the rapidly ageing population would result in a growing client base that was likely to comprise the majority of future clients.

Following lengthy consultation with stakeholders, the organisation undertook a rebranding process. The result was a change to its name from *The Independent Living Centre* to *LifeTec Queensland.* In addition, it was relocated from a 1950s era, former children's hospice to a more accessible, vibrant inner-city shopping precinct. The goal of this process was to integrate the organisation, and by extension its services and the assistive technology itself, into an everyday community environment accessible to the existing clientele, while at the same time introducing assistive technology to the broader population of emerging assistive technology users. Three years later, our data show that these changes have impacted positively upon both client groups. LifeTec's client base is now more diverse and more representative of the community of need.

Although LifeTec's evolution has resulted in it being better able to deliver client services, the health system in which it operates remains very fragmented. This segregation of services can lead to ineffective and inconvenient services for clients who may otherwise benefit from a more holistic and consistent level of care. This chapter highlights the potential of assistive technology to aid in the general wellbeing of people. It also addresses some of the limitations of the current assistive technology programs in Australia, and proposes a holistic and more effective assistive technology program to facilitate sustainable preventative health strategies.

AN EMERGING DEMAND FOR ASSISTIVE TECHNOLOGY

The correct application of assistive technology aims to improve the independence and quality of life of people with disability and chronic disease. However, assistive technology is no longer the preserve of only those who identify as having a disability, although disabled people account for 20 per cent of the Australian population (Australian Bureau of Statistics, 2004).

The ageing of the population is one of the most significant changes in Australia's demographics.

Changes in the rates of fertility, migration, and life expectancy over decades have combined to increase the proportion of Australians in older age brackets. The nation's median age is projected to change from 35.4 in 2000 to 46.7 in 2050 (Australian Bureau of Statistics, 2004). Some projections show that one in four Australians will be aged 65 years and over by 2056 (Australian Bureau of Statistics, 2008).

While its social and policy implications are far-reaching, this change in population is expected to have an immediate and observable impact on the demand for assistive technology. Today, on average, people can expect to live with a disability for almost 20 years (Australian Institute of Health and Welfare, 2006). This figure will rise substantially with population ageing and, by extension, will place significant demands on all aspects of the assistive technology industry.

A new group of assistive technology users is emerging from the ageing population surge, that is those who are past working age, who are self-funded, and who enjoy generally good health. These people may require assistance with some activities of daily living such as walking, reading, safety in the home, or perhaps something as simple as opening food jars. However, they do not identify these needs as disabilities. Wessels (2003) has shown that those who acquire disability have a very different view of assistive technology compared to those born with disability. The latter see assistive technology as a means to attain new levels of independence and quality of life, whereas people with acquired disabilities see the same devices as reminders that function and quality of life have been lost. Similarly, people with slower-developing, progressive conditions more frequently tend to view technology as evidence of limitations (Hocking, 1999). Similar psychology may explain attitudes to assistive technology among people who do not identify as having a disability at all. Any stigma associated with disability extends to assistive technology devices which can lead to its abandonment.

ABANDONMENT AND CURRENT ASSISTIVE TECHNOLOGY FRAMEWORKS

Australia presently lacks a coordinated and cohesive approach to assistive technology prescription and provision. State based funding schemes focus on providing standardised solutions from existing technologies. Each scheme also places minimum requirements for all technology preselected for prescription. For example, all assistive technology must meet a particular Australian standard. Walker (2008) argues that this emphasis on standardisation stifles local innovators and leaves local manufacturers vulnerable to being overtaken by international companies.

We would contend that such schemes also stifle innovation and holistic service delivery at the time of prescription. While funding schemes ensure minimum standards of safety are in effect for prescribed devices, they also restrict assistive technology prescribers to a fixed selection from a predetermined range. Essentially, prescribers choose their solutions 'off-the-shelf'.

While 20 years of research has shown that assistive technology can greatly improve both function in activities of daily living and quality-of-life, it is also subject to high rates of abandonment (Wessels, 2003). A review of literature, primarily in the UK and USA, showed abandonment rates as high as 30 to 50 per cent (Scherer, 1997). The appearance of a device and the presence of a supportive social environment are major considerations for the acceptance of assistive technology (Wessels, 2003) yet these factors are often overlooked in the current prescription and funding models.

Another important consideration is misprescription, whether by a health professional, carers or salespeople, or by clients themselves. Misprescription of assistive technology can result from several factors including a lack of clinical reasoning, lack of relevant knowledge, equipment-centric rather than people-centric provision of options, the limited range of options available, and commercial bias.

Wessels (2003) identifies the most important factors in a client's acceptance of a device as the level of communication during prescription, consideration of the user's opinion, and the quality of ongoing instruction, training, and maintenance.

A HOLISTIC ASSISTIVE TECHNOLOGY PROGRAM

The rapid growth in the ageing population and associated increase in disability indicate the importance of shaping Australia's future health services around people, equity, prevention and wellbeing. The following holistic and people-centric program for assistive technology is a possible model which can assist government in creating a future focused health framework suited to both present and future generations. Such a program would see practical solutions funded by government and offered to individuals in the form of assistive technology to enable them to self care more effectively and more safely. Using a consultative model between health professionals and the end user, with minimal provision restrictions as well as high emphasis on ensuring the appropriateness of the recommended solutions, services could be provided to people through different mediums, including face-to-face, over the telephone, or via the Internet.

Ideally the proposed assistive technology program would:

- Take into consideration the different contextual factors involved.
- Take a holistic approach to individuals' needs and goals.
- Provide solutions through a health professional consultative model.
- Integrate with other primary and secondary health processes.
- Minimise restrictions in the provision of assistive technology.
- Provide services to people with no commercial bias.

Each of these ideas will be discussed in turn.

Context Factors

For the proposed program to be effective and truly holistic, it needs to take into consideration a multitude of settings and contexts for the end user. Some of these contextual factors include general settings, and physical, emotional, social and cultural contexts.

General context evaluates the person's home, work, school and greater community settings, while the physical context includes factors associated with the person's direct environment including regional and seasonal factors such as terrain and weather. A person's emotional context includes their attitude and feelings towards different elements in their environment. This includes their view of assistive technology, which will directly impact on how a piece of equipment is received and whether or not it is used to its full potential. The social and cultural context relates to human elements including family members, support groups, peers and carers. Cultural contexts are those related to customs and practices, religious beliefs, and personal and communication etiquette.

Holistic Approach

The traditional biomedical approach to healthcare primarily addresses a person's physical health, which risks a "one size fits all" approach. This approach can lead to a situation where a person with a particular physical need may be given a specific treatment regime which does not take into account his/her emotional, social and even spiritual features. As such, it does little to address issues such as non-compliance and abandonment of assistive technology. The goal of a holistic approach is to provide effective solutions to a person's needs in their entirety, rather than different areas in isolation. A holistic approach has successfully underpinned the LifeTec service provision model for years. The complementary approaches provided by the LifeTec health professionals take into account the person's wants, needs, support systems, contextual factors and resources. LifeTec staff also considers the client's psychosocial as well as his/her physical wellbeing before making their recommendations.

One widely used holistic model is the HAAT (Human, Activity and Assistive Technology) program (De Jonge & Rodger, 2006). This model identifies important areas that are essential in the correct application of assistive technology. To illustrate the importance of a holistic view, the different components of the HAAT model are explained as follows.

Human Component

This area focuses on and assesses the person's health, goals and motivation, and closely examines physical, social, and emotional factors. Physical factors such as the person's age, medical history, physical ability and their environment are examined to assist in making daily activities easier and safer. Social factors include integrating the person with their family, friends, peers, and ultimately with their community. The emotional aspect aims to improve self-esteem and reduce social stigmas associated with disability while minimising practical limitations.

Activity Component

This component addresses the requirements of specific activities undertaken by the person. It takes into account the different needs of domestic, work, educational, and recreational activities. Activity factors take into account self care activities such as personal hygiene, eating and dressing, as well as daily activities including socialising, shopping, getting to work and cleaning. Activity factors are also extended to incorporate vocational, educational and recreational pursuits.

The way people complete activities can be adapted to better match their abilities and contextual factors. A health professional may recommend that a person completes a task in a different manner, or that a person uses a specific piece of assistive technology in order to make that task safer and easier. Using a shower chair and sitting down to shower is one example of how an activity can be altered in order to match abilities.

Assistive Technology Components

The adoption of assistive technology solutions can depend on specific features of the assistive technology. The importance of these factors is easily overlooked and can make a significant difference to the successful adoption of assistive technology. Some of these factors include appropriateness, ease of functionality, aesthetics, cost, transportability, shape, weight, maintenance requirements as well as specifications and capacities.

Health Professional Consultative Model

The correct application of assistive technology is essential for a preventative health strategy to be successful. This is best achieved in a setting that determines people's needs through clinical reasoning, such as the health professional consultative model. A health professional can determine a person's holistic needs, analyse the daily tasks that are meaningful for them, assess different assistive technology options, and, by using clinical reasoning, align the person's needs with the most appropriate solution. A health professional is also able to provide continuity of care through education and training of carers, improving the odds of a successful outcome.

The correct application of assistive technology through health professional intervention can have other significant benefits. It can help minimise the abandonment of assistive technology by specifically addressing the factors outlined above, most importantly in the level of communication between prescriber and client, and by ensuring the client's needs are balanced with clinical reasoning. LifeTec has adopted a health professional model for provision of its services for many years. Its continued success means this approach is the recommended one for the proposed assistive technology model.

Integration with Other Health Processes

Current government programs for the providing assistive technology are restrictive and segregated at best. Providers can be dependent on a range of funding sources and need to conform to different reporting formats. For example, some programs limit their application to domestic use only and will only assess the domestic environment. However, a person's needs are not confined to the home environment. Other programs limit the application of assistive technology for education purposes to strict curriculum based purposes even though a student's educational needs are not restricted to the classroom.

A successful holistic assistive technology program needs to be an integrated component of a primary and secondary care health model. Such a program would ideally operate in parallel with other health programs and solutions, and address a person's needs in a multidisciplinary setting. This approach would alleviate limitations imposed by segregated services.

Minimise Provision Restrictions

The aim of the proposed program is to provide practical assistive technology solutions to as many qualifying individuals as possible, to enable them to self care more effectively and more safely. Improvements in wellbeing at the individual level would have the flow-on effect of giving rise to more healthy communities, which in turn would feed back into greater opportunities for improvements in wellbeing at the individual level. For this to occur, appropriate assistive technology solutions would need to be funded by government, without means testing, to any qualifying person based on their holistic requirements.

Under the proposed assistive technology program, any person with a permanent, impaired functional capacity could qualify for the provision of solutions prescribed within the holistic model described. Impaired functional capacity refers to a person's inability to meet the expectations and demands placed upon that person by their daily activities and environment. Other criteria such as residency status and qualifying periods are of a bureaucratic nature, and are not discussed here.

Removing Commercial Bias

Growing demand for assistive technology can be expected to lead to a greater variety of suppliers and retailers of assistive technology. Because of their commercial nature, suppliers may have restrictions on the range of available options, due to manufacturer-to-agency arrangements and exclusivity agreements. The proposed assistive technology program described here incorporates a holistic health professional model to make recommendations based on clinical reasoning rather than product marketing. The possibility of commercial bias could be overcome by developing an independent body to administer the program and source assistive technology solutions from hundreds of suppliers.

A Model

Figure 2 is a diagrammatic representation of the proposed holistic assistive technology program described in this chapter. Central to a holistic approach are the client needs and objectives at the top of the flowchart.

The proposed model is an evolution of the thinking from Cook and Hussey (2002). Cook

Figure 2. The holistic assistive technology model

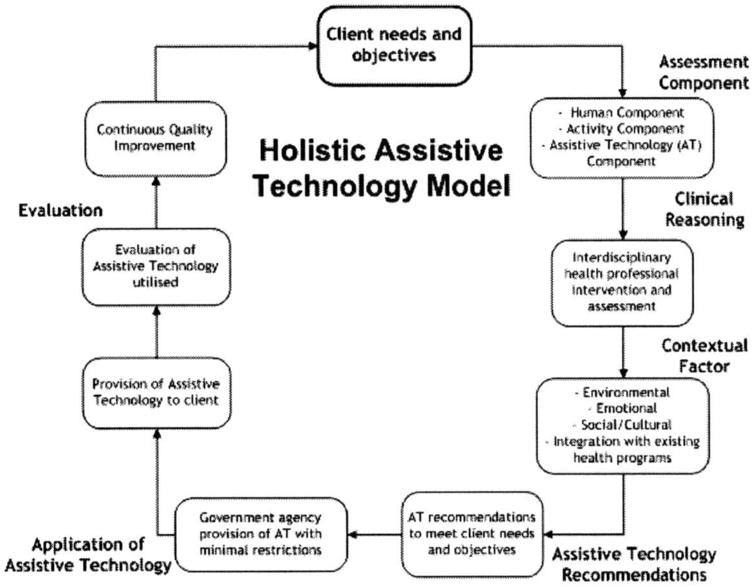

and Hussey have identified that a holistic assistive technology program may present many benefits desirable in a preventative health strategy for the future. Such a program could promote individual independence and safety whilst alleviating future demand on the health system. Some of the potential benefits of a holistic assistive technology approach specifically identified by Cook and Hussey (2002) include:

- *Promoting wellbeing.* Assistive technology solutions can greatly improve an individual's physical and psychosocial wellbeing. The collective wellbeing of individuals can similarly be expected to lead to vibrant and healthy communities.
- *Increasing independence and the ability to self care.* Assistive technology aimed at improving independence would be an effective strategy for preventable and premature admission to health care.
- *A focus on people.* Health professional intervention, combined with an extensive range of solutions, means this model could be responsive to both simple and complex client needs. The provision of services to clients, whether face to face, over the phone, or via email, means all people could have better equity of access to valuable services.
- *Specialist service.* Clinical reasoning by health professionals could further promote the correct application of assistive technology that aims at producing positive health outcomes and minimising the abandonment of recommended items.
- *Economic benefits.* Healthy people can better contribute to healthy communities. Healthy and dynamic communities can similarly be expected to contribute to employment and business opportunities.

The introduction of a holistic assistive technology program, such as the one proposed in this chapter, can provide an alternative preventative health strategy aimed at addressing the wellbeing of Australians and their communities. The proposed program incorporates all the above benefits identified by Cook and Hussey (2002). It incorporates a health professional consultative model designed to provide people who qualify with appropriate government funded assistive technology options to assist with their physical, social, and emotional needs in a people-friendly, and future focused manner. In particular, it can help to minimise inappropriate and premature admissions to hospitals and other institutional care, giving rise to important social and economic benefits.

CONCLUSION

This chapter discusses LifeTec and the environment for assistive technology services including issues such as the high rate of abandonment. Significant growth in the ageing population suggests that unless Australia's current health services are redesigned in the near future, they are likely to become unsustainable. A new health framework for assistive technology can ameliorate these pressures. The proposed holistic service delivery model discussed in this chapter has been refined from the observations and experiences of LifeTec staff over many years as providers of consultative services on assistive technology solutions.

REFERENCES

Australian Bureau of Statistics. (2004, June 16). *4102.0 - Australian Social Trends, 2004.* Retrieved February 15, 2009, from http://www.abs.gov.au/

Australian Bureau of Statistics. (2004, June 5). *4446.0 - Disability, Australia, 2003.* Retrieved February 10, 2009, from http://www.abs.gov.au/

Australian Bureau of Statistics. (2008). *Population Projections, Australia, 2006–2101.* Canberra: Australian Bureau of Statistics.

Australian Intitute of Health and Welfare (AIHW). (2006). *Life Expectancy and Disability in Australia 1988 to 2003.* Canberra: AIHW.

Blake, D. J., & Bodine, C. (2002). An overview of assistive technology for persons with multiple sclerosis. *Journal of Rehabilitation Research and Development, 39*(2), 299–312.

Cook, A. M., & Hussey, S. M. (2002). *Assistive technologies: Principles and practice.* St Louis: Mosby.

De Jonge, D., & Rodger, S. (2006). Consumer-identified barriers and strategies for optimizing technology use in the workplace. *Disability and Rehabilitation. Assistive Technology, 1*(1-2), 79–88. doi:10.1080/09638280500167324

Hocking, C. (1999). Function or feelings: Factors in abandonment of assistive devices. *Technology and Disability, 11*, 3–11.

Livneh, H. (2009). Denial of chronic illness and disability: Part I. Theoretical, functional, and dynamic perspectives. *Rehabilitation Counseling Bulletin,* (52): 225–236. doi:10.1177/0034355209333689

McCreadie, C., & Tinker, A. (2005). The acceptability of assistive technology to older people. *Ageing and Society, 25*(9), 1–110.

Parette, P., & Scherer, M. (2004). Assistive technology use and stigma. *Education and Training in Developmental Disabilities Journal, 39*(3), 217–226.

Queensland Health. (2002). Smart State 2020: A Vision for the Future. *Directions Statement* (pp. 6-11).

Scherer, M. (1997). The impact of assistive technology on the lives of people with disabilities. In Gray, D. Q. (Ed.), *Designing and using assistive technology: The human perspective.* Baltimore, Maryland: Brookes Publishing Co.

Scherer, M. (2002). The change in emphasis from people to person: Introduction to the special issue on assistive technology. *Disability and Rehabilitation*, *24*(1-3), 1–4. doi:10.1080/09638280110066262

Walker, L. (2008). Equipment funding schemes — blocking innovation? In *Proceedings ARATA 2008*. Australian Rehabilitation and Assistive Technology Association.

Wessels, R. D. (2003). Non-use of provided assistive technology devices: A literature overview. *Technology and Disability*, (15): 231–238.

Wielandt, T. A. (2000). Compliance with prescribed adaptive equipment: A literature review. *British Journal of Occupational Therapy*, *63*(2), 65–75.

Section 3
Innovations Supporting the Frail Elderly and Aged Care Providers

Chapter 15
Attitudes toward Intelligent Technologies:
Elderly People and Caregivers in Nursing Homes

Lorenza Tiberio
Institute for Cognitive Sciences and Technologies (ISTC-CNR), Italy

Massimiliano Scopelliti
Libera Università Maria Ss. Assunta (Lumsa), Italy

Maria Vittoria Giuliani
Institute for Cognitive Sciences and Technologies (ISTC-CNR), Italy

ABSTRACT

Nursing homes provide long-term care services and can help preserve the quality of life of elderly people subject to physical and cognitive impairments. In this chapter, we explore the role of intelligent technologies as a supplement to human care-giving and the potential to improve quality of life for both older adults and their caregivers in nursing homes. A study was conducted on elderly people's and caregivers' attitudes toward the use of intelligent technologies in nursing homes, with the aim of understanding in which domains of everyday activities the application of intelligent technologies can be more suitable. Results showed that attitude toward the application of intelligent technologies in nursing homes is positive, although multifaceted. Elderly people and caregivers considered intelligent technologies as relevant devices for the improvement of quality of life in different domains. Nonetheless, differences related to the role that technologies played in nursing homes clearly emerged.

INTRODUCTION

In the last decades, the increase in life expectancy has been evident especially in industrialised countries. Eurostat data (Giannakouris, 2008) forecast that the elderly population (older than 65) in Europe will be about 30% of the total in 2060; by the same period, elderly people aged 80, or older, will be about 12%. This phenomenon has tangible consequences for families, health-related services, and society. The huge increase in the total number of elderly people is associated

DOI: 10.4018/978-1-61520-825-8.ch015

with a higher incidence of physical and cognitive impairments. The older the population is, the higher the occurrence of disability, and chronic and degenerative diseases (Strandberg & Pitkälä, 2007). The consequences of the loss of competence of the elderly are manifold, ranging from social to economic, and involving different contexts of everyday life: overall, less autonomous persons are highly demanding, in terms of both human assistance and practical resources.

Frailty in elderly people has been a burden of families for decades. More recently, the change in social customs has affected family roles and practices, thus leading to a fall in informal caregiving to frail elderly, and the need for alternative solutions to this problem. Therefore, the role of an integrated network of healthcare services for the ageing population is becoming more and more important. Nursing homes are conceived as a service providing both support and rehabilitation after an incident or illness and long-term medical, nursing and social/recreational assistance to elderly people. Their aim is to promote the overall quality of life of users, which implies a focus on both physical and psychological needs (Haas, 1999; Janse et al., 2004). Several studies show that both objective (environmental, functional, and organisational features of the nursing homes) and subjective (physical, psychological, social, and cultural characteristics of people) factors – from the two-fold perspective of elderly residents and caregivers – may affect the perception of quality of life in nursing homes (Ball et al., 2000; Faulk, 1988; Kane et al., 2003; Mitchell & Kemp, 2000).

The aim of quality of life could be better achieved through the use of intelligent technologies (IT). Recently, concern about and interest in the application of IT in everyday life of older people has arisen. The huge increase in conferences and projects on this topic and the proliferation of technological solutions emphasise the potential contribution of IT to reducing elderly people's dependence on others (Cook & Hussey, 1995; Haigh & Yanco, 2002; Labelle & Mihailidis, 2006). In addition, the role of IT in alleviating the burden of and facilitating long-term assistance for caregivers has been underlined (Czaja & Rubert, 2002).

IT are innovative devices that are highly relevant in the management of activities related to health and well-being for the elderly in nursing homes, thus promoting quality of life (Charness, Czaja, Fisk & Rogers, 2002). Haigh and Yanco (2002) have identified different factors that may lead to institutionalisation of frail elderly, and discuss the advantages of many pioneering technologies which are capable of supporting the elderly with physical, cognitive and psychological disabilities, thus reducing the negative effects of impairments in their relationship with the domestic and assistive environment.

On the one hand, IT can be a useful means to promote "ageing in place", which is highly preferred by elderly people and is related to life satisfaction and well-being (Costa-Font, Elvira & Mascarilla-Mirò, 2009; Horner & Boldy, 2008); on the other hand, IT can also be important in nursing homes, but their use should encompass a comprehensive analysis of the two-fold perspective of elderly guests and caregivers, in which both practical and psychological aspects are to be taken into account.

To this aim, in this chapter we address the issue of the potential role of IT in promoting quality of life in nursing homes from a psycho-social perspective. We first discuss the role of environmental and social factors influencing well-being in nursing homes, and current applications of IT in healthcare settings. We then propose an integrative framework for the use of IT in healthcare settings, and present our study on elderly people's and caregivers' attitudes toward the use of IT for improved quality of life.

BACKGROUND

Quality of Life in Nursing Homes

The relocation of elderly people from their everyday environment to a residential facility can be a highly distressing event, requiring adaptation to a new and demanding situation. A successful adaptation process is related to a variety of factors, including the characteristics of people involved, the features of the old and new environment and people-environment transactions. Environmental psychology (Bechtel & Churchman, 2002) identifies specific issues to be considered: among them, the affective bond – or attachment – with the old environment (Giuliani, 1991, 2003), also relevant in the definition of self (Proshansky, Fabian & Kaminoff, 1983; Twigger-Ross & Uzzell, 1996), the loss of socialisation (Qassis & Hayden, 1990) and the management of privacy and territoriality, implying personal control over the environment (Altman, 1975). Lawton (1989) describes three different functions of the environment for the elderly: maintenance (environmental aspects may support self-identity and continuity in later life); stimulation (environmental features may provide opportunities for new experiences); and support (environmental characteristics may compensate for lost competences). Nursing homes, which are conceived to promote quality of life of elderly residents, should ensure not only appropriate care services but also social and environmental well-being.

The literature about potential factors influencing quality of life in nursing homes is limited; nonetheless, some studies underline the multidimensional aspect of this concept binding together objective and subjective components (Kane et al., 2003). Lawton (1991, 1994) defines quality of life in terms of objective environment, psychological well-being, behavioural competence, and perceived quality of life; accordingly, Kane et al. (2003) identify ten domains of quality of life in nursing homes: comfort, functional competence, autonomy, dignity, privacy, individuality, meaningful activity, relationships, enjoyment, security, and spiritual well-being.

Among objective components, the spatial organisation of the physical environment in nursing homes was found to promote physical, mental and functional health of residents (Gutheil, 1991; Kruzich, Clinton & Kelber, 1992). Among subjective components, the positive effect of social support on physical and psychological well-being of the elderly consistently emerged: social contact with family members and friends has a positive impact on life satisfaction of older people, and contributes to avoiding the risk of social isolation and depression (Drageset et al., 2009; Kahn, 1994; Street, Burge, Guadagno & Barrett, 2007). Faulk (1988) discusses the importance of social relationships among elderly residents; Cummings (2002) stresses the role of nursing homes in encouraging social contact not only among elderly residents, and with their relatives and friends, but also with formal and informal caregivers. In addition, several studies show that factors such as expression of decision-making capabilities and personal control are indicators of quality of life, in that they are related to emotional and mental well-being, and satisfaction (Kasser & Ryan, 1996; Mancini, 1980; Perlmutter, Monty & Chan, 1986; Reid & Ziegler, 1980). Elderly people in residential care settings often complain about a loss of personal control and choice in their life because the internal organisation of nursing homes imposes limitations and rules that influence life satisfaction of residents.

Nursing homes should afford environmental and social conditions promoting at the same time feelings of security and expression of autonomy, in both mental (e.g., active participation in self-related choices) and bodily (e.g., mobility and physical self-maintenance) domains. Meeting the needs of elderly people in nursing homes therefore should take into account a variety of aspects, ranging from physical to social, organisational and psychological. Far from being unrelated domains, they should be considered within a comprehensive framework. This suggests the need for innovative directions for development of healthcare settings oriented to the maintenance of personal skills, the stimulation of residual abilities, and the compensation for functional limitations of elderly people.

Trends in IT and their Role in Nursing Homes

The use of IT is a suitable way to improve the environment, thus pursuing the goals of maintenance, stimulation, and support, both in domestic settings and in nursing homes. In the domestic environment, IT are found to reduce the effects of physical and cognitive decline due to ageing in different domains: aids such as the *Digital Family Portrait* (Mynatt, Rowan, Craighill & Jacobs, 2001) make it easier to promote elder person-family interactions; cognitive orthotics such as *Autominder* (Pollack, 2005) provide physical assistance for walking and offer mnemonic support for activities of daily living. There are many intelligent monitoring and control systems in domestic settings to detect activity levels and behaviour of older adults in a non-obtrusive way. Inada et al. (1998) implemented a home care support information system for health evaluation of the elderly in the domestic environment. Yamaguchi, Ogawa, Tamura and Togata (1998) developed one of the first passive monitoring systems for collecting data (e.g., hours of sleep, physiological habits, body weight) for the use of caregivers.

In addition, some intelligent devices show a significant influence on quality of life in terms of reduction in the level of loneliness and perceived stress, and improvement in psycho-social well-being (Cody, Dunn, Hoppin & Wendt, 1999; Loges & Jung, 2001; White et al., 1999). More sophisticated intelligent systems, such as the *Personal Emergency Response System*, the *Automated Track Activity and Analysis System* and *Smart Houses,* have been developed through the integration of various technological components (Parker & Sabata, 2004). For example, *Smart Houses* are residences equipped with computing and information technology which respond to the needs of the elderly and people with disabilities, guaranteeing safety and support to their independent lifestyle (Dewsbury, Taylor & Edge, 2001; Morini & Biocca, 2004; Stefanov, Zeungnam & Bang, 2004).

In healthcare settings, IT can have many different applications, and help develop more liveable environments, for both the elderly and their caregivers; in addition, they can improve the efficiency in healthcare management (Liu & Castle, 2009). In a recent review of the literature about the use of technological supports in care settings, Topo (2009) identifies a variety of employed technologies. The majority of the studies reported a wide range of physical and psychological benefits for elderly people with dementia and their caregivers.

Research on the implementation of IT in nursing homes is mainly focused on monitoring and multi-agent robotic systems for rehabilitation and entertainment. A multidisciplinary research project at Carnegie Mellon University in Pittsburgh has created Pearl, a mobile robot assistant for elderly people living in different settings, particularly those with mild cognitive impairment (Pollack et al., 2002). Pearl can perform two main functions: reminding people to take medicine or go to the bathroom etc., and guiding them through the environment; and assisting them to interact with the outside world through mapping technology that allows them to become familiar with the environment and to navigate autonomously. The robot interacts with the user through a touch screen and different modes of interaction (speech, visual displays, facial expressions and physical motion). In different experimental sessions carried out in a nursing home, Pearl has successfully executed its functions.

The *Tiger Place Project* describes an intelligent system capable of improving communication between the elderly person and his family, thus encouraging the independence of the elderly and, in general, promoting quality of life (Tyrer et al., 2006). Other experiments in a nursing home show an improvement in the mood of the elderly and a reduction in the levels of stress as a consequence of interaction with Paro, a robotic baby seal (Taggart, Turale & Kidd, 2005). Results also show a decrease in the level of stress of caregivers, due to a reduced amount of supervision required by patients when they were engaged with the robot.

The advantages for caregivers can be multifaceted. IT can help detect critical situations and emergencies in the environment, lightening the workload of caregivers (Parker & Sabata, 2004). In particular, many studies report an improvement in terms of perceived support to social contacts, reduction of stress and workload, and ease of access to information and care services (Bank, Arguelles, Rubert, Eisdorfer & Czaja, 2006; Beauchamp, Irvine, Seeley & Johnson, 2005; Chang, Nitta, Carter & Markham, 2004).

THE STUDY

Open Issues and Aims of the Study

The use of IT in healthcare settings implies consideration of different aspects referring to the people-environment relationship to do with self-efficacy, perceived autonomy, and personal identity. IT may be perceived as a mid-point between environmental demands and personal resources of elderly people; on the other hand, their use may be associated with perceived loss of personal competence, thus leading to psychological discomfort. What about the caregivers' perspective? What can the role of IT be in their activities?

The use of IT should be integrated in comprehensive framework for quality of life. Baltes and Baltes (1990) put forward a model of successful ageing, in which the issues of selection of relevant competence domains, optimisation of related capabilities and compensation for previously available resources are of importance. Environmental modifications may support successful aging, as stated by Lawton (1989). Does the implementation of IT in nursing homes help promote successful ageing as well? Recently, Lindenberger, Lövdén, Schellenbach, Li and Krüger (2008) discuss the potential role of IT in successful ageing. Forlizzi, Di Salvo and Gemperle (2004) analysed the use of products by the elderly from an ecological perspective, and argued how robotic products can support the maintenance of personal identity, dignity and independence. The issue of acceptability presumably plays a central role in this debate (McCreadie & Tinker, 2005): we still need to understand to what extent elderly users, and caregivers as well, perceive congruence between the characteristics of IT and personal needs.

The analysis of elderly people's and caregivers' attitudes toward the use of IT in nursing homes seems to be highly relevant in this respect. Social psychology consistently stresses the role of attitudes in understanding behaviour (Fazio & Olson, 2003): the possibility for IT to be accepted or, conversely, to go unused in nursing homes, has much to do with the evaluations expressed by people. As a consequence, the aim of this study was to analyse the attitudes toward IT and their role in supporting quality of life of elderly residents in nursing homes, from the two-fold perspective of elderly people and caregivers. Our analysis was developed in order to understand suitable domains for the application of IT. From the caregivers' viewpoint, a further aim was to analyse the attitudes toward IT with reference to the potential improvement in the quality of their activities at a nursing home.

Methods

Context of the Study

The study was conducted in a nursing home near Bergamo, a city in Northern Italy. The nursing home provides residential, assistive, medical, rehabilitative and leisure/socialisation services to 60 elderly guests with different levels of cognitive impairment and motor disability. Among the values and principles inspiring the assistive activity at the nursing home, the idea of guests who are to be hosted and treated as whole and unique persons (not simply for their impairment), the personalisation of activities and services, the flexibility and monitoring/revision of programs, and the importance of socio-environmental integration to overcome marginality, are stressed.

Participants and Procedure

We first asked for an authorisation for data collection through questionnaires, and received ethics approval from the manager of the nursing home. The aims of the study were clarified in a pre-administration meeting with all the staff of the nursing home. We assured all participants that the data to be collected would be used anonymously and only for scientific purposes, and that feedback based on our results would eventually be given to the nursing home manager, as a possible contribution for improving the organisation.

At the end of the meeting, procedures, times, and modes of data collection were agreed upon in order to avoid negative interferences with everyday activities at the nursing home. Elderly guests with no severe cognitive impairment were selected through the analysis of scores at the Mini Mental State Examination (MMSE), as described in the clinical reports of the nursing home. In addition, caregivers working at the nursing home and friends/relatives or other unpaid caregivers were involved in the data collection. A total of 80 persons were finally asked to participate in the study by filling in a questionnaire. Participants were:

- 40 elderly residents, with no severe cognitive impairment (MMSE ≥ 24, as stated by scientific literature). The majority of them were women (N = 34). Elderly residents age ranged from 67 to 97 (M = 82.28, SD = 7.91). The educational level was low: 34 respondents attended only primary school.
- 20 internal caregivers - 18 women and 2 men, aged from 30 to 48 (M = 35.50, SD = 5.76). Internal caregivers were long-term, paid workers at the nursing homes, with a specific medical, technical and/or assistive training and background (M = 10.71, SD = 7.04). Their professional profile (doctors, nurses, rehabilitation technicians, animators, etc.), duties and working schedule are distinct. They provide for basic medical, rehabilitative, and personal and environmental care assistance, as stated by the law regarding nursing homes.
- 20 external caregivers - 16 women and 4 men, aged from 31 to 72 (M = 51.88, SD = 13.49). External caregivers are non-paid workers, with no specific assistive training background, and a shorter experience at the nursing home (M = 4.93, SD = 3.13). Their activities and working schedule are much more flexible, but basically they provide for social and leisure assistance. They may be enrolled in non-profit associations devoted to assistive activities, or simply be relatives of elderly people residing at the service.

Internal caregivers were involved in the data collection as both respondents and assistants for elderly residents filling in the questionnaire, as suggested in the pre-administration meeting. In fact, elderly residents were not easily able to express their own evaluations, and the presence of a person they knew well made it easier to gather the data, and to reduce mistrust toward strangers. Caregivers were also instructed to give examples of intelligent devices and their potential use at the nursing home, to support elderly understanding of IT. The presence of researchers during the administration improved the reliability of answers.

Table 1. The questionnaire sections

Section	Number of items	Measure
1. Perceived importance of autonomy in activity	20	Likert-type scale 1-5 ("very little" - "very much")
2. Improvement in quality of life of the elderly if assisted by IT	20	Likert-type scale 1-5 ("very little" - "very much")
3. Preference for human vs. technological help	20	Closed-ended item (Human - IT - No preference)
4. Improvement in the quality of care-giving through IT (caregivers only)	20	Likert-type scale 1-5 ("very little" - "very much")
5. Socio-demographics (gender, age, educational level) and caregivers experience (role, duration)	5	Various

Tools

We took as a starting point the literature on the evaluation of the level of autonomy for elderly people suffering from cognitive impairment and/or physical disabilities: namely, Activities of Daily Living (ADL) (Katz, Down, Cash & Grotz, 1970), and Instrumental Activities of Daily Living Scale (IADL) (Lawton & Brody, 1969). We identified a list of 20 basic activities referring to four different domains that play a key role in quality of life of elderly people:

- **Personal care:** this domain refers to everyday activities such as washing oneself, using the toilet, shaving (for men) or making up (for women), wearing clothes;
- **Basic physiological needs and health:** this domain refers to eating/drinking, controlling urinary and faecal discharge, taking medicines, alerting caregivers in the case of an emergency, keeping in good shape;
- **Autonomy of movement:** this domain refers to autonomy of movement in the environment at different levels of scale (the room, the floor, the building, the external environment);
- **Socialisation:** this domain refers to activities that have to do with leisure and social interaction among elderly residents at the nursing home, and with other people outside it.

With reference to these activities, we developed a questionnaire with the aim of exploring the potential role of IT in the improvement of quality of life of elderly residents in nursing homes. Two different versions of the questionnaire were developed, in order to address this issue from the two-fold perspective of elderly residents and caregivers. The caregiver version also included a section on the potential improvement in the quality of their activity through the use of IT. The final section collected socio-demographic and caregiver experience data. The questionnaire sections are reported in Table 1.

Analyses

Data were used to perform different analyses through the software SPSS 13.0, in line with the objectives of the study. Two Factor Analyses (FAs) were carried out with reference to Sections 1 and 2 of the questionnaire respectively, in order to identify the dimensions of attitude referring to both Perceived importance of autonomy and Improvement in quality of life of elderly people if assisted by IT. The internal consistency of factors extrapolated through FAs was then assessed

Table 2. Factor Analysis – Perceived importance of autonomy

	Factor 1	Factor 2
Item	Self-expression and relations with the socio-physical world	Basic physiological and personal needs
Autonomy in walking near the nursing home	.824	
Autonomy in talking to people outside the nursing home	.769	
Autonomy in keeping in good shape	.745	
Autonomy in going to the courtyard outside the nursing home	.687	
Autonomy in knowing what's going on in the world	.672	
Autonomy in cultivating interests	.626	
Autonomy in talking to other guests	.621	
Autonomy in using the toilet		.845
Autonomy in washing		.798
Autonomy in moving from floor to floor		.741
Autonomy in wearing clothes		.684
Autonomy in alerting caregivers in the case of an emergency		.603
Autonomy in taking a bath		.492
Eigenvalues	4.53	2.47
Explained variance	34.8	19.0
Cronbach's alpha	.84	.81

(Cronbach's alpha). Finally, mean aggregate scores for each factor were calculated and the dimensions of attitude of elderly guests and caregivers toward IT in nursing homes were analysed and compared through a series of Analyses of Variance (ANOVA). Preferences for human vs. technological help were assessed through a series of Chi-square analyses. The Improvement in the quality of care-giving through the use of IT was assessed through descriptive statistics and a repeated measure ANOVA.

Results

Results showed that the attitude toward IT in nursing homes is positive, although multifaceted. Elderly people and caregivers identify different domains of autonomy which are of importance for the quality of life of the former. Moreover, they identify different areas of potential improvement in their quality of life. With reference to potential improvement, the role of IT was found to be relevant, even though more suitable for some areas than others. Significant differences emerged between elderly people and caregivers, in terms of both attitudes and preference for a human vs. technological assistance in everyday activities. Finally, in the analysis of the quality of their care-giving, caregivers identified areas in which the use of IT to support the needs of elderly people seems to be more relevant.

More details on these specific issues are given in the following result sections.

Perceived Importance of Autonomy: Dimensions of Attitude

The first FA was performed with reference to the items of Perceived importance of autonomy. The analysis yielded a 2-factor solution, with Varimax rotation, explaining 53.8% of the variance (see Table 2). The factors did not show a significant correlation. Thirteen out of the initial twenty items entered the final solution, while seven items were removed because of a low factor loading (<.40).

The first factor, explaining 34.8% of the total variance, refers to personal control over self-expression activities, involving both a physical and a cognitive relationship with the world outside the nursing home. It was labelled "Self-expression and relations with the socio-physical world". The analysis of the internal consistency showed a high level of reliability (Cronbach's alpha = .84).

The second factor, explaining 19.0% of the total variance, refers to everyday basic activities which have to do with personal care and hygiene, movement throughout the nursing home, and alerting caregivers. It was labelled "Basic physiological and personal needs". The analysis of the internal consistency showed a high level of reliability (Cronbach's alpha = .81).

Improvement in Quality of Life of Elderly People: Dimensions of Attitude

The second FA was performed with reference to the items of Improvement in quality of life of elderly people through the use of IT. The analysis yielded a 3-factor solution, with Oblimin rotation, explaining 75.1% of the variance (see Table 3). The factors showed a moderate correlation (Pearson's r ranging from .36 to .53, $p < .01$). Eighteen out of the initial twenty items entered the final solution, while two items were removed because of a low factor loading (<.40).

The first factor, explaining 53.9% of the total variance, refers to everyday basic activities which have to do with personal care, hygiene and administration of medicine. It was labelled Basic physiological and personal needs. The analysis of the internal consistency showed a high level of reliability (Cronbach's alpha = .89).

The second factor, explaining 12.3% of the total variance, refers to everyday activities which involve socialisation and leisure, the cultivation of personal interest, and contact with the world outside; interestingly, also items referring to health and safety related activities showed a significant factor loading in this factor. It was labelled Socialisation and personal well-being. The analysis of the internal consistency showed a high level of reliability (Cronbach's alpha = .93).

The third factor, explaining 8.9% of the total variance, refers to activities involving movement, both into the nursing home and outside. It was labelled Easiness of movement. The analysis of the internal consistency showed a high level of reliability (Cronbach's alpha = .95).

Mean aggregate scores of the dimensions of attitude referring to both Perceived importance of autonomy and Improvement in quality of life of elderly people through the use of IT were then calculated. No significant correlation between the dimensions of Perceived importance of autonomy and the dimensions of Improvement in quality of life of elderly people was found (Pearson's r ranging from .03 to .22, *ns*).

Perceived Importance of Autonomy and Improvement in Quality of Life Provided by IT: Attitude of and Differences between Elderly People and Caregivers

Mean aggregate scores of the two dimensions of attitude referring to Perceived importance of autonomy showed that both domains identified through FA are highly relevant for quality of life of guests (Self-expression and relations with the socio-physical world: $M = 4.13$, $SD = .74$; Basic physiological and personal needs: $M = 4.25$, $SD = .69$).

A 3 x 2 repeated measure ANOVA (general linear model), considering the Group (Elderly guests vs. Internal caregivers vs. External caregivers) as a between subjects factor, and the domains of Perceived importance of autonomy (Self-expression and relations with the socio-physical world vs. Basic physiological and personal needs) as a within subject factor, was then performed.

Table 3. Factor Analysis: Improvement in quality of life of elderly people

	Factor 1	Factor 2	Factor 3
Item	Basic physiological and personal needs	Socialisation and personal well-being	Easiness of movement
Improvement in washing	.860		
Improvement in taking a bath	.814		
Improvement in using the toilet	.805		
Improvement in shaving/making up	.758		
Improvement in wearing clothes	.685		
Improvement in taking medicines	.541		
Improvement in sharing leisure time at the nursing home		.941	
Improvement in making leisure activities accessible		.893	
Improvement in alerting caregivers in the case of an emergency		.769	
Improvement in keeping in good shape		.768	
Improvement in cultivating interests		.753	
Improvement in eating/drinking		.664	
Improvement in knowing what's going on in the world		.428	
Improvement in going to the courtyard outside the nursing home			.958
Improvement in walking near the nursing home			.949
Improvement in moving from room to room			.914
Improvement in moving inside the room			.866
Improvement in moving from floor to floor			.767
Eigenvalues	9.70	2.20	1.61
Explained variance	53.9	12.3	8.9
Cronbach's alpha	.89	.93	.95

No significant difference in the overall relative importance of the two domains emerged ($F_{(1, 79)} = 1.61$, *ns*). Conversely, significant interactions were found. In the comparison among groups in nursing homes, a significant difference in the evaluation of the importance of autonomy in both Self-expression and relations with the socio-physical world ($F_{(2, 77)} = 3.42$, $p < .05$) and Basic physiological and personal needs ($F_{(2, 77)} = 5.93$, $p < .01$) was found (see Table 4a). Post hoc analyses (Bonferroni, $p < .05$) showed that external caregivers give a higher importance to autonomy in Self-expression and relations with the socio-physical world than internal caregivers; conversely, elderly guests attribute a higher importance to autonomy in Basic physiological and personal needs than external caregivers.

In the comparison between domains of Perceived importance of autonomy, a significant interaction effect ($F_{(2, 77)} = 8.58$, $p < .001$) was found (see Table 4b).

Post hoc analyses (Bonferroni, $p < .05$) showed that both elderly guests and internal caregivers attribute a higher importance to autonomy in Basic physiological and personal needs than in Self-expression and relations with the socio-physical world; conversely, external caregivers give a higher importance to autonomy in Self-expression and relations with the socio-physical

Table 4a. ANOVA: Perceived importance of autonomy. Differences among groups

Perceived importance of autonomy	Group	*N*	*M*	*SD*	$F_{(2, 77)}$	*p*
Self-expression and	Elderly guests	40	$4.16^{a,b}$	.84		
relations with the	Internal caregivers	20	3.79^{b}	.62	3.42	< .05
socio-physical world	External caregivers	20	4.38^{a}	.51		
Basic physiological and personal needs	Elderly guests	40	4.48^{a}	.73		
	Internal caregivers	20	$4.16^{a,b}$	.69	5.93	< .01
	External caregivers	20	3.88^{b}	.36		

Table 4b. ANOVA: Perceived importance of autonomy. Differences between domains

Group	Perceived importance of autonomy	*N*	*M*	*SD*	$F_{(2, 77)}$	*p*
Elderly guests	Self-expression and relations with the socio-physical world	40	4.16^{b}	.84		
	Basic physiological and personal needs		4.48^{a}	.73		
Internal caregivers	Self-expression and relations with the socio-physical world	20	3.79^{b}	.62	8.58	< .001
	Basic physiological and personal needs		4.16^{a}	.69		
External caregivers	Self-expression and relations with the socio-physical world	20	4.38^{a}	.51		
	Basic physiological and personal needs		3.88^{b}	.36		

world than in Basic physiological and personal needs.

Mean aggregate scores of the three dimensions of attitude referring to Improvement in quality of life of elderly people through the use of IT showed that all domains identified through FA are deemed to be pertinent to the use of a technological help (Basic physiological and personal needs: $M = 3.26$, $SD = 1.12$; Socialisation and personal well-being: $M = 3.45$, $SD = 1.10$; Easiness of movement: $M = 4.04$, $SD = 1.14$).

A 3 x 3 repeated measure ANOVA (general linear model), considering the Group (Elderly guests vs. Internal caregivers vs. External caregivers) as a between subjects factor, and the domains of Improvement in quality of life of elderly people (Self-expression and relations with the socio-physical world vs. Basic physiological and personal needs) as a within subject factor, was performed.

A significant difference in the expected improvement in the three domains emerged ($F_{(2, 154)} = 19.64, p < .001$). Post hoc analyses (Bonferroni, $p < .05$) showed that the domain of Easiness of movement was considered more suitable for an improvement through the use of assistive IT than the domains of Basic physiological and personal needs and Socialisation and personal well-being. Also significant interactions were found.

In the comparison among groups in nursing homes, a significant difference in the evaluation of the Improvement in quality of life through the use

Table 5a. ANOVA: Improvement in quality of life of elderly people. Differences among groups

Improvement in quality of life of elderly people	Group	N	M	SD	$F_{(2, 77)}$	p
Basic physiological and personal needs	Elderly guests	40	2.85[b]	1.15		
	Internal caregivers	20	3.94[a]	1.05	7.48	< .01
	External caregivers	20	3.38[a,b]	.76		
Socialisation and personal well-being	Elderly guests	40	2.94[b]	1.16		
	Internal caregivers	20	4.08[a]	.64	10.86	< .001
	External caregivers	20	3.84[a]	.87		

Table 5b. ANOVA: Improvement in quality of life of elderly people. Differences among domains

Group	Improvement in quality of life of elderly people	N	M	SD	$F_{(4, 154)}$	p
Elderly guests	Basic physiological and personal needs	40	2.85[b]	1.15		
	Socialisation and personal well-being		2.94[b]	1.16		
	Easiness of movement		3.85[a]	1.43		
Internal caregivers	Basic physiological and personal needs	20	3.94[a]	1.05	2.65	< .05
	Socialisation and personal well-being		4.08[a]	.64		
	Easiness of movement		4.29[a]	.73		
External caregivers	Basic physiological and personal needs	20	3.38[b]	.76		
	Socialisation and personal well-being		3.84[a,b]	.87		
	Easiness of movement		4.18[a]	.72		

of IT, for both Basic physiological and personal needs ($F_{(2, 77)} = 7.48$, $p < .01$) and Socialisation and personal well-being ($F_{(2, 77)} = 10.86$, $p < .001$) was found (see Table 5a). Post hoc analyses (Bonferroni, $p < .05$) showed that internal caregivers expect a higher improvement in Basic physiological and personal needs than elderly guests; conversely, both internal and external caregivers expect a higher improvement in Socialisation and personal well-being than elderly guests. With reference to Easiness of movement ($F_{(2, 77)} = 1.19$, *ns*) no significant difference among groups in the expected improvement in quality of life of elderly people emerged.

In the comparison among domains of Improvement in quality of life of elderly people through the use of IT, a significant interaction effect ($F_{(4, 154)} = 2.65$, $p < .05$) was found (see Table 5b). Post hoc analyses (Bonferroni, $p < .05$) showed that elderly guests expect a higher improvement in Easiness of movement than in both Basic physiological and personal needs and Socialisation and personal well-being; external caregivers expect a higher improvement in Easiness of movement than in Basic physiological and personal needs. Conversely, internal caregivers expect the same level of Improvement in quality of life of elderly people in the comparison among domains.

Preference for Human vs. Technological Help

Independently of the role of respondent, a human caregiver was preferred over IT for the assistance

Figure 1. Improvement in the quality of care-giving: Highest and lowest mean scores

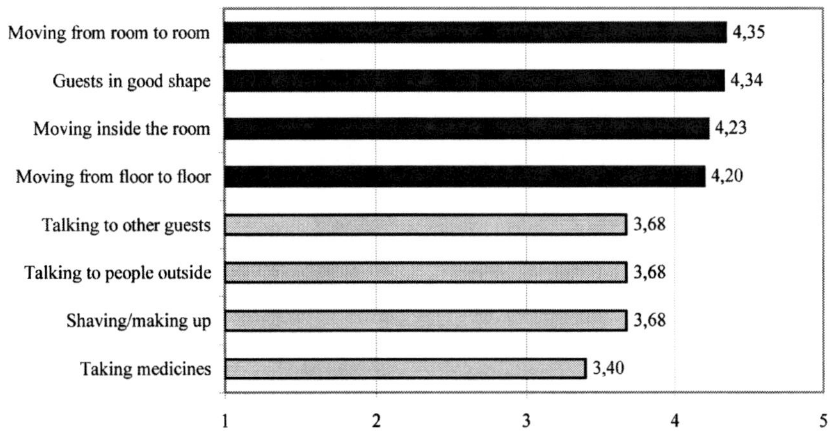

of elderly guests in 16 out of the 20 activities considered; the exception is related to the 4 activities implying movement. However, even in this case, a preference x role interaction emerged: elderly people prefer the help of a human caregiver much more than caregivers, be the movement inside the room (*Chi-square* = 9.54, $df = 4$, $p < .05$), from room to room (*Chi-square* = 14.92, $df = 4$, $p < .01$), from floor to floor (*Chi-square* = 11.82, $df = 4$, $p < .05$), or outside the nursing home (*Chi-square* = 9.57, $df = 4$, $p < .05$). The preference for the human assistance was particularly strong as regards activities implying personal care and well-being (wearing clothes: 83.8% of respondents; shaving/making up: 71.3%; eating/drinking: 70%; taking a bath: 60%), and social interaction (talking to other guests: 76.3%; talking to people outside the nursing home: 72.5%). For some of these activities (eating/drinking: *Chi-square* = 9.57, $df = 4$, $p < .05$; keeping in good shape: *Chi-square* = 32.27, $df = 4$, $p < .001$; leisure: *Chi-square* = 10.03, $df = 4$, $p < .05$), a role-oriented opposition emerged, with elderly guests expressing a stronger preference for a human assistant, external caregivers showing a preference for IT, and internal caregivers not expressing a preference.

Improvement in the Quality of Care-Giving

The analysis of caregivers' attitude toward the use of IT in nursing homes has also taken into account their own perspective as potential users of such devices. In other words, we explored not only the potential effects of IT on quality of life of elderly guests, but also whether or not, from the perspective of caregivers, IT are supposed to improve the quality of their care-giving. Results showed that Improvement in the quality of care-giving through the use of IT was expected with reference to all activities, but especially for activities requiring physical effort and, to a lesser extent, for activities referring to health, care, and socialisation, in which a physical effort is not required (see Figure 1).

We also explored if the four areas of activities identified through IADL and ADL (Personal care, Basic physiological needs and health, Autonomy of movement, and Socialisation) were identified also by caregivers as effective dimensions of assistive activity in nursing home. Reliability analyses of items referring to each areas showed a good internal consistency for Personal care (Cronbach's alpha = .83), Autonomy of movement

Table 6. ANOVA – Improvement in Quality of care-giving. Differences among areas of activity

Area of activity	*N*	*M*	*SD*	$F_{(3, 117)}$	*p*
Personal care	40	3.88[b]	.79		
Basic physiological needs and health	40	3.96[a,b]	.68	3.85	< .05
Autonomy of movement	40	4.20[a]	.74		
Socialisation	40	3.80[b]	.84		

(Cronbach's alpha = .84), and Socialisation (Cronbach's alpha = .87), and a moderate internal consistency for Basic physiological needs and health (Cronbach's alpha = .64). Aggregate scores for each area were calculated and a repeated measure ANOVA was performed to identify areas in which the use of IT seems to be more suitable (see Table 6). The analysis showed a significant difference in the expected Improvement of the quality of care-giving in the four areas ($F_{(3, 117)}$ = 3.85, $p < .05$). In post hoc analyses (Bonferroni, $p < .05$), Autonomy of movement emerged as the area in which the support of IT would better improve the quality of care-giving.

Discussion

This study was focused on attitudes toward the potential role of IT to support both the needs of guests and the activities of the staff members in nursing homes. We considered as a starting point the frameworks of ADL and IADL, which identify different areas of everyday activities in which autonomy of elderly people is related to quality of life and well-being (Katz et al., 1970; Lawton & Brody, 1969). We analysed how the autonomy in these areas of activities is conceived by all people who have to do – from the specific perspective of their role – with nursing homes, and how IT can improve these domains.

Elderly residents and caregivers in nursing homes do not seem to perceive the areas of personal care, basic physiological needs and health, autonomy of movement and socialisation as distinct domains; rather, these domains are merged together when people are asked to think about how important it is to be autonomous. In their representation, autonomy has to do with two distinct domains: a more basic one, which refers to primary/physiological needs and personal care; and a more high-level one, which involves self-expression, socialisation, and the connection with the world outside the nursing home. These results are consistent with the definition of quality of life put forward by Kane et al. (2003). Although both domains emerged as key determinants of personal autonomy, the different role played by people at the nursing home (guest, internal caregiver, external caregiver) showed a clear influence on their relative importance.

This finding confirms the need of assuming a psycho-social perspective when studying people's evaluations, as group membership becomes a key variable. For elderly guests, both are of great importance, but basic activities are perceived as the fundamental domain in which autonomy should be maintained. How can they consider themselves as autonomous persons if they are able to keep in touch with the world outside, but they cannot perform basic everyday activities? To be autonomous is important anyway, but the elderly seem to identify a path starting from primary to secondary needs and activities; this is in line with classical models of human development (Maslow, 1971). The same pattern emerged for internal caregivers, but presumably because basic activities are the most demanding for them, and the autonomy of the elderly in this respect would make better the quality of their job. Only for external caregivers the autonomy in self-expression, socialisation, and the connection with the world outside the nursing home is more important, probably because it involves activities which are pertinent to their own assistance.

When the role of IT for the improvement of quality of life of the elderly at nursing homes was considered, three distinct domains of potential application were found. All of them were considered by research in IT for the implementation of assistive devices, thus showing a good consistency between technological developments and people's representations. First is the domain of basic physiological and personal needs, involving primary activities (Labelle & Mihailidis, 2006). Second is the domain of leisure, well-being and socialisation, involving secondary needs (Taggart et al., 2005; Tyrer et al., 2006). Third is the domain of movement and physical activities, which can be recognized as a mid-point between primary and secondary needs: on the one hand, it allows performing basic activities; on the other hand, it is highly relevant to keep in touch with the world outside the nursing home (Pollack et al., 2002).

However, IT supporting elderly people in nursing homes were found to be more suitable for a specific area, namely the domain of movement and physical activities. This is the only domain for which elderly guests' and caregivers' attitude agrees, when they are asked to evaluate the perceived improvement in quality of life of the elderly if supported by IT. With reference to the other domains, the role played at the nursing homes was found to be important. As regards activities related to leisure, well-being and socialisation, caregivers are more confident than the elderly about the improvement in quality of life of guests if IT should assist them. In performing activities related to physiology and basic personal needs, the improvement in quality of life is expected by internal caregivers above all. These findings suggest that caregivers may perceive quality of life in terms of quality of their care-giving: the higher the improvement in autonomy of the elderly, the better the perception of the role of IT in reducing their stress and burden (Bank et al., 2006; Beauchamp et al., 2005; Chang et al., 2004). Conversely, elderly people seem to identify specific domains of activities whose meaning is chiefly social, and IT do not seem to be suitable devices in this respect. The analysis of preference for a human vs. technological help gives further support to this idea, as the elderly clearly prefer human assistance when compared to caregivers, also for those activities involving movement, for which the suitability of IT was found to be highest independently of role. The importance of social interaction for elderly people was consistently shown in the literature on quality of life in nursing homes (Cummings, 2002; Drageset et al., 2009). On the other hand, they may simply be unaware of the "social" potential of IT (Taggart et al., 2005). Interestingly, the attitude toward the domains of autonomy and the domains of potential improvement in quality of life did not show any relationship. This seems to suggest that, although people recognize in which areas of everyday activities autonomy is important, they are not influenced in the evaluation of the potential role of IT in nursing homes by their wishes.

Finally, if we consider the perspective of caregivers, they clearly identify the area of assistance in which the use of IT would best improve the quality of their care-giving: the domain of movement and physical activities, which also emerged as the most suitable from the perspective of the elderly. This domain should probably be considered as the more demanding for caregivers, especially if compared to the assistive activities related to personal care, medicine administration, leisure, and socialisation (Menzel, Brooks, Bernard & Nelson, 2004).

FUTURE RESEARCH DIRECTIONS

This study provided some hints on the potential use of IT in nursing homes. However, some limitations should be acknowledged, thus giving indications for future research. First, we stressed the importance to address the role of users' attitudes toward IT when studying acceptability. Attitudes, however, always develop within a specific social and cultural context; our analysis emerged from a very specific context (a nursing home near a middle-sized city in Northern Italy), and both elderly guests and caregivers showed specific socio-demographic characteristics. To give an example, the educational level of elderly guests was low, and attitudes toward the use of IT is affected by this variable (Giuliani, Scopelliti & Fornara, 2005; Scopelliti, Giuliani & Fornara, 2005). In order to gain a more comprehensive understanding of the representation and attitudes toward IT in nursing homes, a greater variety of locations and a larger sample is undoubtedly needed.

Second, our study showed that some domains of activities seem to be more suitable for the use of IT than others. However, it may depend, at least to some extent, on a biased representation of technology by users, who are not completely aware of the wide array of possibilities provided by recent developments in such a dynamic field. Some areas of implementation may appear more reasonable because the support of technologies is easier to imagine (e.g. in the domain of physical activities and rehabilitation), but when users are able to actually see what IT can do in real environments, their evaluations may be different (Cesta et al., 2007). As a consequence, the issue of the respondents' understanding of IT may be raised in our study, even though the procedure we adopted was developed to avoid this problem. So, future research should probably address the issue of use and acceptability of IT in nursing homes through different approaches, also including field experiments allowing the analysis of users' attitudes toward devices whose capabilities can be clearly recognized.

CONCLUSION

The role of IT in nursing homes can be highly relevant in preserving autonomy and promoting quality of life of the elderly. Caregivers can also benefit from the implementation of IT. Beyond practical advantages, the use of IT in nursing homes should be investigated within the systemic framework of person-environment relationships, in which psychological aspects are of importance. Far from being mere tools, IT are filled with meaning, and have to be considered in the light of personal needs and goals of final users. Future research on the role of IT in nursing homes should address more directly the issue of acceptability, by including in its agenda a thorough analysis of attitudes, needs, and preferences of people who have to use them. Moreover, beyond the idea of a "general user", also group differences should be better taken into account in this analysis. Our study showed that elderly residents, paid caregivers and volunteer helpers have different ideas on the importance for the elderly to be autonomous in different domains of activities, and different attitudes toward the use of IT in those domains. This suggests the relevance of considering the role people have in nursing homes when studying their evaluations.

REFERENCES

Altman, I. (1975). *The environment and social behavior: Privacy, personal space, territoriality and crowding*. Monterey, CA: Brooks/Cole.

Ball, M. M., Whittington, F. J., Perkins, M. M., Patterson, V. L., Hollingsworth, C., King, S. V., & Combs, B. (2000). Quality of life of assisted living residents: Viewpoints of residents. *Journal of Applied Gerontology*, *19*, 304–325. doi:10.1177/073346480001900304

Baltes, P. B., & Baltes, M. M. (1990). Psychological perspectives on successful aging: The model of selective optimization with compensation . In Baltes, P. B., & Baltes, M. M. (Eds.), *Successful aging: Perspectives from the behavioral sciences* (pp. 1–34). New York: Cambridge University Press. doi:10.1017/CBO9780511665684.003

Bank, A. L., Arguelles, S., Rubert, M., Eisdorfer, C., & Czaja, S. J. (2006). The value of telephone support groups among ethnically diverse caregivers of persons with dementia. *The Gerontologist*, *46*, 134–138.

Beauchamp, N., Irvine, A. B., Seeley, J., & Johnson, B. (2005). Worksite-based Internet multimedia program for family caregivers of persons with dementia. *The Gerontologist*, *45*, 793–801.

Bechtel, R., & Churchman, A. (Eds.). (2002). *Handbook of environmental psychology*. New York: Wiley.

Cesta, A., Cortellessa, G., Giuliani, M. V., Pecora, F., Rasconi, R., Scopelliti, M., & Tiberio, L. (2007). Proactive assistive technology: An empirical study. *Lecture Notes in Computer Science*, *4662*, 255–268. doi:10.1007/978-3-540-74796-3_25

Chang, B. L., Nitta, S., Carter, P. A., & Markham, Y. K. (2004). Perceived helpfulness of telephone calls. *Journal of Gerontological Nursing*, *30*, 14–21.

Charness, N., Czaja, S., Fisk, A. D., & Rogers, W. (2002). Preview gerontechnology 2002: Creative use of technology for better aging. *Gerontechnology (Valkenswaard)*, *1*, 198–202. doi:10.4017/gt.2001.01.03.008.00

Cody, M. J., Dunn, D., Hoppin, S., & Wendt, P. (1999). Silver surfers: Training and evaluating Internet use among older adult learners. *Communication Education*, *48*, 269–286. doi:10.1080/03634529909379178

Cook, A. M., & Hussey, S. M. (1995). *Assistive Technologies: Principles and Practice*. Saint Louis: Mosby.

Costa-Font, J., Elvira, D., & Mascarilla-Mirò, O. (2008). "Ageing in place"? Exploring elderly people's housing preferences in Spain. *Urban Studies (Edinburgh, Scotland)*, *46*(2), 295–316. doi:10.1177/0042098008099356

Cummings, S. M. (2002). Predictors of psychological well-being among assisted living residents. *Health & Social Work*, *27*(4), 293–302.

Czaja, S. J., & Rubert, M. P. (2002). Telecommunications technology as an aid to family caregivers of persons with dementia. *Psychosomatic Medicine*, *64*, 469–476.

Dewsbury, G., Taylor, B., & Edge, M. (2001). Designing safe smart home systems for vulnerable people. *Health Informatics Journal*, *8*, 104–110. doi:10.1177/146045820200800208

Drageset, J., Nygaard, H. A., Eide, G. E., Bondevik, M., Nortvedt, M., & Natvig, G. K. (2009). The impact of social support and sense of coherence on health-related quality of life among nursing home residents - a questionnaire survey in Bergen, Norway. *International Journal of Nursing Studies*, *46*, 65–75. doi:10.1016/j.ijnurstu.2008.07.005

Faulk, L. (1988). Quality of life factors in board and care homes for the elderly: A hierarchical model. *Adult Foster Care Journal*, *2*(2), 100–117.

Fazio, R. H., & Olson, M. A. (2003). Attitudes: Foundations, functions, and consequences . In Hogg, M. A., & Cooper, J. (Eds.), *The Handbook of Social Psychology* (pp. 139–160). London: Sage.

Forlizzi, J., Di Salvo, C., & Gemperle, F. (2004). Assistive robotics and an ecology of elders living independently in their homes. *Human-Computer Interaction*, *19*, 25–59. doi:10.1207/s15327051hci1901&2_3

Giannakouris, K. (2008). Ageing characterises the demographic perspectives of the European societies. *Eurostat Statistics in Focus 72/2008* from http://epp.eurostat.ec.europa.eu.

Giuliani, M. V. (1991). Towards an analysis of mental representations of attachment to the home. *Journal of Architectural and Planning Research*, *8*, 133–146.

Giuliani, M. V. (2003). Theory of attachment and place attachment . In Bonnes, M., Lee, T., & Bonaiuto, M. (Eds.), *Psychological theories for environmental issues* (pp. 137–170). Aldershot: Ashgate.

Giuliani, M. V., Scopelliti, M., & Fornara, F. (2005). Elderly people at home: Technological help in everyday activities. *Proceedings of 14th IEEE International Workshop on Robot and Human Interactive Communication* (August 13-15, 2005, Nashville, Tennessee U.S.A.), (pp. 365-370). Helsinki: Omnipress.

Gutheil, I. (1991). The physical environment and quality of life in residential facilities for frail elderly. *Adult Residential Care Journal*, *5*(2), 131–145.

Haas, B. K. (1999). A multidisciplinary concept analysis of quality of life. *Western Journal of Nursing Research*, *21*, 728–742. doi:10.1177/01939459922044153

Haigh, K. Z., & Yanco, H. (2002). Automation as caregiver: A survey of issues and technologies . In *Automation as caregiver: The role of intelligent technology in elder care* (pp. 35–53). AAAI Workshop.

Horner, B., & Boldy, D. P. (2008). The benefit and burden of "ageing-in-place" in an aged care community. *Australian Health Review*, *32*(2), 356–365. doi:10.1071/AH080356

Inada, H., Horio, H., Nakazawa, K., Sekita, Y., Yamanaka, T., & Harasawa, E. (1998). A study on a home health care support information system for health evaluation. *Journal of Medical Systems*, *22*(2), 69–75. doi:10.1023/A:1022639001300

Janse, A., Gemke, R., Uiterwaal, C., van der Tweel, I., Kimpen, J., & Sinnema, G. (2004). Quality of life: Patients and doctors don't always agree: A meta-analysis. *Journal of Clinical Epidemiology*, *57*(7), 653–661. doi:10.1016/j.jclinepi.2003.11.013

Kahn, R. (1994). Social support: Content, causes and consequences . In Abeles, R., Gift, H., & Ory, M. (Eds.), *Aging and quality of life* (pp. 163–184). New York: Springer Publishing Company.

Kane, R. A., Kling, K. C., Bershadsky, B., Kane, R. L., Giles, K., & Degenholtz, H. B. (2003). Measuring quality of life of nursing home residents. *Journal of Gerontology: Medical Sciences*, *58*, 240–248.

Kasser, V. G., & Ryan, R. M. (1999). The relation of psychological needs for autonomy and relatedness to vitality, well-being, and mortality in a nursing home. *Journal of Applied Social Psychology*, *29*(5), 935–954. doi:10.1111/j.1559-1816.1999.tb00133.x

Katz, S., Down, T. D., Cash, H. R., & Grotz, R. C. (1970). Progress in the development of the index of ADL. *The Gerontologist*, *10*(1), 20–30.

Kruzich, J., Clinton, J., & Kelber, S. (1992). Personal and environmental influences on nursing home satisfaction. *The Gerontologist*, *32*, 342–350.

Labelle, K. L., & Mihailidis, A. (2006). The use of automated prompting to facilitate hand washing in persons with dementia. *The American Journal of OccupationalTtherapy: Official publication of the American Occupational Therapy Association*, *60*, 442-450.

Lawton, M. P. (1989). Three functions of the residential environment. *Journal of Housing for the Elderly*, *5*, 35–50. doi:10.1300/J081V05N01_04

Lawton, M. P. (1991). A multidimensional view of quality of life . In Birren, J. E., Lubben, J. E., Rowe, J. C., & Deutchman, D. E. (Eds.), *The concept and measurement of quality of life in the frail elderly* (pp. 3–27). New York: Academic Press.

Lawton, M. P. (1994). Quality of life in Alzheimer's disease. *Alzheimer Disease and Associated Disorders*, *8*, 138–150.

Lawton, M. P., & Brody, E. M. (1969). Assessment of older people: Self-maintaining and instrumental activities of daily living. *The Gerontologist*, *9*(3), 179–186.

Lindenberger, U., Lövdén, M., Schellenbach, M., Li, S.-C., & Krüger, A. (2008). Psychological principles of successful aging technologies: A mini-review. *Gerontology*, *54*, 59–68. doi:10.1159/000116114

Liu, D., & Castle, N. G. (2009). Health information technology in nursing homes. *Journal of Applied Gerontology*, *28*(1), 38–58. doi:10.1177/0733464808321887

Loges, W. E., & Jung, J. Y. (2001). Exploring the digital divide: Internet connectedness and age. *Communication Research*, *28*(4), 536–542. doi:10.1177/009365001028004007

Mancini, J. (1980). Effects of health and income on control orientation and life satisfaction among aged public housing residents. *International Journal of Aging & Human Development*, *12*, 215–220.

Maslow, A. H. (1971). *The farther reaches of human nature*. New York: Penguin.

McCreadie, C., & Tinker, A. (2005). The acceptability of assistive technology to older people. *Ageing and Society*, *25*(1), 91–110. doi:10.1017/S0144686X0400248X

Menzel, N. N., Brooks, S. M., Bernard, T. E., & Nelson, A. (2004). The physical workload of nursing personnel: Association with musculoskeletal discomfort. *International Journal of Nursing Studies*, *41*, 859–867. doi:10.1016/j.ijnurstu.2004.03.012

Mitchell, J. M., & Kemp, B. (2000). Quality of life in assisted living homes: A multidimensional analysis. *Journal of Gerontology*, *55*, 117–127.

Morini, A., & Biocca, L. (2004). Il contributo della domotica . In Micheli, G. A. (Ed.), *La questione anziana. Ridisegnare le coordinate di una società che invecchia* (pp. 166–177). Milano: Franco Angeli.

Mynatt, E. D., Rowan, J., Craighill, S., & Jacobs, A. (2001). Digital family portraits: Providing peace of mind for extended family members. In *Proceedings of the ACM Conference on Human Factors in Computing Systems* (pp. 333-340). CHI 2001; Seattle, Washington. New York: ACM Press.

Parker, M. H., & Sabata, D. (2004). Home, safe home: Household and safety assistive technology . In Burdick, D. C., & Kwon, S. (Eds.), *Gerotechnology Research and Practice in Technology and Aging* (pp. 145–160). New York: Springer Publishing Company.

Perlmutter, L., Monty, R., & Chan, F. (1986). Choice, control and cognitive functioning . In Baltes, M., & Baltes, P. (Eds.), *The psychology of control and aging* (pp. 91–118). Hillsdale, NJ: Lawrence Erlbaum Associates.

Pollack, M., Engberg, S., Matthews, J. T., Thrun, S., Brown, L., Colbry, D., et al. & Roy N. (2002) Pearl: A mobile robotic assistant for the elderly. In *Proceedings of Workshop on Automation as Caregiver: the Role of Intelligent Technology in Elder Care (AAAI)*. Edmonton, AB.

Pollack, M. E. (2005). Intelligent technology for an aging population: The use of AI to assist elders with cognitive impairment. *AI Magazine*, *26*(2), 9–24.

Proshansky, H. M., Fabian, A. K., & Kaminoff, R. (1983). Place-identity: Physical world socialization of the self. *Journal of Environmental Psychology*, *3*, 57–83. doi:10.1016/S0272-4944(83)80021-8

Qassis, S., & Hayden, D. C. (1990). Effects of environment on psychological well-being of elderly persons. *Psychological Reports*, *66*(1), 147–150. doi:10.2466/PR0.66.1.147-150

Reid, D., & Ziegler, M. (1980). Validity and stability of a new desired control measure pertaining to psychological adjustment of the elderly. *Journal of Gerontology*, *35*, 315–402.

Scopelliti, M., Giuliani, M. V., & Fornara, F. (2005). Robots in a domestic setting: A psychological approach. *Universal Access in the Information Society*, *4*(2), 146–155. doi:10.1007/s10209-005-0118-1

Stefanov, D. H., Zeungnam, B., & Bang, W.-C. (2004). The smart house for older persons and persons with physical disabilities: structure, technology arrangements, and perspectives. *Neural Systems and Rehabilitation Engineering . IEEE Transactions on Rehabilitation Engineering*, *12*(2), 228–250. doi:10.1109/TNSRE.2004.828423

Strandberg, T. E., & Pitkälä, K. H. (2007). Frailty in elderly people. *Lancet*, *369*, 1328–1329. doi:10.1016/S0140-6736(07)60613-8

Street, D., Burge, S., Guadagno, J., & Barrett, A. (2007). The salience of social relationships for resident well-being in assisted living. *The Journals of Gerontology. Series B, Psychological Sciences and Social Sciences*, *62*, 129–134.

Taggart, W., Turale, S., & Kidd, C. D. (2005). An interactive robot in a nursing home: Preliminary remarks . In *Toward Social Mechanisms of Android Science*. Stresa, Italy: Cognitive Science Society.

Twigger-Ross, C. L., & Uzzell, D. L. (1996). Place and identity processes. *Journal of Environmental Psychology*, *16*, 205–220. doi:10.1006/jevp.1996.0017

Tyrer, H. W., Alwan, M., Demiris, G., He, Z., Keller, J., Skubic, M., & Rantz, M. (2006). Technology for Successful Aging. In *Proceedings, IEEE 2006 International Conference of the Engineering in Medicine and Biology Society* (pp. 3290-3293). New York.

White, H., McConnell, E., Clipp, E., Louise, B., Teague, C., & Navas, L. (1999). Surfing the net in later life: A review of the literature and a pilot study of computer use and quality of life. *Journal of Applied Gerontology*, *18*(3), 358–378. doi:10.1177/073346489901800306

Yamaguchi, A., Ogawa, M., Tamura, T., & Togata, T. (1998). Monitoring behavior in the home using positioning sensors. In *Proceedings of the 20th annual IEEE Conference on Engineering in Medicine and Biology*.

ADDITIONAL READING

Baruch, J., Downs, M., Baldwin, C., & Bruce, E. (2004). A case study in the use of technology to reassure and support a person with dementia. *Dementia (London)*, *3*, 372–377.

Bates, D. W., Cohen, M., Leape, L. L., Overhage, J. M., Shabot, M. M., & Sheridan, T. (2001). Reducing the frequency of errors in medicine using information technology. *Journal of the American Medical Informatics Association*, *8*(4), 299–308.

Burdick, D. C., & Kwon, S. (Eds.). (2004). *Gerotechnology: Research and Practice in Technology and Aging*. New York: Springer Publishing Company.

Chan, M., Bocquet, H., Campo, E., Val, T., & Pous, J. (1999). Alarm communication network to help carers of the elderly for safety purposes: A survey of a project. *International Journal of Rehabilitation Research. Internationale Zeitschrift fur Rehabilitationsforschung. Revue Internationale de Recherches de Readaptation*, *22*(2), 131–136. doi:10.1097/00004356-199906000-00008

Charness, N., & Schaie, K. (Eds.). (2003). *Impact of technology on successful aging*. New York: Springer.

Dang, S., Bank, S. L., Harris, J., Malphurs, J., Maymi, E. M., & Portales, A. (2004). Utilization of TLC technology by dementia family caregivers. *The Gerontologist*, *44*, 604–604.

Engström, M., Ljunggren, B., Lindqvist, R., & Carlsson, M. (2005). Staff perceptions of job satisfaction and life situation before and 6 and 12 months after increased information technology support in dementia care. *Journal of Telemedicine and Telecare*, *11*, 304–309. doi:10.1258/1357633054893292

Fozard, J., Rietsema, J., Bouma, H., & Graafmans, J. (2000). Gerontechnology: Creating enabling environments for the challenges and opportunities of aging. *Educational Gerontology*, *26*(4), 331–344. doi:10.1080/036012700407820

Haigh, H. Z., Kiff, L. M., Myers, J., Guralnik, V., Kirschbaum, K., & Phelps, J. Plocher, T., & Toms, D. (2003). *The independent lifestyle assistant (ILSA): Lessons learned* (Tech Rep ACSPO3023). Honeywell Laboratories.

Hanson, E. J., & Clarke, A. (2000). The role of telematics in assisting family carers and frail older people at home. *Health & Social Care in the Community*, *8*, 129–137. doi:10.1046/j.1365-2524.2000.00232.x

Harrington, T., & Harrington, E. L. (2000). *Gerontechnology why and how*. Maastricht: Shaker.

Kart, C., Kinney, J., Murdoch, L., & Ziemba, T. (2002). *Crossing the digital divide: Family caregiver's acceptance of technology (Tech Rep)*. Oxford, Ohio: Scripps Gerontology Center, Miami University.

LoPresti, E. F., Mihailidis, A., & Kirsch, N. (2004). Assistive technology for cognitive rehabilitation: State of the art. *Neuropsychological Rehabilitation*, *14*(1/2), 5–39. doi:10.1080/09602010343000101

Mahmood, A., Yamamoto, T., Lee, M., & Steggell, C. (2008). Perceptions and Use of Gerotechnology: Implications for Aging in Place. *Journal of Housing for the Elderly*, *22*(1/2), 104–126. doi:10.1080/02763890802097144

Mann, W. C., & Helal, A. (Eds.). (2006). Promoting independence for older persons with disabilities. *Selected Papers from the 2006 International Conference on Aging, Disability and Independence, 18*. Assistive Technology Research Series.

Mann, W. C., Ottenbacher, K. J., Fraas, L., Tomita, M., & Granger, C. V. (1999). Effectiveness of assistive technology and environmental interventions in maintaining independence and reducing home care costs for the frail elderly: A randomized controlled trial. *Archives of Family Medicine*, *8*, 210–217. doi:10.1001/archfami.8.3.210

Mihailidis, A., Boger, J., Craig, T., & Hoey, J. (2008). The efficacy of the COACH prompting system to assist older adults with dementia through activities of daily living: An intervention study. *BMC Geriatrics*, *8*(28).

Mihailidis, A., Cockburn, A., Longley, C., & Boger, J. (2008). The acceptability of home monitoring technology among community-dwelling older adults and baby boomers. *Assistive Technology*, *20*(1), 1–12.

Mihailidis, A., Fernie, G. R., & Barbenel, J. (2001). The use of artificial intelligence in the design of an intelligent cognitive orthosis for people with dementia. *Assistive Technology*, *13*, 23–39.

Mynatt, E., Melenhorst, A., Fisk, A., & Rogers, W. (2004). Aware technologies for aging in place: Understanding user needs and attitudes. *Pervasive Computing*, *3*(2), 36–41. doi:10.1109/MPRV.2004.1316816

Pew, R., & Hemel, S. V. (Eds.). (2004). *Technology for Adaptive Aging*. Washington, D.C.: National Academies Press.

Roy, N., Baltus, G., Fox, D., Gemperle, F., Goetz, J., Hirsch, T., et al. (2000). Towards Personal Service Robots for the Elderly. *Workshop on Interactive Robots and Entertainment* (WIRE). Pittsburgh, PA.

KEY TERMS AND DEFINITIONS

Analysis of Variance (ANOVA): A statistical technique used to evaluate the association between a categorical independent variable (IV) and a continuous dependent variable (DV). It is based on the comparison between the variability of data between conditions (the levels of the IV) and within the cases (the subjects on which the DV is measured).

Attitude: A central construct in social psychology, referring to the evaluations of an object through the expression of some degree of favor or disfavor. Attitudes are traditionally considered to have a cognitive, affective, and behavioural component.

Chi-Square Analysis: A statistical technique used to evaluate the association between categorical variables. It is based on the comparison between expected and observed frequencies of cases in each cell of a table, in which columns represent the levels of the first variable, and rows represent the levels of the second variable.

Cronbach's Alpha: A measure of scale reliability referring to internal consistency. It expresses how well a set of items measures a latent construct. It is assessed through the evaluation of the average correlation of each item with all the other included in the scale.

Factor Analysis: A statistical technique used to reduce a list of variables to a smaller number of latent constructs. It is based on the measurement of intercorrelations observed in the data.

Quality of Life: A multidimensional construct concerning the subjective evaluation of satisfaction of individual needs, goals and desires, and the perception of well-being in different domains of everyday life.

Self-Efficacy: Trust in personal ability to reach specific goals.

Successful Ageing: A process based on the identification of personal resources, the stimulation of residual competences, and the support to lost capabilities in ageing people, with the aim of promoting life satisfaction.

Chapter 16

Supporting Family-Based Care for Aged Patients with Chronic Illness

Lemai Nguyen
Deakin University, Australia

ABSTRACT

Family carers play an important role in care for aged patients with chronic illness, particularly in home and community settings. The information needs of these family carers and their patients are poorly understood and current health information systems do not adequately support their needs. This chapter describes current models in understanding patient and family carer information needs and analyses technology solutions in a new field of consumer health informatics. The analysis shows that current technology solutions in consumer health informatics fail to effectively support aged people in their own management of chronic illness and as well failing to support their family carers. The chapter also identifies key research issues in developing technologies that support aged patients and family carers in chronic illness management.

INTRODUCTION

About 13 per cent of our Australian population is aged 65 years or older (Department for Health and Ageing, 2008). This is projected to rise to 18 per cent by 2021 and to 26 per cent (around 7 million people) in 2051. Healthy ageing and aged care have increasingly become an important, national issue. There is a wide range of social, health and economic aspects in ageing and aged care. One of many challenging aspects is how to cope with and manage the increasing incidence of chronic illness, for example depression, diabetes, heart disease, asthma, and various types of cancer. Morbidity and mortality related to major chronic diseases increase after 65 years of age (AIHW, 2006). Chronic illness, if not well managed, can become an expensive challenge (WHO, 2002). For optimum chronic illness management, an integrated hospital and home continuous care programme is required (ITTA-eHealth, 2004).

Hospital care involves high costs and is an inefficient use of care resources compared with preventative, primary or community care. Family carers play an important role in reducing costs

DOI: 10.4018/978-1-61520-825-8.ch016

associated with aged patients with chronic illness. Better understanding of and addressing the information needs of family carers is expected to provide significant benefits in providing chronic illness care for aged patients (Clayton, Butow, & Tattersall, 2005). Family carers not only provide home-based continuous care for aged patients but also often act as their proxy information seeker (Williamson & Asla, 2009). In addition to having a rich understanding of the patient-specific care needs, the family carer also has his/her own needs, for example, access to patient's health information, knowledge about the patient's illness and care instructions, and how to cope with emotions and stress associated with care (Docherty, et al., 2008). Inclusion of the information needs and information behaviours of the family carers in health information strategies and systems can be expected to provide significant benefits.

Consumer health informatics is a relatively new field that aims to understand and address the information needs of patients and their families, and empower them in health care planning, delivery and decision making (Altinkemer, De, & Ozdemir, 2006; Hersey, Matheson, & Lohr, 1997). Based on an analysis of the information needs of patients and family carers, especially in the context of home-based aged care, this chapter reviews and discusses current technologies used in consumer health informatics. A research programme will be described to support family-based care by addressing the information needs of aged patients and family carers.

INFORMATION NEEDS OF AGED PATIENTS WITH CHRONIC ILLNESS AND THEIR CARERS

What is Consumer Health Informatics?

Traditional health informatics, also referred to as medical informatics, tends to focus on the information needs of the healthcare provider, as opposed to the healthcare consumer (see Figure 1). Consumer health informatics can be described as "*the study, development, and implementation of computer and telecommunications applications and interfaces designed to be used by health consumers*" (Ferguson, 1993).

Eysenbach (2000, p. 1715) offers a more comprehensive definition using five dimensions:

- *Analysing and modelling consumer preferences, information needs, and information use;*
- *Developing and evaluating methods and applications to support consumers in obtaining and using health information;*
- *Developing and evaluating methods and applications to integrate consumer needs and preferences into information management systems in clinical practice, education, and research;*
- *Investigating determinants, conditions, elements, models, and processes to design, implement, and maximise the effectiveness of computerised information and telecommunication and network systems for consumers; and*
- *Studying the effects of these systems on public health, the patient-professional relationship, and society.*

This chapter focuses on the first dimension in Eysenbach's (2000) definition and addresses the information needs and behaviours of a specific group of health consumers, that is aged patients and family carers in chronic illness management. Key research directions will be outlined with a view to addressing the second dimension, that is to develop and evaluate methods and applications to support these information needs and behaviours of this group of health consumers.

The following three sub-sections discuss three topic areas in the literature: chronic illness care, aged care, and the information needs of health

Figure 1. Customer Health Informatics – Focus of new medical informatics (adapted from Eysenbach, 2000)

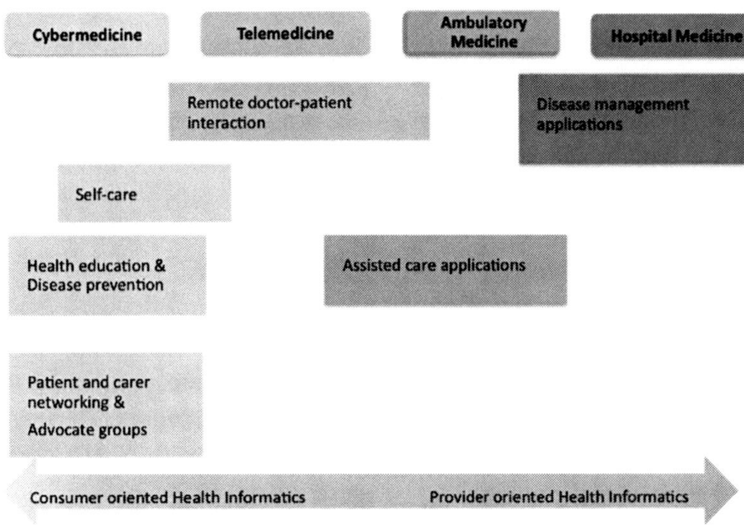

consumers, particularly patients and their family carers.

Chronic Illness Care

Chronic illnesses are difficult to diagnose often due to multiple factors leading to their onset and a long period of development with unclear symptoms. Major chronic illnesses include different types of cancer (especially lung cancer, colorectal cancer), chronic kidney disease, depression, diabetes, arthritis, asthma, heart disease, and osteoporosis. Dimensions of chronic care include survival, quality of care, patient wellness and satisfaction, and cost-effectiveness (Kattlove & Winn, 2003). Chronic illness requires continuous care involving long term interactions between multiple parties including patients, family carers and various healthcare professionals.

Consequently, the care process often involves high costs over long timeframes (for diagnosis, treatment, and follow-up procedures), and continuous communication and sharing of health information between patients, their family carers and the healthcare team (Von Korff, Gruman, Schaefer, Curry, & Wagner, 1997). Chronic care is an information intensive process. Traditional approaches to health information systems focus on the provision of information services to various healthcare specialists and heath care providers through using applications such as electronic patient records, appointment booking, ambulance dispatch, hospital admission and discharge information systems, ePrescribing, supply chain management, and so on (Ayres, Soar, & Conrick, 2006; Felkey, Fox, & Thrower, 2006; Soar, 2004). Such systems, however, provide limited information support for patients and their families to equip them with knowledge about illness and treatment, allow them access to their health records, and enable them to undertake self-care. Therefore, current health information systems do not effectively support the patient and their family carer in care decision-making and home-based care management. Consequently, the current systems are limited in their efficiency, quality and outcome of care provision through the lack of interfaces for patients and their family carers.

The Chronic Care Model was developed to improve chronic care outcomes (Bodenheimer,

Wagner, & Grumbach, 2002; Wagner, et al., 2005). According to this model, more effective interactions between the healthcare team and their informed and activated patients can play a key role in improving care outcomes. The model proposes a set of six components: a system to coordinate care activities within and across the care provider organisations; a structured delivery system to support evidence-based care; a decision support system that is consistent with scientific evidence and patient preferences; clinical information systems to facilitate individual patient care planning, enable access to patient information, and send reminders to the involved care providers; self-management tools to support the patient in health assessment and goal-setting, action planning, problem-solving and follow-up; and community resources to support collaborative care to the outpatient as well as outpatient self-management. Recently, Coleman and her colleagues (2009) examined 82 research papers describing the implementation of CCM mostly in the U S, and international settings such as Europe, Canada and Australia since 2000. Their examination shows increased quality of care and improved outcomes, such as more informed patients, better adherence to care management plans, fewer hospital visits and shorter stays in hospital, reduced risk of cardiovascular disease in diabetic patients, and improved quality of life. Coleman et al. (2009) also found that many care providers implemented different components of CCM at different levels of sophistication. For example, the implementation of the self-management component ranged from formal (a hospital-led programme), semi-formal (community-based nurse educator), to informal (motivating interviews). Although CCM was not seen as an immediately replicable solution in the short term, evidence of cost-effectiveness in the long term was beginning to emerge (Coleman, et al., 2009).

This chapter will expose the self-management component of CCM in terms of assisting outpatients and their families in acquiring skills and confidence to support self-care and assess their healthcare needs routinely. The active participation by the patient and their family carer, such as the acquisition and interpretation of health information, specific illness information and patient records, personalised self-care instructions, and information communication and sharing, is critical.

Aged Care

Aged care covers a range of settings including community care, residential care, and palliative care (see for example, Abbey, 2005; Gray, 2003; Zimmerman, et al., 2003). Community care refers to services to aged people who live at home, such as home visits by community nurses, home maintenance, meal delivery, assistance with shower and laundry, assistance with dressing, shopping and other activities of daily living. Residential care refers to a range of services to patients who can no longer live at home. Residential care services are provided at residential aged care facilities, such as hostels, retirement villages and nursing homes. Residential care services can be low care or high care. Low care includes accommodation, personal care, social activities, and occasional nursing care. In addition to such services, high care provides continuous nursing care to aged people with high frailty. Palliative care refers to supportive end-of-life care and aims at reducing suffering, identifying and addressing physical, psychological, social, cultural and spiritual needs of the patient, family and care staff. Amongst these, community-based care (that is home-based care) has been described as a strong trend in aged care in Australia (Gray, 2003; Productivity Commission, 2008) due to an increasing number of elderly people who wish to stay at home as long as possible. In response to this, a number of programmes, for example, the Home and Community Care (HACC) and Community Aged Care Packages (CACP), were introduced in Australia to provide basic maintenance and support services to older people wishing to live independently at home (Productivity Commission, 2008).

There is a wide range of issues associated with ageing covering independence, clinical, psychosocial and other dimensions. Clinical issues include chronic illness management, with dementia and mental illnesses and fall prevention and fall detection being important components (Nay & Garratt, 2005). Over 80% of people over 65 years old have three or more chronic illnesses (AIHW, 2006). Recently, assisted independent living using technology intervention has emerged as a focus in community care (Soar & Croll, 2007). This includes the use of monitoring devices, for example detecting falls or tracking locations of dementia patients at risk of wandering.

Psychosocial issues are recognised as an important aspect in healthy ageing and aged care (Gallant, Spitze, & Prohaska, 2007; Keleher, 2006). Family, friends, and social networking can significantly influence the quality of life of older adults. In their studies into chronic illness care for aged patients, Gallant and colleagues (2007) conducted 13 focus groups and identified positive as well as negative influences by family and friends. Positive influences are associated with disease management activities, medications and testing, doctor visits and consultations, information sharing with the doctor, care decision-making, and psychosocial coping. Negative influences can be differences in dietary, unwanted advice, lack of understanding, and depressing talks. Understanding and addressing the health information needs of elderly people and their family carers will increase in importance to support the desire of elderly people with chronic illnesses to receive care in their home.

Information Needs of Patients and Family Carers

Human information needs and behaviours are subject to many previous studies in information science. Wilson (2000) provided an overview of the area and described different stages of needs initiation, information seeking, processing and using. This author also highlighted various contextual and individual factors influencing human information behaviours. In a recent analysis (Logan & Tse, 2007), general human information behaviours were integrated in the context of healthcare with a view to facilitating further studies into consumer health informatics. In this analysis, a cyclic model of information behaviours (consisting of need, access and evaluate) was linked to the information source (informal to formal) through a channel (characterised with interactivity, modality, and accessibility). This section describes findings specific to information needs of patients and family carers to refine such general models and relate the findings to aged patients with chronic illness.

Patient information needs studied in the literature have included those for cancer and palliative care. A systematic review of 18 studies (Ankem, 2005) reported that two types of information, about illness and about treatment, are most important to cancer patients. In addition, other factors such as age, time since diagnosis, and patient decision making style were found to influence patient information needs.

Patient information behaviours have been described using a three stage information journey model: (i) information need identification, (ii) information search, and (iii) information interpretation (Adams & Blandford, 2005; Adams, Blandford, & Attfield, 2005). During the first stage, the patient identifies his/her information needs, which can be direct (such as a specific illness) or passive (such as a disease outbreak announcement in the media). During the second stage, the patient searches for information. This stage is associated with various factors such as information sources, search tools and time, and information presentation formats. During the third stage, the patient makes sense of information, evaluates and applies it for decision making. Adams and her colleagues (Adams & Blandford,

2005; Adams, et al., 2005) also highlighted that the family plays an important role in all the stages and that information needs vary prior to and after the consultation with doctors.

Nguyen and Shanks (2007) refined and extended the information journey of the family carer and identified four stages: information needs identification, searching, interpreting, and sharing. This model confirms the dynamic changes in information needs of the family carer over time. Second, it highlights the ad-hoc and on-going learning process of information searching and interpreting due to the lack of formal medical knowledge on the part of most family carers. The family carer sought information from different sources: doctors, specialists, web sites, friends and other patients and carers, on the Internet and face-to-face with clinicians. Integrating and interpreting the information from different sources was a challenge for him or her. Third, the extended information sharing stage includes collaboration with doctors to confirm information interpretation and information content creation to share with other patients and families. Nguyen, Shanks, Vetere and Howard (2008) also identify social needs (emotional, financial, cultural values etc) as an important factor in care decision-making by the family carer. A shared understanding about cultural values among the patient, family carer, and the healthcare professional was found to be important in enabling the family carer to access the patient's clinical information and health records. The family carer in this study reported feeling empowered and more positive when sharing his information, observations, and experiences with other patients and family carers. The family carer is identified as a key stakeholder in healthcare provision. Technologies that assist family carers in accessing health information and sharing their rich patient information with doctors and their experiences with other patients and families can be expected to result in positive health outcomes.

Although the Nguyen extended information model for family carers was developed from a case study of a family carer for a young cancer patient, its implications are in line with findings from a systematic review of the literature in information needs of the family carer in palliative care (Docherty, et al., 2008). Docherty and colleagues (2008) undertook a systematic review and analysis of 34 research papers, published during the period from January 1994 to November 2006, discussing information needs of family carers (informal carers) in palliative care. They noted a trend to providing more palliative care in patients' homes. They highlighted differences between information needs by the patient and family carer: different perceptions about the level of access to the patient's clinical information, carer' instructions, and different emotions and experiences with the illness. Their analysis stresses the importance of understanding and addressing the information needs of informal carers (family and friends) and suggests a need to support complex triadic interactions between the patient, family carer and care provider.

Williamson and Asla (2009) specifically studied information needs and information behaviours of aged people. These authors analysed aged factors such as physical limitations, loss of senses, declined cognitive abilities, and reduced social networks and strongly argued for the importance of incidental information acquisition through social networks, social engagement and communication. Amongst their suggestions were compensating for the reduced information literacy of aged patients through better supporting their proxy information seekers, that is carers, and encouraging greater use of the Internet as a potential information tool in improving health literacy for aged people. They also suggested that portable technology and social networking software can be used more to search for aged care and chronic care information and to communicate and interact with care providers and clinicians.

In summary, the information needs and behaviours of the patient as well as of the family carer need to be better understood and supported. The three information stages described in Adam et al. (2005) are consistent with information behaviours described by other authors (Logan & Tse, 2007; Wilson, 2000). These encourage more support for information interpretation by the patient and to extend information systems beyond the information needs of professional carers. The fourth stage of information (creation and) sharing described in Nguyen et al. (2008) extends the previous information behaviours and recognises a new behaviour of the information user: information creation and collaboration. Any model of information behaviours of the information users needs to be placed within a specific context and within an information environment (Logan & Tse, 2007). The specific context can be understood through a number of contextual factors, for example family situation and culture, as well as individual factors, for example physical limitations, loss of senses, cognitive ability. The information environment includes information sources, media, accessibility, search and presentation tools, social networks, modes (on-line vs. face-to-face, synchronous vs. asynchronous). Further, information needs of the patient and his/her carer can be different and need to be better understood.

Synthesis

With respect to providing support for family-based care for aged patients with chronic illnesses, this section draws and relates findings from the literature in chronic care, aged care and information science. The shift towards home-based care and recognition of the significant role of family carer suggest a need for providing more information for family-based care. The family carer has a specific patient and holds rich information about that patient. This information could potentially be made available to support the professional care process and enable better continuous care. Access to outpatient and inpatient data is important to family carers just as it is for professional carers. Family carers need to learn and understand care instructions and be included in the care communication loop with the clinical care team(s).

The discussion in the above sub-sections suggests the following focus areas in developing a tool to address the information needs of aged patients and their family carers:

- *Identifying relevant parties involved in care services and an appropriate information access level for each party.* The literature in aged care and palliative care tend to suggest three parties including the patient, the family carer, and the care provider. However, there are different individual professionals and care teams behind the concept of a 'care provider party'. The chronic care model (Bodenheimer, et al., 2002; Wagner, et al., 2005) also suggests utilising community based resources (for example community nurse educators and counsellors). The levels of access to patient's clinical information may be different across different parties and need to be negotiated.
- *Supporting relevant and on-going information provision and updates (about illness, treatment options, treatment plans, patient records, monitoring and care guides) to the patient as well as family carer.* As explained earlier in this chapter, chronic care is an information intensive process. The self-management component of the chronic care model (Bodenheimer, et al., 2002; Wagner, et al., 2005) promotes an informed and activated patient. When applying this model in chronic care for an aged patient, it is important to not only recognise and support a family carer's role in providing continuous care to the patient but also support his/her role in acting as a proxy health information user. The patient and family carer need case-specific and relevant information to enable family-based care. As chronic care is also an on-going process, the informa-

tion needs are continuous. A plan for long-term interactions is important, as opposed to one-off information provision such as handing health brochures and leaflets.

- *Supporting information interpretation (for example accessing and communicating with healthcare experts).* Previous studies (Adams & Blandford, 2005; Nguyen & Shanks, 2007) stress the importance of information interpretation of the patient and family carer through the activities of sense making, relating the retrieved information to their specific situation, and evaluating information for decision making. Not being equipped with medical knowledge, it is important to provide the patient and family carer with access to quality and relevant information, and support their information integration and interpretation for decision making. In addition, it is important to recognise and support their learning processes through different illness stages and health events in on-going chronic care. The inclusion of the patient and family carer in the communication loop with healthcare experts can improve their information interpretation and decision making.
- *Supporting content creation and information sharing (social networking tools and community resources).* Patients and family carers create and share health information, emotions, illness and treatment experiences, and cultural value (see for example Nguyen & Shanks, 2007). They find emotional and social support from each other. Moreover, they feel empowered when sharing with others their newly acquired knowledge. It is common that the community of patients and family carers lies largely outside the world of health professionals. Therefore, it is important to assist the patient and family carer in networking, creating and sharing as well as in safely and effectively using the information created and shared within their community.

The next section reviews current technologies and assesses their support for the information needs of health consumers.

TECHNOLOGIES TO SUPPORT THE AGED CARE INFORMATION NEEDS OF FAMILY CARERS

Desktop Applications

Desktop applications refer to a range of PC-based or kiosk-based computer programmes which typically use hypertext or hypermedia. These applications often provide topic-based health education, health promotion, and/or tutorials with multiple-choice questions for the public or a specific patient to learn about his/her illnesses and care plan. For example, the Grampian asthma study of integrated care (GRASSIC) provides computer based health education for asthma patients. Based on computer based patient records, GRASSIC generates personalised and interactive questionnaires for patients. This enhanced patient education programme was found useful in reducing hospital admissions and improving patient mobility (Osman, et al., 1994). CardioPharm is another example. It is a kiosk-based touch screen multimedia programme designed for health promotion (Hariri, Goodyer, Meyer, & Anderson, 2000). This interactive programme collects information about the patient's health information (weight, height, blood pressure, etc) and health behaviours, assesses their risk to heart diseases, and provides them with suggestions for how to change their lifestyle habits and health behaviours to reduce the risk. The programme was found useful in disseminating health information and increasing health promotion activities in community pharmacies (Hariri, et al., 2000). A number of desktop applications make use of patient medical records to retrieve health information relevant to the patient's specific situation (Bental, Cawsey, Pearson, & Jones, 2000).

Computer games have also been explored as interactive media in health education, disease prevention and intervention. ReMission (http://www.re-mission.net), HopeLab (http://www.hopelab.org) and The Cancer Game (http://www.cancergame.org) are examples of computer games to assist young cancer patients in learning about cancer and chemotherapy, promoting self-care and adherence to cancer medications, and improving their sense of power and control in living with cancer. Great Detective, Space Inhalers, and The Wheezing Wizard (http://www.myonlinewellness.com/topic/asthmagames) are games to disseminate information to children with asthma and their parents about causes of asthma, how to use inhalers, and developing an asthma plan. The Magi and The Sleeping Star (http://themagigame.net) is an example of games to disseminate health information about diabetes and knowledge to control the disease. Peng (2009) conceptually examined approaches to computer games, video games, television and radio entertainment-education programmes and pointed out key issues for further development in this area. Identification, a concept describing how players relate themselves to game characters, can be seen as essential in leveraging the effect of attitude and behaviour modification of health computer games. Interactivity and narrative are ambivalent but are equally important features of computer games. Interactivity needs to be matched with individual differences of users to increase engagement and effectiveness of health related games. Narrative can be essential in identification. Degrees of interactivity and narrative need to be better understood and optimised in developing computer games to disseminate health information and lead to intended change in life style and behaviours. Another issue, pointed out by Peng (2009), is gender differences in length and frequency of game playing, that is males tend to play longer and more often than females and some games, associated with a certain illness, can be relevant to one gender, but not the other. An underlying assumption is that the target audience is young users.

It has been reported that elderly patients were generally satisfied with computer based health education although there were age-related issues, for example sensory, especially visual deficits (Lewis, 1999). This author conducted an analysis of 66 articles including 21 research-based reports published from 1971 to 1998. Findings from this analysis suggested that computer based health education appeared to be both effective and efficient, however knowledge acquisition over time could be an issue for future research. Further, computer based health education should be flexible and customised to adapt to the dynamics of the patient's information needs and social circumstances. What is relevant to our discussion in this chapter is that the interface design and health education materials should be age-sensitive.

Desktop consumer health informatics applications tend to support individual health information acquisition and improve patient health literacy. However, such applications do not support patient content creation and information sharing with involved care teams, nor support on-going provision of updated information about illness, treatment and follow-up activities. Further, the carers' information needs, such as care instructions for carers, access to the patient's clinical information, and interactions with care teams, are not explicitly supported in parallel with information needs of the patient. An appropriate computer interface for elderly patients is also required.

Health Web Sites

The information service providers of content for health information web sites can be classified as government, community, and private organisations, such as hospitals and specialists. Hospital web sites, such as Mercy Health (see http://www.mercyhealth.net), and various NSW hospitals, such as Prince of Wales and Royal Hospital for Women, (http://www.sesiahs.health.nsw.gov.au/Hospitals/index.asp) tend to use their web sites as a marketing tool rather than providing health services specific to their patients. MDKiosk (http://www.mdkiosk.com), VirtualMedicalCentre (http://www.virtualmedicalcentre.com), and WebMD (http://www.emedicinehealth.com) are examples of health consumer information web sites whose information is provided and edited by different groups of medical professionals. These web sites are highly interactive and provide multimedia rich health information across a large range of health topics. Health consumers can search for information about illnesses based on symptoms or classification of illnesses. Different treatment methods are explained at these web sites. WebMD also offers self-care instructions and facilities to locate a doctor and book an appointment on-line. Such health information provides patients and their carers with medical knowledge and supports their decision making, whether to self-care at home or go to see a doctor. Such web sites tend to address a general audience rather than being specifically designed around the needs of aged people. Although they provide a Sign-In option, such sites still provide information services and health education to the general public rather than tailoring information to a specific patient and his/her care team. Their sign-in members can post questions and exchange information with other members in an on-line forum. However, the level of interactivity is rather low. This could be due to two factors: the low number of messages generated daily and asynchronous responses to messages posted by sign-in members. Currently, there is no support for private medical consultations between the patients, carers and medical professionals at such health education web sites.

In addition to providing information about public health, diseases and self-care instructions, some web sites also provide fee based consultation services to web patients. Such information and interactions are offered by private healthcare providers using software provided by technology vendors such as HotHealth by Global Health. Recently, an Intelligent Disease Management Service has been developed as a collaborative effort between the Western Australia Department of Health, Diabetes Australia, and other parties. The Intelligent Disease Management Service involves different hospitals, general practitioners, specialists and care teams, and health insurance companies and is delivered via broadband network to support collaborative care for patients with diabetes (Georgeff & Hilton, 2009). This project aims at improving communication between medical practitioners, providing health information, and supporting patients' self-care and increasing their adherence to monitoring and medications.

There is an increasing number of community and social applications (Powell, Lowe, Griffiths, & Thorogood, 2005). Web 2.0 provides a vehicle for WWW applications and services which support social networking, collaboration and information sharing between Web users. Numerous web 2.0 applications, such as blogs, wikis, chat, web forums, and social networking sites (e.g. Twitter and Facebook) provide information services to health consumers. Such web sites allow users to share their experiences and provide emotional support to each other. Virtual environments have recently emerged and allow interactions between health consumers and specialists, for example MD kiosk or HealthInfo islands on Second Life. SecondLife (http://www.secondlife.com) is a three-dimensional virtual world where people meet and interact with each other using their avatars.

In summary, many health web sites tend to provide general information rather than tailored illness information and care plans. Interactions between patients and health professionals are often asynchronous. Social networking and information sharing web sites become popular and adopted by health consumers.

Mashup Applications to Public Health

Mashup is an emerging type of application that integrates information services from different applications and delivers them on the Internet for different purposes, such as education, business, and healthcare. For example, Healthmap Global Disease Alert (http://www.healthmap.org/en) provides facilities to search for and check disease outbreak notices in different countries, cities and towns. Healthmap Global Disease Alert aggregates multiple data sources including Program for Monitoring Emerging Diseases, World Health Organisation, EuroSurveillance, Goggle News and Google Maps, commercial news feed Moreover, and Global Wildlife Disease News Map. MC+A Physician Finder is another example. It is a mashup of Google Search and Google Maps to allow users to search for doctors in their area.

Mashup applications offer potential benefits through integrating data and services provided by different care teams. Nevertheless, support for interactions between care providers and collaborative care for specific aged patients and their family carers should also be included. At present, customised health information, self-care instructions, or their social networking are not well supported.

Tele-Health

Tele-health applications provide flexible care delivery to patients in remote areas via electronic means (Whetton, 2005). Hence, such applications can be useful in providing home-based care services for aged patients in the community. For example, Smart Home includes electronic and computer-based devices to support frail elderly, chronic illness sufferers and people with disabilities and promote their independence (Soar & Croll, 2007). Other examples include interactive voice response (IVR) systems and remote monitoring devices for patients with cardiovascular diseases and diabetes (Black, et al., 2004; Jacobus, 2003). Tele-health offers potential benefits in providing home-based care services for aged patients in the community through information provision and updating, remote consultation and monitoring, and information communication and sharing. While technologies are available, major adoption concerns include access, quality, cost efficiency, and provider selection (see for example a report by Demiris, Edison, & Vijaykumar, 2005). Although family carers and patients are the primary adopters of tele-health, the family context (family carers and social context) is often neglected and not discussed in this report. Longitudinal evaluative studies on a large scale are required (Whetton, 2005). In addition, there is a lack of a solid business model to enable the remote monitoring of clinical data supplied from using tele-health devices and technical support for the patients and their carers (Soar & Croll, 2007). Therefore, tele-health technologies are still at an early adoption stage.

Discussion

Current technologies can be seen as useful in providing health education information, promoting self care and adherence to medication and care plan, searching for clinics, assisting patients in decision-making (e.g. whether to undertake self-care or see a doctor, which treatment options are appropriate), or receiving paid private consultations and tele-health care.

The following observations can be made:

- Many consumer health informatics applications provide general knowledge rather than customise their information services to specific patients based on their health records.
- Many health information web sites provide patients and their carers with medical information about illnesses, assist them in locating a doctor, but do not support an ongoing process of diagnosis, treatment and

follow-up for patients and their family carers according to a chronic care plan.

- The triadic interactions between the medical professional, patient and family carer as discussed in section 2.4, are not explicitly supported. Many desktop applications, health web sites, tele-health and marshup applications tend to address the information needs of the patient with an assumption that the carer will act as a proxy information seeker. Different needs of the patient and carer are not supported. This is important because aged patients with chronic illness require continuous care, which often takes place in a family context.
- While some web sites provide on-line consultations, there is lack of synchronous access to medical experts to support their information interpretation and validation in a timely manner. This could be due to different time zones and asynchronous responses when a medical professional, often acting as a health forum moderator, responds to a message posted by the forum member.
- There is a lack of integration and decision-making tools. Patients and family carers receive information from different web sites and other sources (books, hospital leaflets, their (often brief) meetings with doctors and specialists…). Patients and family carers search for information from different web sites, from different medical professionals and other patients and carers. A challenge for them and their family carers is how to interpret and integrate information and make decisions.
- Social networking and information sharing web sites are popular and widely adopted by patients and carers. Carers may act as a proxy information seeker on behalf of aged patients.
- Further, an appropriate user interface is required to increase useability and accessibility for aged patients.

RESEARCH AGENDA

Based on the discussion in the previous sections, a research programme is proposed with a view to developing and evaluating technologies to support family-based care for aged patients with chronic illness management. The programme extends the patient-based view into the family context. Relevant care teams and participants, for example doctors, specialists, district nurses, aged care providers, and family carers, will be identified. Relevant access levels will be designed and assigned in designing a care programme to support specific needs of individual aged patient. Age-related factors, such as cognitive load limitation, visual deficit, and physical constraints and impediments of aged patient and their family carer will be identified and taken into account when developing a suitable user interface for aged patients. Based on the information needs of patients and family carers and a review of current technologies, the research programme includes the following four components.

1. Reducing the clinical knowledge gap through information provision to patients and family carers:
   - Topic based knowledge system including health education with references to clinical knowledge systems and recommended information sources such as useful, endorsed web sites;
   - Customising information provision based on patient's specific illness and health records;
   - Customising information presentation and delivery methods to suit aged patients and their carers' needs and information behaviours.

   - Patient and family carer access to their electronic health records (their access levels are subject to the patient's consent and discussion with the clinician);
   - Web based knowledge systems, accessible with mobile and desktop technologies.
2. Providing patients and families with care instructions:
   - Personalised care instructions;
   - Monitoring and note-taking capabilities;
   - Encouraging electronic diary use and sharing.
3. Enhancing communication and collaboration with healthcare specialists:
   - Multiple communication channels (asynchronous and synchronous) with general practitioners, specialists, care teams and other healthcare professionals;
   - Mechanism to locate and communicate with specialists as a patient or a carer;
   - Providing reminders and supporting on-going interactions and information flows between the care professional, patient and carer.
4. Community support:
   - Access to communities including other patients and their families using social software such as Web forums and social networking systems (profiles and networks of friends);
   - Experience sharing – public and private communication.

This proposed programme has led to the development of several research projects. Currently, a funded project is underway conducting a focus group and a series of case studies to explore and model information and social needs as well as information behaviours of the elderly and their carers. The research participants include elderly who reside in the community, their informal carers, and community aged care staff. Research findings will be published later.

In conclusion, the above proposed research will empirically enhance current models of information needs of the patient and family carer (Adams & Blandford, 2005; Nguyen, et al., 2008), the self-management component of the Chronic Care Model (Bodenheimer, et al., 2002) and aged care literature (Nay and Garratt, 2005; Gallant et al., 2007; Williamson and Asla, 2009). Based on findings from this research, technologies will be developed and incorporated within a clinical care and aged care plan. The four components outlined in this research programme should be integrated within a clinical chronic care model to support care services provided by healthcare professionals. Family and cultural factors will be taken into account when implementing and evaluating the technologies in order to improve care outcomes and quality of life for the patient or the elderly person. In addition, as aged patients often have multiple illnesses requiring complex chronic care and at times acute care, complex information needs and behaviours of the patient and their family carer will need to be examined thoroughly and supported.

The proposed research will support healthy ageing through providing an integrated web based environment to provide health information, communication channels with doctors, and social networking for patients and families. In future, this web environment can incorporate mobile phone applications, virtual (3D) and interactive voice capabilities for tele-health.

ACKNOWLEDGMENT

The author would like to thank Professor Graeme Shanks, the University of Melbourne, for sharing his thoughts and insights, and for his great mentorship, support and encouragement in conducting research in health informatics and information analysis.

REFERENCES

Abbey, J. (2005). Palliative Care. In R. Nay & S. Garratt (Eds.), *Nursing older people – Issues and innovations* (2nd ed., pp. 259-275). Churchill Livingstone: Elsevier.

Adams, A., & Blandford, A. (2005). Digital libraries' support for the user's information journey. *IEEE and ACM Joint conference of digital libraries ACM/IEEE JCDL 2005.*

Adams, A., Blandford, A., & Attfield, S. (2005). Implementing digital resources for clinicians' and patients' varying needs. *BCS Healthcare Computing 2005.*

AIHW. (2006). *Chronic diseases and associated risk factors in Australia (No. AIHW Cat. No. PHE 81.)*. Canberra: Australian Institute of Health and Welfare.

Altinkemer, K., De, P., & Ozdemir, Z. (2006). Toward a Consumer-to-Healthcare Provider (C2H) electronic marketplace. *Communications of the AIS*, *18*, 413–430.

Ankem, K. (2005). Types of information needs among cancer patients: A systematic review. *Library & Information Science Research, 15*(2).

Ayres, D., Soar, J., & Conrick, M. (2006). Health information systems. In Conrick, M. (Ed.), *Health informatics: Tranforming healthcare with technology* (pp. 197–211). Thomson, Social Science Press.

Bental, D., Cawsey, A., Pearson, J., & Jones, R. (2000). Adapting web-based information to the needs of patients with cancer. In *Proceedings of International Conference on Adaptive Hypermedia and Web-based systems*, Trento, Italy.

Black, L.-A., McTear, M., Black, N., McMeel, C., Harper, R., & Lemon, M. (2004). Talking telemedicine: Is the interactive voice-logbook evolving into the cornerstone of diabetes healthcare? *AAAI Fall Symposium, Dialogue Systems for Health Communication*, Menlo Park, California.

Bodenheimer, T., Wagner, E. H., & Grumbach, K. (2002). Improving primary care for patients with chronic illness. *Journal of the American Medical Association*, *288*(14), 1775–1779. doi:10.1001/jama.288.14.1775

Clayton, J. M., Butow, P. N., & Tattersall, M. H. N. (2005). The needs of terminally ill cancer patients versus those of caregivers for information regarding prognosis and end-of-life issues. *Cancer*, *103*(9), 1957–1964. doi:10.1002/cncr.21010

Coleman, K., Austin, B. T., Brach, C., & Wagner, E. H. (2009). Evidence on the chronic care model in the new millennium. *Health Affairs*, *28*, 75–85. doi:10.1377/hlthaff.28.1.75

Demiris, G., Edison, K., & Vijaykumar, S. (2005). A comparison of communication models of traditional and video-mediated health care delivery. *International Journal of Medical Informatics*, *74*(10), 851–856. doi:10.1016/j.ijmedinf.2005.03.018

Docherty, A., Owens, A., Asadi-Lari, M., Petchey, R., Williams, J., & Carter, Y. H. (2008). Knowledge and information needs of informal caregivers in paliative care: a qualitative systematic review. *Palliative Medicine*, *22*(2), 153–171. doi:10.1177/0269216307085343

Eysenbach, G. (2000). Consumer health informatics. *BMJ (Clinical Research Ed.)*, *320*(7251), 1713–1716. doi:10.1136/bmj.320.7251.1713

Felkey, B. G., Fox, B., & Thrower, M. R. (2006). *Health care informatics: A skill-based resource.* Washington, D.C.: American Pharmacists Association.

Ferguson, T. (1993). What is consumer health informatics? Retrieved May 2008 from http://www.fergusonreport.com/articles/tfr07-03.htm.

Gallant, M. P., Spitzc, G. D., & Prohaska, T. R. (2007). Help or hindrance? How family and friends influence chronic illness self-management among older adults. *Journal of Research on Aging*, *29*, 375–409. doi:10.1177/0164027507303169

Georgeff, M., & Hilton, J. (2009). *The use of a web based chronic disease management service (CDMS) for collaborative care*. Retrieved from www.hisa.org.au/system/files/u2233/hic09-2_MGeorgeffJHilton.pdf.

Gray, L. C. (2003). 2020: A vision for aged care in Australia. *Australian Society for Geriatric Medicine Newsletter, 6*(6).

Hariri, S., Goodyer, L. I., Meyer, J., & Anderson, C. (2000). Assessment of a touch-screen promotion system in independent community pharmacies. *Health Education Journal*, *59*(1), 99–107. doi:10.1177/001789690005900109

Hersey, J. C., Matheson, J., & Lohr, K. N. (1997). *Consumer health informatics and patient decision making* (No. Report NR AHCPR - Publication No.98-N001). Rockville.

ITTA-eHealth. (2004). *Chronic care improvement: How medicare transformation can save lives, save money, and stimulate an emerging technology industry* (No. An ITAA E-Health White paper): A Product of the ITAA E-Health Committee.

Jacobus, C. (2003). *The billing, cost, and outcome benefits from remote patient monitoring (Whitepaper)*. Cybernet Medical Systems.

Kattlove, H., & Winn, R. J. (2003). Ongoing care of patients after primary treatment for their cancer. *CA: a Cancer Journal for Clinicians*, *53*(3), 172–196. doi:10.3322/canjclin.53.3.172

Keleher, H. (2006). Promoting healthy ageing. In Keleher, H., & Murphy, B. (Eds.), *Understanding health – A determinants approach*. Oxford: Oxford University Press.

Lewis, D. (1999). Computer-based approaches to patient education: A review of the literature. *Journal of the American Medical Informatics Association*, *6*(4), 272–282.

Logan, R. A., & Tse, T. (2007). A multidiscipline conceptual framework for consumer health informatics. *Studies in Health Technology and Informatics*, *29*(Part 2), 1169–1173.

Nay, R., & Garratt, S. (2005). *Nursing older people – Issues and innovations* (2nd ed.). Churchill Livingstone: Elsevier.

Nguyen, L., & Shanks, G. (2007). Families as carers - Information needs in a cultural context. In *Proceedings of 18th Australasian Conference on Information Systems*, Toowoomba, Australia.

Nguyen, L., Shanks, G., Vetere, F., & Howard, S. (2008). Information systems and healthcare XXVIII: The information needs of family carers in collaborative healthcare. *Communications of the Association for Information Systems*, *23*(10).

Osman, L. M., Abdalla, M. I., Beattie, J. A. G., Ross, S. J., Russell, I. T., & Friend, J. A. (1994). Reducing hospital admission through computer supported education for asthma patients. *BMJ (Clinical Research Ed.)*, (308): 568–571.

Peng, W. (2009). Theoretical guidance for using computer and video games for health intervention. *Paper presented at the annual meeting of the International Communication Association*, Sheraton New York.

Powell, J. A., Lowe, P., Griffiths, F. E., & Thorogood, M. (2005). A critical analysis of the literature on the Internet and consumer health information. *Journal of Telemedicine and Telecare, 11 Suppl*(1), 41-43.

Productivity Commission (2008). *Trends in aged care services: Some implications*.

Soar, J. (2004). Improving health and public safety through knowledge management. *Thailand International Conference on Knowledge Management*, Bangkok, Thailand.

Soar, J., & Croll, P. (2007). Assistive technologies for the frail elderly, chronic illness sufferers and people with disabilities - A case study of the development of a smart home. In *Proceedings of 18th Australasian Conference on Information Systems*, Toowoomba, Australia.

Von Korff, M., Gruman, J., Schaefer, J., Curry, S. J., & Wagner, E. H. (1997). Collaborative Management of Chronic Illness. *Annals of Internal Medicine*, *127*(12), 1097–1102.

Wagner, E., Bennett, S., Austin, B., Greene, S., Schaefer, J., & Vonkorff, M. (2005). Finding common ground: Patient-centeredness and evidence-based chronic illness care. *The Journal of Alternative and Complementary Medicine*, *11*(Supplement 1), S7-0S15.

Whetton, S. (2005). *Health informatics: a socio-technical perspective*. South Melbourne: Oxford University Press.

WHO (2002). *Innovative care for chronic conditions: Building blocks for action* (No. WHO/MNC/CCH/02.01 - NLM classification: WT 31).

Williamson, K., & Asla, T. (2009). Information behaviour of people in the fouth age: Implications for the conceptualisation of information literacy. *Library & Information Science Research*, *31*, 76–83. doi:10.1016/j.lisr.2009.01.002

Wilson, T. (2000). Human Information Behaviors. *Informing Science, Special Issue on Information Science Research, 3*(2).

Zimmerman, S., Gruber-Baldini, A., Sloane, P. D., Eckert, J. K., Hebel, J. R., & Morgan, L. A. (2003). Assisted living and nursing homes: Apples and oranges? *The Gerontologist*, *43*, 107–117.

Chapter 17
Telenursing in Aged-Care:
Systematic Evidence of Practice

Sisira Edirippulige
University of Queensland, Australia

Rohana Basil Marasinghe
University of Sri Jayewardenepura, Sri Lanka

ABSTRACT

The rapidly growing aged population is challenging conventional methods of care provision. Global ageing, combined with other challenges, has compelled health systems to explore new methods for providing health care. Telenursing, providing nursing care at a distance using new technologies, is identified as one alternative. The lack of evidence for the effectiveness of telenursing in aged care is a drawback for its wider use. The aim of this chapter is to review the evidence of randomised controlled trials (RCT) in geriatric telenursing practices. We performed a systematic literature review using the Ovid Medline and Pubmed databases on telenursing. A total of 62 articles were retrieved and 18 studies were selected for comprehensive analysis. The review found that the RCTs were conducted in different areas of geriatric telenursing and various information and communication technologies (ICT) were used in the interventions. Although robust evidence, based on RCTs in aged care telenursing is yet to emerge, the majority of current studies suggest that telenursing is an effective tool.

INTRODUCTION

Providing care for the rapidly growing aged population has challenged the health systems in both the developed and developing world. The cost associated with aged care is predicted to increase steadily. The lack of healthcare professionals to provide appropriate care for the ageing population has compelled governments to rethink traditional care systems. The solutions to these problems require significant financial investment and long term policy implementation. Evidence is emerging that if used in the right context, telehealth may offer some solutions to these critical problems. Telenursing in aged care is one of the emerging areas. This chapter sets out to report on a systematic review of literature on the use of telenursing techniques in aged care.

DOI: 10.4018/978-1-61520-825-8.ch017

BACKGROUND

Elderly people are more likely to suffer from conditions of disability, chronic disease, and multiple impairments, and are therefore more likely to require care. Research shows that almost 75% of elderly (aged 65 and over) have at least one chronic illness (Calkins, Boult, & Wagner, 1999). The cost associated with treating the elderly with chronic conditions is high and continuing to grow. The World Health Organization (WHO) predicts that chronic disease will be the leading cause of disability by 2020 and will be the most expensive problem facing health care systems (Belfield & Colin-Thome, 2004). For example, studies show that caring for people with chronic diseases consumes approximately 78% of all health care spending in the United States – more than $USD 1 trillion annually (ITAA e-Health Committee, 2004).

One serious obstacle to providing care to the growing number of aged people is the lack of health professionals. The difficulty of recruiting and retaining quality health care workers has been well documented (Cooper, Getzen, McKee & Laud, 2002; Blumenthal, 2004). Nurses traditionally play an important role in aged care. According to the projections of the Health Resources and Services Administration (HRSA), the shortage of nurses in the US could escalate to one million by 2020 (HRSA, 2006). Australia projects a shortage of 40,000 nurses by 2010 (International Council of Nurses, 2005). The lack of nurses is a critical issue in developing countries too. According to WHO statistics, Sub Saharan Africa is short of 60,000 nurses to meet Millennium Development Goals (World Health Report, 2006).

Governments and health systems around the world are in search of solutions to the problems posed by global ageing. Logic dictates that the optimal solution would be the producing of more doctors, nurses and other health professionals. However, this requires long-term policy changes, funding and infrastructure development. Therefore, among other alternative solutions, the role of telehealth to address some critical issues in aged care has been identified.

What is Telenursing?

Telenursing is the use of information and communication technologies to provide nursing services at distance (Edirippulige et al., 2007). Telenursing can be used in both healthcare settings and non-institutional settings – that is at home or in an assisted-living facility (Wootton, Kvedar, & Dimmick, 2006). Telenursing applications may include real time techniques, (for example videoconferencing or telephony) and store-and-forward techniques, (for example email or web-based applications).

The use of real time and store-and-forward telenursing applications is becoming popular in providing health services to remote patients. Devices such as videoconferencing equipment help health professionals to make 'virtual visits' to deliver services to their patients. Such applications are becoming commonplace in both institutional and non-institutional settings. Studies have shown that real time transmission of audio and video data is sufficient to facilitate a quality online consultation. Telenursing applications provide access to nursing care for remote patients while offering numerous benefits to the care givers. Figure 1 depicts the use of videoconferencing for gait assessment by a geriatric specialist involving a patient at a remote location.

In addition to interactive video techniques, various devices such as alarms, sensors and monitoring equipment are being used in telenursing applications (Darkins, Dearde, & Rocke, 1996). The use of these systems allows nurses to monitor physiological parameters such as blood pressure, blood glucose and respiratory peak flow. Telenursing techniques help provide accurate and timely information for making critical decisions relating to care processes. Telenursing can also

Figure 1. Telenursing in aged care

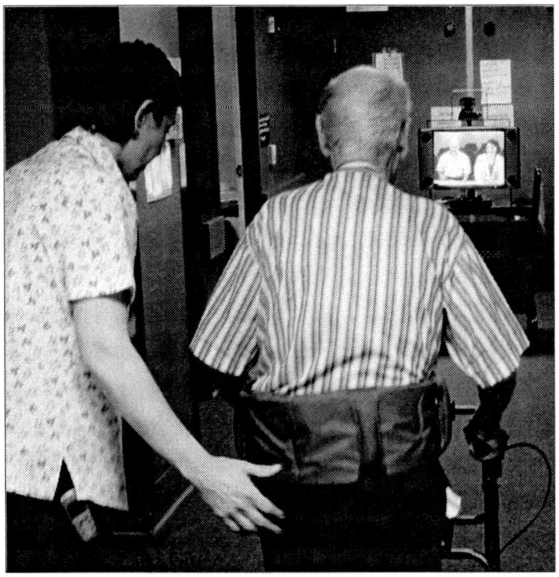

offer alternative ways for more frequent contact with clients, avoiding traditional home visits.

Interest in telenursing is increasing. Data shows that nearly 40% of American-based home health agencies employ some kind of telehealth in their day to day operations (Wootton, Kveda, & Dimmick, 2006). The last few years have seen an increase in the number of manufacturers of home telehealth equipment, mainly in the US. It is believed that in the United States almost half of the on-site nursing visits could be replaced by telenursing (AHRQ, 2000). The situation is similar in Europe and other developed countries. There is a significant increase in the number of home telehealth episodes. During 2001-2003 the number of Medicare home health users increased to 2.6 million and the number of episodes rose to 36 million in the US (Wootton, Kvedar, & Dimmick 2006).

THE OBJECTIVE

The objective of this chapter is to report on a systematic review of literature in telenursing in aged care. Considering that randomized controlled trials (RCT) are the gold-standard in best evidence, this study sets out to analyze the RCTs in telenursing in aged-care. The study examined the following areas:

1. dominant health areas of telenursing
2. technologies used in telenursing practices
3. evidence for feasibility and effectiveness of telenursing

METHODOLOGY OF THE REVIEW

This literature search was conducted in December 2008 using the electronic database of Ovid Medline and Pubmed. The search terms used were: "nurs*.mp" and "age*.mp" or "Geriatr*.mp" and "random*.mp" in combination with the search term "tele*.mp" or "Distanc*.mp" or "mobile*.mp" or "video*.mp" or "VC.mp".

The Pubmed search was performed using the following Mesh terms. ("Nursing"[Mesh] AND ("Telephone"[Mesh] OR "Telenursing"[Mesh] OR "Cellular Phone"[Mesh] OR "Computer Communication Networks"[Mesh])) AND ("Geriatric Nursing"[Mesh] OR "Homes for the Aged"[Mesh]) AND Random*.

Titles, abstracts and keywords were scanned for every record retrieved. Full articles were retrieved for further assessment if the primary information suggested that the study:

1. involved any telehealth technique
2. involved nurses or nursing care
3. had a randomized allocation of patients with a clearly defined control group

If there were doubts about these criteria (in title, key words or abstract) the full article was retrieved for clarification. By examining the cited references in the retrieved papers, past reviews were performed to obtain papers that are relevant to the study. Using the cited reference search of the Web of Science, a forward search was also performed. This was to obtain any studies which cite the retrieved article. Articles with duplicate publications and incomplete data were excluded.

RESULTS

A total of 62 articles were retrieved from the selected databases, and 18 RCTs in aged care-telenursing were selected for detailed analysis. The studies included research work relating to therapy, education, administration and research in telenursing in aged care. Therapeutic studies included interventions in follow up care, counseling and health promotion. Several studies have attempted to examine the effectiveness of telehealth techniques in providing education for nurses and patients. The effectiveness of ICT in health administration has also been the focus of research. Meanwhile, evidence shows that information and communication technologies are becoming useful tools in health and medical research. The following table summarizes the selected RCTs in aged-care telenursing.

As Table 1 demonstrates, the technology used in telenursing studies has been diverse; studies have tested the effectiveness of a variety of technologies (both real-time and store-and-forward) ranging from telephone, email, and interactive web tools to videoconferencing. The following section will provide a more detailed description of RCT studies in aged-care telenursing.

Providing Therapy

A study conducted by Heyn-Billipp (2001) tested the effectiveness of an interactive computer program in providing mental health aged services. Randomized groups of elderly people were provided with an interactive computer program with a combination of nurse visits, no nurse visits and no computer terminals. The study showed that a combination of nurse visits with interactive computer use was capable of improving self-esteem and reducing depression among elders. A combination of nurse substitute visit with the interactive computer use showed a significant effect on improving self-esteem, but had no effect on depression. However, interactive computer use without a nurse or a substitute did not show a significant effect on either improving self-esteem or depression.

McDonald, Thomas, Livingston, and Severson (2005) conducted a study to test the effect of a videotape on post operative pain management in elderly patients. The intervention group watched a videotape about communication and management of postoperative pain while the control group watched a videotape about managing postoperative pain only. Outcome measures were pain relief (i.e. patient's perception that pain has decreased over time), and pain interference (i.e. the degree to which pain had interfered with daily activities). The intervention group reported greater pain relief and less pain interference on postoperative day 1. The control group reported greater pain relief on postoperative day 2 after attaining a pain interference level similar to the intervention group.

Camberg et al. (1999) used store-and-forward messages over the telephone (in the form of continuously playing audio messages) in the context of a simulated presence (SP). Simulated Presence (SP) is a technique used to provide a personalized intervention for a person especially with moderate to severe cognitive impairment. This is done by obtaining some of the best loved memories of the person's lifetime, and then introducing those memories to the patient. In this study, those memories have been introduced in the format of a telephone conversation using a continuous play audio tape system. This study compared three groups. The intervention group (SP) was able to listen to the best-loved memories of the person's lifetime in the format of a telephone conversation. The placebo group was provided with an audio tape of a person reading the newspaper. The control group received the usual care. The outcomes

Table 1. Summary of randomized controlled trials in aged-care telenursing

Study	Intervention	Control	Effect on Condition
Providing therapy			
Heyn-Billipp (2001)	(a) weekly nurse visits to teach interactive computer use with telecommunications terminals (NV+ICU) (b) interactive computer with substitute nurse trainer (SN+ICU) over 3 months	weekly nurse visits, but no computer terminal use. (NoICU)	*Over 3 months,* Rosenberg Self-Esteem Scale (NV+ICU) > NoICU; (SN+ICU) > NoICU; (ICU) = NoICU Geriatric Depression Scale (NV+ICU) > NoICU; (SN+ICU) = NoICU; (ICU) = NoICU
McDonald et al. (2005)	Communication group watching a videotape about communicating and managing postoperative pain (C+M)	videotape about managing postoperative pain only (TAU)	*Postoperative Days 1 and 2, and 1 and 7 days after hospital discharge* C + M = TAU
Camberg et al. (1999)	(a) simulated Presence (SP) (b) placebo audio tape of a person reading the newspaper (PL)	TAU	Direct observations SP = TAU > PL overall agitation or mood aspects of withdrawal SP = TAU
Hiltunen et al. (2005)	Home visit and telephone calls at 2, 6, and 10 weeks after an face- to-face meeting by an advanced practice nurse (APN)	TAU	*Over 12 weeks,* APN = TAU
Follow up care			
Kauh et al. (2005)	Geriatric Rehabilitation Unit (GRU) (a) comprehensive geriatric assessment (b) weekly interdisciplinary team rounds with a geriatrician + geriatric nurse practitioner (GNP) (c) followed up with telephonic case management over 1 year	TAU	*At discharge,* Length of stay GRU < TAU *At 1 year,* Hospital readmissions GRU < TAU
Mahoney et al. (2007)	(a) two in-home visits from a trained nurse/ physical therapist (b) recommendations to the subject and their primary physician, (c) referrals to physical therapy and other providers (d) 11 monthly telephone calls and a balance exercise plan (HV& TC)	Home safety assessment (HSA)	Rate of falls HV & TC = HSA Nursing home days HV & TC < HSA
Gaugler et al. (2008)	Enhanced counselling and support (ECS) (a) 6 sessions of individual and family counselling (b) support group participation (c) continuous availability of ad hoc telephone counselling over 16 years	TAU	*over 2 years* (Mittelman et al., 2007) Self-Rated Health (SRH) ECS <TAU *Over a 9.5-year period,* Burden (modified Zarit Burden Interview) Depressive symptoms (Geriatric Depression Scale). ECS <TAU

TAU - Treatment As Usual
SMAF- Functional Autonomy Measurement System
SPS - Social Provisions Scale

were measured either by direct observation or by weekly reports of overall agitation or mood aspects of withdrawal. On direct observation, the study found that the simulated presence (SP) and the usual care were equally effective when compared with the placebo. However, there was no significant difference found on overall agitation or mood aspects of the withdrawal.

Hiltunen et al. (2005) reported a community based clinical trial among cardiac elders. The efficacy enhancement of nursing intervention was based on social, cognitive and bio-psycho-behavioural domains. This intervention was delivered by advanced practice nurses (APN) to 110 cardiac elders who were recovering from myocardial infarction and coronary artery bypass grafting. The intervention was designed to have an initial meeting and follow up visits by an APN, including telephone calls at 2, 6, and 10 weeks after discharge. Over 12 weeks, the intervention showed no differential effectiveness, but it showed the feasibility of the intervention to enhance the recovery process of cardiac elders.

Follow Up Care

Some studies utilised telehealth applications purely for follow up care. Kauh, Polak, Hazelett, Hua, & Allen (2005) conducted a telephonic case management study. This was a multidisciplinary study to compare discharge outcomes, post-discharge health care use, and death rates among geriatric patients. The intervention consisted of comprehensive geriatric assessment and weekly interdisciplinary team-rounds with a geriatrician and a geriatric nurse practitioner together with telephone case management. A year-long study reported that the length of stay at discharge and hospital admissions significantly improved in the intervention group compared with the usual care group.

Mahoney et al. (2007) conducted a community based RCT to reduce the rate of falls in high-risk community-dwelling older adults. In this intervention, regular (monthly) telephone contacts were made in combination with home visits by a nurse/physical therapist over 11 months. Results revealed that there was no difference with the primary outcome measure (rate of falls) when compared with the usual care. However, there was a decline in number of days spent in nursing homes.

Byles et al. (2004) conducted a RCT on health assessments for older Australian veterans and war widows. The intervention consisted of annual or 6 monthly home-based health assessments by health professionals, with telephone follow-ups, followed by a written report submitted to a nominated general practitioner. The outcomes such as quality of life, hospital admission rates or deaths were not significantly different to that of usual care over 3 years.

The comparative study mentioned previously (Hiltunen et al. 2005) evaluating the effect of home visits by an advanced practice nurse (APN) with the usual care for cardiac elders can also be considered as a follow-up study. The intervention was designed to have an initial meeting together with follow up visits by APN, including telephone call follow ups at 2, 6, and 10 weeks after discharge. Over 12 weeks, the intervention showed no differential effectiveness, but it showed the feasibility of the intervention to enhance the recovery process of cardiac elders.

Counseling and Support

Counseling and support is an area where telehealth has played an active role. Gaugler, Roth, Haley, and Mittelman (2008) reported a study to determine whether counseling and support reduce the burden and depressive symptoms of spouse-caregivers of patients with Alzheimer's disease (AD) during the transition to institutional care. An enhanced counseling and support intervention consisted of six sessions of individual and family counseling, support group participation, and continuous availability of ad hoc telephone counselling sessions. The outcome measures included burden (modified Zarit Burden Interview) and depressive symptoms (Geriatric Depression Scale). Results revealed that burden and depressive symptoms were significantly lower for caregivers in the treatment group compared to the controls receiving usual care at the time and after institutionalization. The study findings were consistent with the study conducted by Mittelman, Roth, Clay, and Haley (2007) that showed an improvement in the parameters of self-rated health measures.

Health Promotion

Liddle et al. (1996) conducted a study to assess whether older people could maintain their quality of life and independence after their homes had been modified as recommended by an occupational therapist. There were three groups: the intervention group was provided with the recommendations of an occupational therapist while the control group was not. The third group did not require any intervention but were followed up by telephone and postal questionnaire. The outcomes were measured using the Sickness Impact Profile, the Philadelphia Geriatric Center Morale Scale, the Life Satisfaction Index, assessment of Activities of Daily Living, the Health Assessment Questionnaire and change in residence. There was no significant difference over a 6 month period on any selected outcomes. The training program followed up by telephone consultations over 3 months did not show a significant difference on program adoption over the absence of such intervention.

Byles et al. (2004) conducted a study to assess the effect of home-based health assessments for older Australians (community-living veterans and war widows) on health-related quality of life, hospital and nursing home admissions, and death. The intervention consisted of annual or 6-monthly home-based health assessments by health professionals, with telephone follow-up and a written report to a nominated general practitioner. Although the intervention-group participants who remained in the study reported a higher quality of life compared to the control group, there was no significant difference in the probability of hospital admission or death between the intervention and control groups over the study period. However, significantly more participants in the intervention group were admitted to nursing homes compared with the control group.

A series of telephone-based sessions was performed by advanced practice nurses in a pilot study conducted by Teel and Leenerts (2005). They assessed a model known as the Self-Care for Health Promotion in Aging (S-CHPA) to provide the basis for promoting health among older adults with dementia and for their carers. Participants reported their understanding of session content (receipt), and their planned use of the information (enactment). Participants also reported an increased awareness about self-care practices and offered specific examples of how they intended to practice better self-care.

Rosenberg et al. (2006) used telephones to follow-up patients at 6-month intervals in a study conducted to examine risk factors for transition from an assisted living to a skilled nursing facility in a random sample of adults residing in assisted living.

Education and Training

A number of studies have assessed the effectiveness of telehealth tools in providing education and training for nurses in aged care. Dunbar, Neufeld, White, and Libow (1996) reported an educational intervention carried out for administrators and clinical nurse coordinators in randomly selected nursing homes. The intervention was mainly a workshop which included telephone communication with other components such as quarterly on-site consultations, regional meetings, a newsletter, and written and audio-visual materials. Participants of this study showed reduced use of physical restraints in nursing homes when managing old patients.

Done and Thomas (2001) carried out a study to investigate the effectiveness of workshop sessions for training in communication skills for care nurses of dementia suffers. The intervention group received training communication skills using video recordings while the control group received only a booklet with the same information. Results found that nurses' awareness of communication skills were superior in the workshop group compared to the control group, but the study did not show a difference in the effect on reducing communication problems or associated level of distress.

Administration

Some studies have attempted to assess the effectiveness of telehealth tools for administrative purposes in aged care settings. Telephone interviews and in-person interviews were conducted to gather the psychosocial status of residents in long-term geriatric care in nursing homes Results indicated that type of facility, resident health conditions, resident race, and facility family orientation were significantly correlated with dimensions of resident psychosocial status (Gaugler, Leach & Anderson, 2004).

Hebert, Robichaud, Roy, Bravo, and Voyer (2001) conducted a study to verify the efficacy of a multidimensional preventive program on the functional decline of older people. The intervention consisted of assessing participants at home by a nurse on 12 different dimensions. Once the assessment was completed, a report was sent to the general practitioner with recommendations for interventions. Subsequently, a monthly telephone contact was made by the nurse for surveillance and to verify if the recommendations had been applied. Results revealed that no significant difference in improvement of functional decline resulted from the intervention.

Nankervis, Schofield, Herrman, and Bloch (1997) reported on an intervention study to identify unmet needs for family carers and their frail or disabled relatives (This carer and care recipient is together labeled as a dyad). The intervention included telephone based services and one-off multidisciplinary home-based assessment of dyad (carer and care recipient) by the research team and regional aged care assessment service. The results showed that needs assessments for carers have the potential to identify needs and engage in new services. The service was also useful for providing emotional support.

Studies have explored the effectiveness of telehealth techniques in reducing hospital readmission in aged care. Kwok et al. (2004) studied the effectiveness of an intensive community nurse (CN)-supported discharge program in preventing hospital readmissions of older patients with chronic lung disease. The intervention consisted of home visits by CNs within 7 days of discharge, then weekly for 4 weeks and monthly until 6 months. Participants were provided with telephone access to CNs during normal working hours from Monday to Saturday. The intervention group reported a higher rate of unplanned readmission within 6 months compared to the control group subjects. There was no significant difference in the number of unplanned readmissions, hospital bed days, accident and emergency room attendance, functional and psychosocial status, and caregiver burden.

A RCT conducted to evaluate the effectiveness of case management provided to a group of home-dwelling, frail elderly patients which included (a) availability for phone assistance to subjects daily from 8am to 9 pm as well as (b) access to the case geriatrician by the case manager for medical support which included telephone consultation found a significant reduction in mean total number of hospital bed-days and mean total number of attendances at the outpatient department (Leung et al., 2004).

Research

Telehealth methods are widely being used as research tools. Telephone, electronic databases, computers and web tools have been useful tools in telenursing research.

Boult et al. (2008) conducted a cluster-randomized controlled trial to assess the effectiveness of comprehensive chronic care to multi-morbid older patients. In this study, the outcomes were assessed by conducting interviews using telephones. Carroll and Rankins (2006) used the telephone to assess the outcomes in an RCT which was conducted to assess the effect of an intervention in older un-partnered adults after myocardial infarction. Schein, Gagno,, Chan, Morin, and Grondines (2005) looked at the association between specific nurse case management interventions and the level of health in elderly people. In this study, outcomes were measured using the telephone in combination with home visit interviews. An exploratory study was undertaken to examine the role of general practitioners (GPs) and public health nurses (PHNs) in prescribing oral nutritional supplements to patients aged 65 years and older. In this study, the telephone was used to administer a questionnaire as a main data gathering tool (Loane, Flanagan, Siun, McNamara, & Kenny, 2004).

In-person and telephone interviews were conducted to gather residents' psychosocial status while providing long-term geriatric care in nursing homes (Gaugler, Leach and Anderson, 2004). In this study, a Principal Investigator (PI) made contact with research subjects over the phone to obtain initial agreement to participate. After conducting in-person interviews, telephone contacts were extended to collect additional data on important dimensions.

Stevens, Holman, Bennett, and de Klerk (2001) conducted a study to evaluate the outcome of an intervention to reduce hazards in the home on the rate of falls in seniors. The intervention was to provide a single home visit from a research nurse followed up for 1 year (after providing a home hazard assessment) with information on hazard reduction, and the installation of safety devices. In this study, telephone interviews were conducted to confirm the results. Gagnon, Schein, McVey, and Bergman (1999) carried out a clinical study to compare the effects of nurse case management with usual care provided to community-dwelling frail older people. The outcomes were assessed either through telephone and/or home interviews. Weinberger et al. (1994) conducted a clinical trial on health-related quality of life in elderly outpatients to compare the differences between telephone and face-to-face administration of outcome tools.

DISCUSSION

Although the results of this systematic review do not provide unequivocal evidence for the effectiveness of telenursing interventions in aged care, a number of randomised controlled trials have shown superior or equal outcomes compared with conventional methods. Studies have shown that telenursing interventions are not inferior to traditional methods. What is evident is that often traditional methods combined with telenursing interventions provide significantly effective outcomes. For instance, the study conducted by Heyn-Billipp using an interactive computer program in combination with a nurse substitute showed significant improvements in self-esteem (Heyn-Billipp, 2001). Similarly, continuously playing audio messages of personal memories combined with nurse-visits had a significant impact on improving the severity of dementia, agitation, mode and interest (Camberg et al., 1999). This may be due to the effect of 'personal and human contact' to augment the role of technology.

The study conducted by McDonald et al. (2005) showed the effectiveness of the additional information on communication of pain. The study showed, however, that the effect is superior on the first post-operative day only .The study suggests that although the post operative patients benefited from the additional information on communication skills, these skills alone are not sufficient for long term pain management. Meanwhile, although telenursing interventions using regular telephone calls have not all shown a superior effect, the evidence is available for the effect of such interventions to enhance the recovery process of the cardiac elders (Hiltunen et al., 2005).

Evidence also shows that even though there is no significant long term benefit of follow-up care over primary outcomes (Byles et al, 2004), telenursing methods are effective in reducing the length of hospital stays, hospital readmissions (Kauh et al., 2005), and nursing home stays (Mahoney et al., 2007).

Telenursing modalities have been particularly useful in providing counselling and support to the elderly and their care-givers. Studies have shown that continuing availability of ad hoc telephone counselling can augment the effect of counselling and support for elderly with depressive symptoms (Gaugler et al., 2008; Mittelman et al., 2007). There is no convincing evidence to say that geriatric telenursing provides superior health promotion over the existing method (Liddle et al 1996; Byles et al., 2004). However, the studies have shown the feasibility of using telenursing methods in aged and the satisfaction of the participants (Rosenberg et al., 2006; Teel et al., 2005) Therefore, it is fair to say that the evidence on the effectiveness of telenursing interventions in clinical and therapeutic areas of aged care is emerging and often the best outcome can be expected when telenursing tools are used in combination with traditional treatment modalities.

RCTs in telenursing for providing education and training have shown extremely positive results. It is evident that the combined use of telephone and audio-visual material produces a superior effect (Dunbar et al., 1996) compared to traditional ways of providing information (i.e. booklet and workshop sessions) (Done et al, 2001).

Evidence is available that telenursing can reduce the length of stay in hospitals and the rate of readmission. These outcomes are associated not only with clinical benefits, but also with the administrative aspects of nursing duties. Studies have shown that the provision of specialist care via telephone has significantly improved the length of hospital stay and reduced readmissions (Leung et al. 2004; Kwok et al., 2004).

The dominant mode of technology used in research relating to nursing care is the telephone, which is increasingly used as a research tool in geriatric telenursing to gather information and conduct interviews. In addition, the standard videoconferencing and web based technologies are also used in research purposes.

CONCLUSION

This literature reviewed shows that there is an attempt to incorporate telehealth tools in nursing practice with the view that these tools may provide opportunities to enhance the care for the elderly. The use of telehealth in aged care is rising. The results of randomized controlled trials have shown satisfactory outcomes from the use of telenursing techniques in providing clinical and therapeutic care to aged people. Telehealth techniques have also been used to complement home visits by nurses saving time and money, and providing services more effectively. Telenursing techniques have been used for enhancing clinical communication between patient and provider. The communication among health professionals has also been positively affected by telenursing. Telehealth tools have also been used in administrative, education and research purposes. The range of telenursing technologies is diverse, and it is expanding.

REFERENCES

Agency for Health Care Research and Quality. (2000). *The characteristics of long-term care users*. Rockville, MD: AHRQ.

Belfield, G., & Colin-Thome, D. (2004). *Improving chronic disease management.* Department of Health, UK National Health Service. Retrieved Sept. 12, 2009 from http://www.dh.gov.uk/en/Publicationsandstatistics/Publications/PublicationsPolicyAndGuidance/DH_4075214.

Blumenthal, D. (2004). New stream from an old cauldron - the physician supply debate. *The New England Journal of Medicine*, *350*(17), 1780–1787. doi:10.1056/NEJMhpr033066

Boult, C., Reider, L., Frey, K., Leff, B., Boyd, C. M., & Wolff, J. L. (2008). Early effects of "Guided Care" on the quality of health care for multimorbid older persons: a cluster-randomized controlled trial. *Biological Sciences & Medical Sciences*, *63*(3), 321–327.

Byles, J. E., Tavener, M., O'Connell, R. L., Nair, B. R., Higginbotham, N. H., & Jackson, C. L. (2004). Randomised controlled trial of health assessments for older Australian veterans and war widows. *The Medical Journal of Australia*, *181*(4), 186–190.

Calkins, E., Boult, C., & Wagner, E. (1999). *New ways to care for older people: Building systems based on evidence*. New York: Springer.

Camberg, L., Woods, P., Ooi, W. L., Hurley, A., Volicer, L., & Ashley, J. (1999). Evaluation of simulated presence: A personalized approach to enhance well-being in persons with Alzheimer's disease. *Journal of the American Geriatrics Society*, *47*(4), 446–452.

Carroll, D. L., & Rankin, S. H. (2006). Comparing interventions in older unpartnered adults after myocardial infarction. *European Journal of Cardiovascular Nursing*, *5*(1), 83–89. doi:10.1016/j.ejcnurse.2005.09.001

Cooper, R. A., Getzen, T. E., McKee, H. J., & Laud, P. (2002). Economic and demographic trends signal an impeding physician shortage. *Health Affairs*, *21*(1), 140–154. doi:10.1377/hlthaff.21.1.140

Darkins, A., Dearde, C. H., Rocke, L. G., Martin, J. B., Sibson, L., & Wootton, R. (1996). An evaluation of telemedical support for a minor treatment centre. *Journal of Telemedicine and Telecare*, *2*(2), 92–99. doi:10.1258/1357633961929853

Done, D. J., & Thomas, J. A. (2001). Training in communication skills for informal carers of people suffering from dementia: a cluster randomized clinical trial comparing a therapist led workshop and a booklet. *International Journal of Geriatric Psychiatry*, *16*(8), 816–821. doi:10.1002/gps.436

Dunbar, J. M., Neufeld, R. R., White, H. C., & Libow, L. S. (1996). Retrain, don't restrain: The educational intervention of the National Nursing Home Restraint Removal Project. *The Gerontologist*, *36*(4), 539–542.

Edirippulige, S., & Wootton, R. (2006). Telehealth and Communication . In Conrick, M. (Ed.), *Health informatics, transforming health care with technology* (pp. 266–278). Melbourne: Thomson.

Gagnon, A. J., Schein, C., McVey, L., & Bergman, H. (1999). Randomized controlled trial of nurse case management of frail older people. *Journal of the American Geriatrics Society*, *47*(9), 1118–1124.

Gaugler, J. E., Leach, C. R., & Anderson, K. A. (2004). Correlates of resident psychosocial status in long-term care. *International Journal of Geriatric Psychiatry*, *19*(8), 773–780. doi:10.1002/gps.1157

Gaugler, J. E., Roth, D. L., Haley, W. E., & Mittelman, M. S. (2008). Can counseling and support reduce burden and depressive symptoms in caregivers of people with Alzheimer's disease during the transition to institutionalization? Results from the New York University caregiver intervention study. *Journal of the American Geriatrics Society*, *56*(3), 421–428. doi:10.1111/j.1532-5415.2007.01593.x

Health Resources and Services Administration (HRSA). (2006). *Physician supply and demand: Projections to 2020*. Retrieved September 10, 2009, from http://bhpr.hrsa.gov/healthworkforce/reports/physiciansupplydemand/default.htm.

Hebert, R., Robichaud, L., Roy, P. M., Bravo, G., & Voyer, L. (2001). Efficacy of a nurse-led multidimensional preventive programme for older people at risk of functional decline. A randomized controlled trial. *Age and Ageing*, *30*(2), 147–153. doi:10.1093/ageing/30.2.147

Heyn-Billipp, S. (2001). The psychosocial impact of interactive computer use within a vulnerable elderly population: A report on a randomized prospective trial in a home health care setting. *Public Health Nursing (Boston, Mass.)*, *18*(2), 138–145. doi:10.1046/j.1525-1446.2001.00138.x

Hiltunen, E. F., Winder, P. A., Rait, M. A., Buselli, E. F., Carroll, D. L., & Rankin, S. H. (2005). Implementation of efficacy enhancement nursing interventions with cardiac elders. *Rehabilitation Nursing*, *30*(6), 221–229.

Information Technology Association of America (ITAA) e-Health Committee. (2004*). Chronic care improvement: How Medicare transformation can save lives, save money and stimulate an emerging technology industry.* ITAA May 2004. Retrieved September 10, 2009, from http://www.itaa.org/isec/docs/choniccare.pdf.

Kauh, B., Polak, T., Hazelett, S., Hua, K., & Allen, K. (2005). A pilot study: post-acute geriatric rehabilitation versus usual care in skilled nursing facilities. *Journal of the American Medical Directors Association*, *6*(5), 321–326. doi:10.1016/j.jamda.2005.04.008

Kwok, T., Lum, C. M., Chan, H. S., Ma, H. M., Lee, D., & Woo, J. (2004). A randomized, controlled trial of an intensive community nurse-supported discharge program in preventing hospital readmissions of older patients with chronic lung disease. *Journal of the American Geriatrics Society*, *52*(8), 1240–1246. doi:10.1111/j.1532-5415.2004.52351.x

Leung, A. C., Yau, D. C., Liu, C. P., Yeoh, C. S., Chui, T. Y., & Chi, I. (2004). Reducing utilisation of hospital services by case management: a randomised controlled trial. *Australian Health Review*, *28*, 79–86. doi:10.1071/AH040079

Liddle, J., March, L., Carfrae, B., Finnegan, T., Druce, J., Schwarz, J., & Brooks, P. (1996). Can occupational therapy intervention play a part in maintaining independence and quality of life in older people? A randomised controlled trial. *Australian and New Zealand Journal of Public Health*, *20*(6), 574–578. doi:10.1111/j.1467-842X.1996.tb01068.x

Loane, D., Flanagan, G., Siun, A., McNamara, E., & Kenny, S. (2004). Nutrition in the community-an exploratory study of oral nutritional supplements in a health board area in Ireland. *Journal of Human Nutrition and Dietetics*, *17*(3), 257–266. doi:10.1111/j.1365-277X.2004.00527.x

Mahoney, J. E., Shea, T. A., Przybelski, R., Jaros, L., Gangnon, R., Cech, S., & Schwalbe, A. (2007). Kenosha County falls prevention study: A randomized, controlled trial of an intermediate-intensity, community-based multifactorial falls intervention. *Journal of the American Geriatrics Society*, *55*(4), 489–498. doi:10.1111/j.1532-5415.2007.01144.x

McDonald, D. D., Thomas, G. J., Livingston, K. E., & Severson, J. S. (2005). Assisting older adults to communicate their postoperative pain. *Clinical Nursing Research*, *14*(2), 109–126, discussion 127–130. doi:10.1177/1054773804271934

Mittelman, M. S., Roth, D. L., Clay, O. J., & Haley, W. E. (2007). Preserving health of Alzheimer caregivers: Impact of a spouse caregiver intervention. *The American Journal of Geriatric Psychiatry*, *15*(9), 780–789. doi:10.1097/JGP.0b013e31805d858a

Nankervis, J., Schofield, H., Herrman, H., & Bloch, S. (1997). Home-based assessment for family carers: a preventative strategy to identify and meet service needs. *International Journal of Geriatric Psychiatry*, *12*(2), 193–201. doi:10.1002/(SICI)1099-1166(199702)12:2<193::AID-GPS580>3.0.CO;2-U

Rosenberg, P. B., Mielke, M. M., Samus, Q. M., Rosenblatt, A., Baker, A., & Brandt, J. (2006). Transition to nursing home from assisted living is not associated with dementia or dementia-related problem behaviors. *Journal of the American Medical Directors Association*, *7*(2), 73–78. doi:10.1016/j.jamda.2005.06.003

Schein, C., Gagnon, A. J., Chan, L., Morin, I., & Grondines, J. (2005). The association between specific nurse case management interventions and elder health. *Journal of the American Geriatrics Society*, *53*(4), 597–602. doi:10.1111/j.1532-5415.2005.53206.x

Stevens, M., Holman, C. D., Bennett, N., & de Klerk, N. (2001). Preventing falls in older people: Outcome evaluation of a randomized controlled trial. *Journal of the American Geriatrics Society*, *49*(11), 1448–1455. doi:10.1046/j.1532-5415.2001.4911236.x

Teel, C. S., & Leenerts, M. H. (2005). Developing and testing a self-care intervention for older adults in caregiving roles. *Nursing Research*, *54*(3), 193–201. doi:10.1097/00006199-200505000-00007

The World Health Report. (2006). Retrieved September 10, 2009, from http://www.who.int/whr/2006/en/.

Weinberger, M., Nagle, B., Hanlon, J. T., Samsa, G. P., Schmader, K., & Landsman, P. B. (1994). Assessing health-related quality of life in elderly outpatients: Telephone versus face-to-face administration. *Journal of the American Geriatrics Society*, *42*(12), 1295–1299.

Wootton, R., Kvedar, J., & Dimmick, S. L. (2006). *Home telehealth: Connecting care within community*. London: Royal Society of Medicine Press.

Chapter 18
Health Insurance Systems as Models for Managing the Increasing Elderly Populations of Japan and Korea

Seungwon Jeong
Nihon Fukushi University, Japan

Yusuke Inoue
Nihon Fukushi University, Japan

ABSTRACT

This chapter looks into the systems and institutions for the elderly population covered by long-term care insurance in Japan and the Republic of Korea (hereafter Korea). It shall discuss the historical changes in policies in these two nations. The Health Care and Welfare Complex elements that make up a single business model for the Health Care and Social Services of the aged in Japan and Korea will also be discussed in this paper. The management environment for medical facilities greatly changed with adjustments in the population structure and the social environment, and this resulted in serious competition between medical facilities for patients. Medical facilities in Japan and Korea showed a rapid increase in comprehensive medical and welfare management. Consequently, there were provisions in both health care and social services through affiliation, chain affiliation and multiplication, before and after the enforcement of long-term care insurance.

THE AGEING SOCIETIES OF JAPAN AND KOREA

In 2008, the ageing ratio in Japan was 22%, the highest in the world. The ratio surpassed 21% in 2007, marking the advent of the super ageing society. In Japan, compared to most other countries, the ageing of society is progressing at a particularly rapid pace. For example, the time taken to change from an ageing to an aged society was 115 years in France, 85 years in Sweden, 47 years in the United Kingdom, and 40 years in Germany compared to 24 years in Japan(National Institute of Population and Social Security Research, 2003; OECD Health Data, 2004; UN, 2008). This rapid increase in the

DOI: 10.4018/978-1-61520-825-8.ch018

ageing rate is due to a longer lifespan resulting from factors such as an increased standard of living and advances in health care, as well as a falling birthrate. In 2006, the total fertility rate in Japan was 1.32. Japanese society will continue to age rapidly, with the ageing ratio projected to reach 29.2% in 2020 and 31.8% in 2030.

The population is also ageing quite rapidly in Korea with the ageing ratio at 10.3% in 2008. Korea became an ageing society in 2000, is predicted to become an aged society in 2018, and a super aged society in 2026(Statistics Korea, 2009). Compared to the time taken for the ageing society in Japan to become an aged society, the time is shorter in Korea, taking just 18 years, and then taking just 8 more years to become a super aged society. The most notable factor behind this is the problem of a falling birthrate, with a total fertility rate of 1.13 recorded in 2006, the lowest among OECD member countries. However, technology has been a big contributor to the prolonged life span in both countries, and ongoing advances in technology look set to extend people's lives even further.

The use and availability of medical technology in Japan and Korea is one of the highest in the world. Technology in these countries is often used for diagnostic and treatment purposes on a larger and wider scale than in most developed countries in the world. This technology is also extensively used in Japan and Korea during the annual medical assessment provided for most of their citizens. It is very much focused on the use of technology. Medical assessment is adopted in Japan and Korea as an important medical practice. As a result, the early detection of diseases has been made possible which, in turn, has increased the effectiveness of treatment methods. Long (2000, p. 124) observes that "the rapid increase in new types of technology and their rapid diffusion into the clinical setting, combined with the rapidly growing elderly population, have led to the common use of advanced life-prolonging treatments in Japan…". Technology is now doing what it is supposed to in these instances: helping to prolong life. However, it has now resulted in an aged population, which, in turn, is costing the country millions of dollars in healthcare and retirement expenses (Pacific Health Summit, 2006).

With the above considerations in mind, this chapter shall assess the systems and institutions for the aged, which are covered by long-term care insurance, and changes in policies in Japan and Korea. In recent years the increase in the aged population has led to changes in the management of long-term care in Japan and Korea. An assessment of the existing elderly healthcare system in these countries implies a clear focus towards adequately serving the needs of the population despite limited resources. Aspects of long-term insurance shall be assessed and evaluated with a view to determining its effectiveness in addressing the problems associated with the elderly health care services of Japan and Korea. The discussions that will follow will help address the question of how the government and private institutions in both countries have managed to come up with solutions to the delivery of health care services. It shall also discuss different healthcare delivery models which have been used and which will be considered in establishing solutions for the challenges posed by an increasingly ageing population.

Long-Term Care Insurance

An ageing population leads to an increased demand for people capable of providing medical treatment and care. When there is a limited availability of such individuals, problems in health care delivery result. In response to the problems of caring for the aged, long-term care insurance has now been introduced in both Japan and Korea.

The Japanese Long-Term Care Insurance System

In Japan, the Long-term care insurance system started in 2000. It is a social insurance system

Figure 1. Levels of certified care (support) need and services available (Long-term Care Insurance, Tokyo Metropolitan Government (2006))

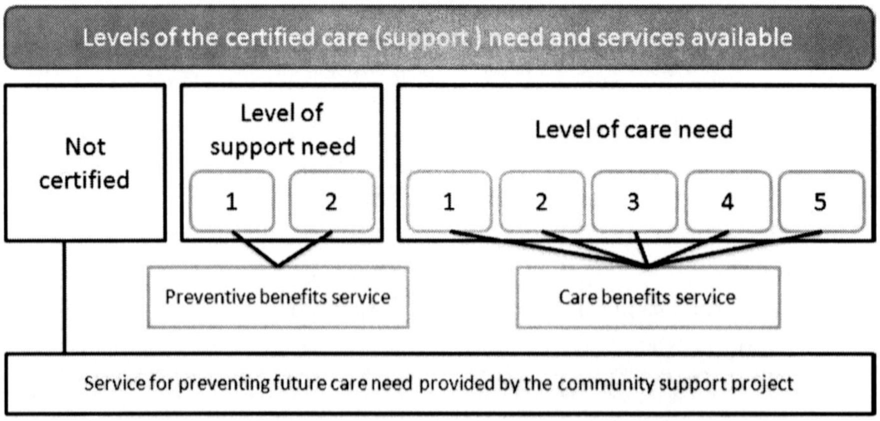

which is financed by tax, insurance premiums and payments by the beneficiaries of care services. The insurers are local authorities. The insured are divided into two categories. The first category consists of people aged 65 years or older; the second category consists of people between the age of 40 and 65. As a rule, however, only people in the first category can receive care services. Care for people in the second category is provided only in cases where a person requires care due to an age-related illness such as early-stage dementia, cerebro-vascular disorder, etc. As of October 2008, the number of people receiving care in the first category was about 12.9% of total population over 65.

The insurance premiums for those in the first and second categories differ. For those in the first category, premiums differ depending on the local authority. They are revised every three years. Long-term care insurance benefits are divided into long-term care and preventive care benefits. Long-term care consists of a service supporting in-home care; three kinds of facility services; 11 kinds of in-home services (as well as an allowance for purchasing equipment for in-home long-term care, and an allowance for home modification for in-home long-term care); and six kinds of services providing allowances for community based long-term care. Preventive care consists of a service supporting in-home care; 11 kinds of in-home services (as well as an allowance for purchasing equipment for in-home long-term care; an allowance for home modification for in-home long-term care); and three kinds of services providing allowances for community based long-term care (See Figure 2.). To be entitled to long-term care insurance services, a person must be certified as in need of care. In addition, the scope of services that a person can receive is limited depending on the degree of care he or she is certified to receive. The need for care is classified as Support Needed categories 1 and 2, and Long-Term Care Needed categories 1 through 5 (Refer to Figure 1). People certified as belonging to Support Needed categories 1 and 2 (those in need of a little care) are entitled to receive preventive care benefits. People certified as belonging to Long-Term Care Needed categories 1 through 5 (those in need of moderate to serious care) are entitled to nursing care benefits. People receiving preventive care benefits receive services after a preventive plan has been drawn up by institution personnel at a community general support center. People receiving nursing care benefits can take advantage of services after a care manager or they themselves draw up a care plan.

Figure 2. Services available from the long-term care insurance system (Care level 1-5) in Japan (Long-term Care Insurance, Tokyo Metropolitan Government (2006))

Type of Service		Description
Preparation of care plan	In-home care management	The care manager will draw up a care plan according to the mental and physical condition, environment, wishes, etc. of the individual in need of care and contact the service provider to make necessary adjustments so that the individual may use in-home care service and other services properly.
Service given at home	Home help service	A caregiver or other staff visits the individual in need of care and looks after them at their home.
	Home help service at night (*)	A caregiver, etc. periodically visits the home of the individual in need of care or the home that requested a visit at night to give them care or to look after them.
	Home-visit bathing service	The staff visits those having difficulty in taking a bath at their bathroom by bathing car and helps them take a bath using, for example, a bathtub brought in the home from the bathing car.
	Home-visit nursing	A nurse, etc. visits the individual in need of care to give them medical care service and supplementary medical examination service needed.
	Home-visit rehabilitation	A physical therapist, etc. visits the individual in need of care to give them training for keeping or recovering their mental or physical functions and for leading daily life independently.
	Management guidance for in-home	A doctor, dentist, pharmacist, etc. gives medical advice and guidance.
Service given at a facility, etc.	Day service	The individual in need of care goes to a facility to have care for taking a bath, having a meal, etc. and function restoring training.
	Day service for the elderly with dementia (*)	The individual in need of care goes to a facility to have the care and function restoring training adapted to the characteristic needs of the elderly with dementia.
	Day rehabilitation service (day care)	The individual in need of care goes to a medical institution, etc. to have training for keeping or recovering their mental or physical functions and for leading daily life independently.
	Short-stay daily-life service (welfare oriented short-stay)	The individual in need of care stays at a special nursing home for the elderly, etc. for a short period of time to have daily-life service and function restoring training.
	Short-stay medical service (medicalcare-oriented short-stay)	The individual in need of care stays at a medical institution, etc. to have medical care service and function restoring training.
	Small-scale and multifunctional in-home care (*)	The individual in need of care goes to or stays at a nearby community facility to have care and function restoring training. They can also have a visit by the staff, etc. of the same facility and when necessary, have care provided in cooperation with an annex facility.
Service given at a place other than the home	Daily-life group care for the elderly with dementia (*) (group home for the elderly with dementia)	Five to nine elderly people with dementia receive care while leading group life.
	Daily-life care service in specified facilities	The individual in need of care receives care while living in a fee-charging home for the elderly, care house, etc.
	Community-oriented daily-life care service in specified facilities (*)	The individual in need of care receives care while living at a small-scale fee-charging home for the elderly.
Service given at a facility	Welfare facility for the elderly requiring care	Those in need of continuous care who find difficulty in home life stay and live at this facility.
	Community-oriented welfare facility for the elderly requiring care (*)	The individual in need of care receives care at a small-scale special nursing home for the elderly.
	Health service facility for the elderly requiring care	This facility receives those who have a stable state of a disease and need both medical and long term care.
	Sanatorium type medical care facilityfor the elderly requiring care	This facility takes in those in need of daily medical care for a relatively long period of time, rehabilitation during the chronic period and long-term care.
Service for assistive devices	Rental of assistive devices	A special bed, wheelchair and other assistive devices are rented.
	Allowance for purchasing assistive devices	The designated service provider is given an allowance in an amount equivalent to 90% of the costs that they needed to buy a sitting-type toilet, chair for bathing, etc.
Home renovation service	Allowance for home renovation	An allowance in an amount equivalent to 90% of the small-scale home renovation (up to ¥180,000 a house), such as installation of handrails and elimination of steps, is paid.

As of July 2008, about 1.2 million people were certified as needing support, and about 3.4 million were certified as needing long-term care (Ministry of Health, Labor and Welfare, 2009). As of January 2009, about 3.0 million people were receiving long-term care benefits and about 810,000 were receiving preventive care benefits. Among those receiving long-term care benefits, facility services were used by about 840,000 people and in-home services by about 2.03 million. After the implementation of long-term care insurance, the number of people using care services rapidly increased while financial conditions deteriorated. As a result, in 2006, the number of Long-Term Care Needed categories was changed from 6 to 7; preventive care services for people needing some support have been limited; long-term care service fees have been reduced; bed and food expenses have been made payable by the beneficiaries; and other steps have been taken to curb long-term care benefit expenses (Ministry of Health, Labor and Welfare, 2009).

Figure 3. Benefits under the Long-term Care insurance in Korea (Ministry for health welfare and family affairs, Korea, http://english.mw.go.kr)

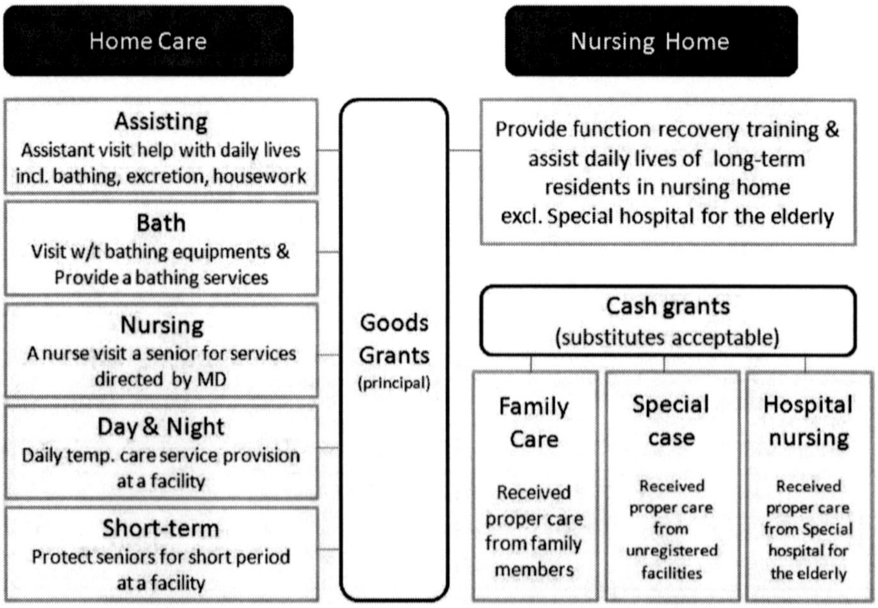

The Korean Long-Term Care Insurance System

In July 2008, a long-term care insurance system for the aged was launched in Korea, equivalent to the long-term care insurance system in Japan. As in Japan, the system is administered by a social insurance system financed by beneficiary payment, insurance premiums, and tax. Since the above system was adopted, there has been a debate on whether or not the insurers should be a *National Health Insurance Corporation* or the local authorities. However, unlike in Japan, health insurers in Korea are integrated. Consequently, for the sake of convenience, the role was filled by a *National Health Insurance Corporation.*

The procedures for certifying whether someone needs long-term care are almost the same as in Japan, with those covered being enrolled in the national health insurance program. Since health insurers in Korea became integrated in 2000, anyone enrolled in a health insurance program is automatically enrolled in the national health insurance program. Beneficiaries of the system are the elderly, aged 65 years or older and others under the age of 65 years with cognitive impairment, cerebrovascular disease and other diseases determined by executive order to be geriatric in nature.

Figure 3 shows the benefits provided under long-term care insurance. Insurance benefits are broadly divided into in-home benefits and facility benefits. In-home benefits apply to home visit long-term care, home visit bathing, home visit nursing, day and night care and short stay care. Facility benefits apply to nursing homes, special facilities for care of the elderly, group homes and other long-term care facilities. There are also monetary benefits such as medical treatment expense benefits for dependent families, expense benefits for special treatment received at care facilities other than long-term care facilities, and expense benefits to provide support when a person is admitted to a geriatric facility or any other hospital. These benefits mainly apply to people living on islands or in remote areas.

Figure 4. The process for receiving benefits under the Long-term care insurance in Korea (Ministry for Health Welfare and Family Affairs, Korea, http://english.mw.go.kr)

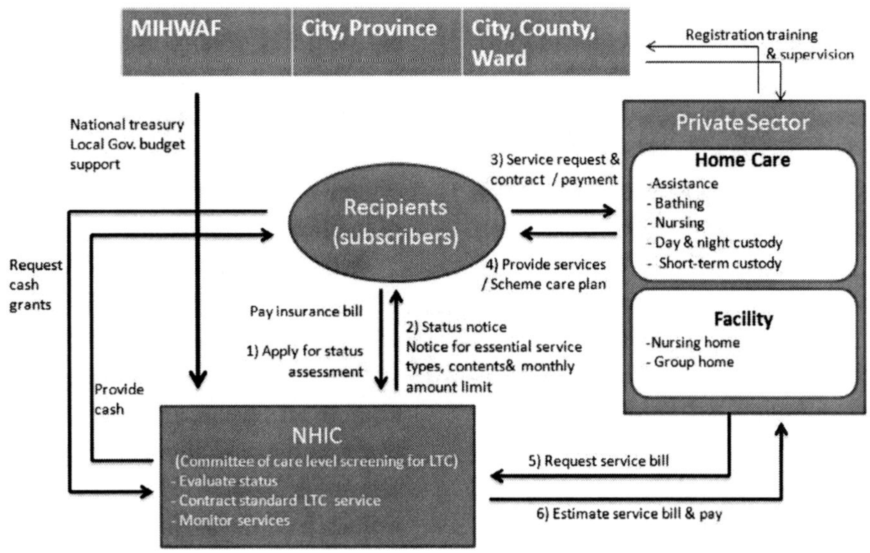

Figure 4 shows the process for receiving benefits under the long-term care insurance in Korea. The procedures for taking advantage of the benefits are almost the same as in Japan. First, the person who wants to use the services has to apply for long-term care certification. A document of the findings of a doctor affiliated with the national health insurance public corporation has to be attached to the certification. An employee of the national health insurance public corporation (social welfare counselor, nurse) will then examine the physical and mental health of the applicant. The findings of the doctor and the results of the examination are then presented to a committee for assessment; the committee will then decide whether the applicant will be allowed to receive long-term care benefits or not. There are three classifications of the degree of need for long-term care. The details of the services, the number of times they are provided, the expenses, and other factors are determined depending on the classification of needs.

The Process Leading to the Introduction of Long-Term Care Insurance

For Japan, the decision to introduce and implement long-term care insurance was made after the infrastructure was more or less in place. In Korea, however, the momentum behind the rapid development of the infrastructure was built after the introduction of long-term care insurance. It could be said that from the point of view of the ageing ratio, long-term care insurance in Korea was introduced earlier than in Japan.

In Japan, prior to the introduction of long-term care insurance, the infrastructure was gradually put in place with various policies and measures such as the Gold Plan in 1989, the New Gold Plan in 1994, and Gold Plan 21 in 1999. In 1994, when the ageing ratio surpassed 14%, full scale debate began concerning the adoption of long-term care insurance which could deal with the potential problems in elderly care. In 1995, the Ministry of Health and Welfare (now the Ministry of Health, Labor and Welfare) formally proposed the establishment of long-term care insurance. After continued debate, the Long-Term Care Insurance Act was eventually enacted in 1997. The Long-Term Care System was then implemented in 2000. The ageing ratio in 2000 was 17.4%. This is the step by step process by which the infrastructure for long-term care insurance was established in Japan in order to implement the long-term care system, six years after the country became an aged society.

In Korea, Kim Dae-jung, the president at the time, proposed the introduction of long-term care insurance in 2001. The next president, Roh Moo-hyun, continued with this policy and the Elderly Long-Term Care Act was enacted in 2007 and was implemented in 2008. After the proposal of long-term care insurance in Korea, there was insufficient infrastructure planned for treatment and welfare facilities for the aged. It was not until the government announced its "10-Year Plan for Health Care and Social Service Facilities for the Aged" in 2005 that efforts were finally begun to set up the infrastructure. After the plan was announced, the number of treatment and welfare facilities for the aged rapidly increased from about 400 in 2005 to about 800 in 2007. However, the ageing rate in Korea in 2007 was 9.9%, rising to over 10.3% in 2008. Such figures were lower than figures for Japan in 2000, when long-term care insurance for the aged was introduced.

The above accounts illustrate the history of long-term insurance for both Japan and Korea. The discussions that now follow will demonstrate possible solutions, both current and recommended for the elderly population in both nations.

Health Care and Welfare Complexes as a Solution

Japan has recently been experiencing deterioration in its national financial state due to the increased expenditures for its ageing society coupled with decreased tax revenues from slow economic growth. For this reason, the Japanese government decreased fee reimbursements several times over the course of medical fee reviews from 2002 to 2008. The management environment for medical facilities greatly changed with adjustments in population structure and social environment, leading to serious competition between medical facilities for patients. This reality necessitated a review of management evaluation and efficiency of medical facilities, in Japan.

In particular, medical facilities in Japan showed a rapid increase in comprehensive medical and welfare management. Such facilities were able to provide both health care and social services through affiliation, chain affiliation and multiplication before and after the enforcement of care insurance in 2000. Niki (1998) defined such medical welfare facilities as *Fukugotai (integrated delivery systems of health care and social services)*. Such facilities are now becoming a business model for small and medium medical facilities in Japan.

Korea is also showing an increase in the unification of medical and welfare services at geriatric hospitals as a result of long term care insurance introduced in July 2008. Jeong (2008) describes how, prior to the enforcement of long term care insurance, there were *Health Care and Welfare Complexes* in Korea, though the absolute number was small. At that time, nine percent of a total of 61 facilities had both medical corporations and social welfare corporations launched, and 36% of all facilities responded that "there is a plan to provide social service for [the] elderly with enforcement of long term care insurance" Jeong (2008, p.139). From these early results, a rapid growth in the number of medical facilities with Health Care and Welfare Complexes is expected in Korea.

Fukugotai (Integrated Delivery Systems of Health Care And Social Services) in Japan

In Japan, a revision of the Medical Service Act in 1985 led to implementation of a mandatory *Medi-*

Figure 5. Profit model of Medical Facilities

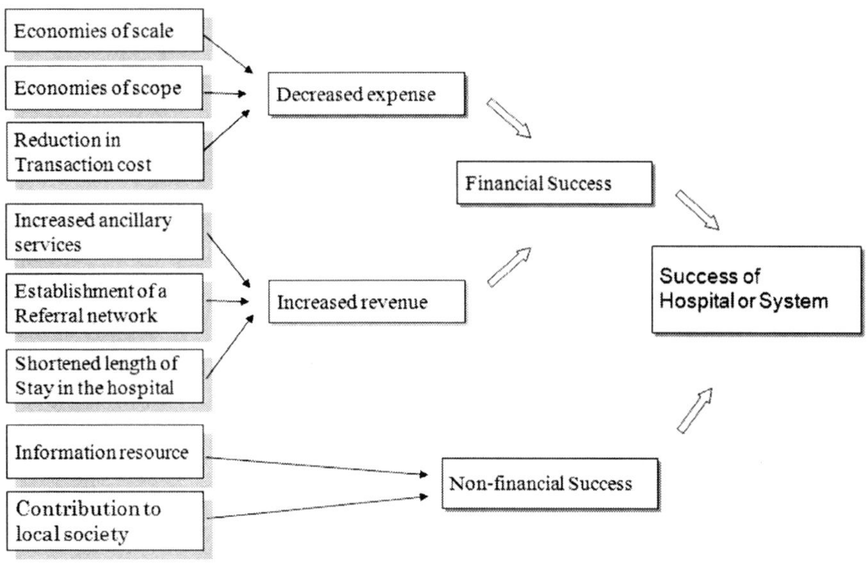

cal Plan. This plan was enforced after it was recognized by the authorities that the excessive supply of hospital beds also increased the cost of medical services. However, the number of elderly patients who were hospitalized indefinitely and who were receiving mainly nursing care rather than medical care, continued to grow as the senior population increased. Because of this growing trend towards long term hospital bed occupancy, the functioning of acute care hospitals and the smooth circulation of hospital beds deteriorated. Serious problems in hospital management were now seen. It was therefore necessary for medical institutions, which were expanding their business by adding hospital beds, to find other ways of growing their business. Since hospitals in over serviced regions were unable to increase their number of beds, they were forced to find additional beds in facilities which were not influenced by the Medical Service Act. Accordingly, medical institutions began to offer special care homes and social service businesses for the elderly population.

Niki (1998) reports in his study that medical facilities in Japan are operating integrated facilities and that 30% of special care homes or welfare facilities are based on medical facilities. He defined *Fukugotai* (integrated delivery systems of health care and social services) as "a group established by medical facilities to singularly (self-fulfillingly) provide health, medical and welfare services by opening related corporations and accompanying health and welfare facilities" (pp.4-5). He refers to groups with a hospital (medical service), elderly health care facility (health care service) and special care home (welfare) as the three parts of *Fukugotai*.

Management Effect of Medical Welfare Complexes

The profit model of service integration in medical facilities shown in Figure 5 is a reorganization of models by Giardina (1990, p.76), Lehman (1998, p.307) and Adachi (2000, p.873). An ultimate measure of the success of reconfiguring medical facilities lies in its contribution to profits. However, overall success is not limited only to financial indices. It includes non-financial factors as well, such as acquisition of information resources and contributions to local society. Fukugotai is one of the most efficient models for managing healthcare and welfare complexes.

Management effects of service integration include realization of *economies of scope*, reduction in *transaction cost*, and an increase in loyalty of customers (Niki, 1998, pp.36-37; Niki, 2000, p.35). Also, Giardina (1990, p.76) and Lehrman (1998, p.303) saw the advancement of acute hospitals in the field of chronic medical service as related diversification of services. They also argued that financial effects can be seen from reduced cost and increased revenue. Shortell et al. (1994, pp.46-64) and Conrad et al. (1996, pp.3-40) argue that IDS (Integrated Delivery System) is advantageous in terms of capital supply, giving it an accounting advantage. It can also explain traditional benefits of vertical and horizontal integration. Coddington et al. (1996, pp.151-164) explained that IDS can change the cost structure, lower the price, and increase market share and profit, thereby creating an opportunity for strategic investment. Such opportunity then leads to re-investment in facilities increases in employees' wages and additional employment.

Jeong et. al.(2009) used financial data from The Health Co-operative Association in Japan (N=106) between 2003 and 2005 to test the effect of *Fukugotai* (integrated medical and social services). In addition, the authors summarized management effects of *Fukugotai* by comparing the data of providing only medical service facilities in two ways (N=213). First, there is an effect of separating the risk from an external factor of medical fee revision. That is, since reduction in profits in either medical fee or care fee can be assisted by guaranteed profit of the other side, integrated services tend to not experience rapid management losses. Second, *Fukugotai* was found to have higher labor productivity and added value compared with medical service facilities.

Health Care and Welfare Complex as a Business Model

Since the 1990s in Japan, local health communities have been formed by existing wealthy medical facilities opening health care and social service facilities.

In contrast, in Korea, survival competition is fierce between small and medium-sized hospitals. As a result, the opening of hospitals and clinics occurs in a relatively liberal environment compared to Japan. Moreover, since medical fees are decided by the government, there are great limitations to management activities becoming similar to normal corporations. Consequently, 10% of their hospitals became bankrupt. A survival strategy for overcoming such difficulty would be a Health Care and Welfare Complex model oriented by local community (See Figure 6).

The Health Care and Welfare Complex would be established by medical facilities in order to provide medical care and social services by opening related corporations and accompanying health and welfare facilities. The Health Care and Welfare Complex would establish a medical service network which integrates a rehabilitation, acute, mental, chronic diseases center; an elderly welfare center; and a home nursing and home rehabilitation center for the local community. These centers would also help maintain the quality of medical services through education courses offered to the members of the community.

These models would also provide convenience and peace of mind to patients by comprehensively and continuously providing diverse medical and welfare services. Also, the establishment of a smooth linked system would help patients efficiently receive hospital, nursing and home care services.

Technology

Just as technology has been a contributory factor to the growth of the elderly population, it can

Figure 6. Health Care & Welfare Complex model

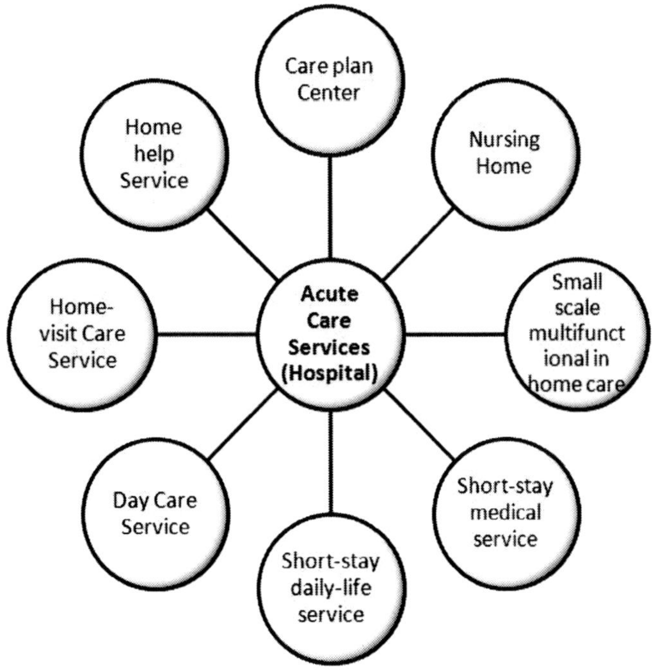

also offer solutions for effectively managing that growth. Technology is now being geared towards making the elderly population more productive and less dependent on their caregivers and on the government health care services. Eizmendi, Azkoitia, and Craddock (2007, pp. 254-255) discuss how technology is actually a tool which can be used to "improve independent living, safety and autonomy of people with dementia and to support the quality of life of such people and their family carers".

Technology Research for Independent Living (2008) points out that, all too often, the ageing population is dependent on their carers and on members of their families in order to perform activities of daily living (ADLs). However, through technology, they can become more independent in their ADLs. They can prepare their own meals, groom themselves, be reminded to take their medication, buy their groceries, and accomplish other tasks safely and efficiently without their family or their caregiver's help. This results in greater freedom for both the elderly and their families. This increased independence brought about by assistive technology, is likely to lead to a decrease in rates of depression among the elderly population who would no longer feel as helpless and dependent as before (Technology Research for Independent Living, 2008).

Various interest groups also envision an increasing role to be played by e-Health or IT (information technology) which can be used to aid the elderly population in coping with their illnesses and other health concerns. For example, a health seminar published online related how IT can help to enhance the quality of life of the elderly population. The seminar discussed how stroke patients can be rehabilitated through virtual reality and how electronic equipment in the homes of the elderly can assist in the monitoring of the elderly population's activities – from measuring their mattresses to the drawing of their baths, and other similar activities (Stalldall et al., 2001).

e-Health also functions as a test and monitoring process. Through a wireless network established in Japan in 2006, it is now possible to remotely monitor elderly health. This network allows the local hospitals to monitor the heart rates of the elderly citizens living alone. The monitoring process is done through sensors patched through a wireless zone where there is less radio wave interference. The sensors will allow local hospitals to provide 24-hour monitoring of the heart rates of elderly people living alone. The sensors in the wireless zone will also track the movement of pedestrians and keep nearby motorists informed (iHealth Beat, 2007).

The bioshirt is an innovation devised by the Korean Ministry of Information and Communication to assist the elderly and disabled. The bioshirt serves as a monitor of a patient's vital signs and consequently signals for help if something is wrong with the patient. The system is known as the 'U-healthcare Service' and mostly targets senior citizens living alone and patients with chronic conditions. This bioshirt also enables options for self-diagnosis while primarily ensuring remote monitoring (Blass, 2006).

Robichon (2004) discusses how technology has created robots to care for the elderly population. The Japanese auto industry has partnered with nursing homes to experiment with robots to care for the aged. In a nursing home run by Matsushita Electric, sensors have been inserted inside a teddy bear. Occasionally, the teddy bear asks the elderly a question. Based on the patient's response time, a nursing assistant is called. Sanyo Electric, on the other hand has come up with a robot bathtub which helps bathe the elderly. This bathtub closes around the elderly person in a wheelchair and the wash and rinse cycles then operate automatically. The nursing aide washes the patient's hair and then towels him off (Robichon, 2004). This technology has helped make the care of the elderly in Japan easier and safer.

Cheong et al., (2007) discuss how the Korean government has been actively promoting the national e-health project in order to help build an integrated health care system. Such a project would lead to an electronic health record system, telemedicine, technology standardization, and technology interoperability shared by hospitals. Through e-health, the accessibility of patient information and medical care is more convenient and much more efficient. It also hopes to eventually improve transparency by exposing inequalities in health care delivery. The system would also ultimately lead to greater cooperation between medical and governmental agencies in the delivery of health care services (Cheong et al., 2007).

CONCLUSION

Due to advances in medical technology, the ageing population of Japan and Korea has increased at unprecedented and currently unmanageable rates. In response to the problems of caring for the aged, long-term care insurance has now been introduced in both Japan and Korea. As a result, health care costs have also increased substantially. The existing health care systems in both countries were overwhelmed by the number of ageing individuals requiring provisions in health care. Models and solutions to health care delivery, such as the health care complex and technology discussed in this chapter, are just some of the solutions being employed by both countries to address their health care problems. Recently in Japan, long-term care insurance support was extended to cover medical supplies and equipment for the elderly including wheelchairs, walkers, protection against bedsores, technology to assist in position changes in bed, and other similar technology. These changes and advances in new technology are continually improving the support, coverage and health care for the elderly.

REFERENCES

Adachi, H. (2000). A study on the effectiveness of integrated health care in California USA. *Hospital.*, *59*(10), 872–879.

Blass, E. (2006). South Korea outfitting elderly disabled with bioshirts. *Engadget.com*. Retrieved September 13, 2009, from http://www.engadget.com/2006/05/15/south-korea-outfitting-elderly-disabled-with-bioshirts/.

Cheong, H. J., Shin, N. Y., & Joeng, Y. B. (2009). Improving Korean service delivery system in health care: Focusing on National E-health System. *International Conference on eHealth, Telemedicine, and Social Medicine* (pp. 263-268).

Coddington, D. C., Moore, K. D., & Fischer, E. A. (1996). *Making integrated health care work*. Englewood, Colorado, USA: Center for Research in Ambulatory Health Care Administration.

Conrad, D. A., & Shortell, S. M. (1996). Integrated health systems: promise and performance. *Frontiers of Health Services Management*, *13*(1), 3–40.

Eizmendi, G., Aztoika, J., & Craddock, G. (2007). *Challenges for assistive technology*. Netherlands: IOS Press.

Enthoven, A., & Vorhaus, C. (2000). *What is a hospital system?* Palo Alto, CA: Graduate School of Business Stanford University.

Giardina, C. W., Fottler, D. F., Shewchuk, R. M., & Hill, D. B. (1990). The case for hospital diversification into long-term care. *Health Care Management Review*, *15*(1), 71–82.

iHealth Beat (2007). Japan to track elderly health via wireless test zone. *iHealth Beat*. Retrieved from http://www.ihealthbeat.org/articles/2007/5/14/Japan-To-Track-Elderly-Health-Via-Wireless-Test-Zone.aspx.

Jeong, S. (2008). *A Study on the efficiency and effectiveness of integrated health care and social services delivery facilities: Special focus on integrating facilities of health care and social services on elderly in Japan and S. Korea*. Nagoya, Japan: The Graduate School of Nihon Fukushi University.

Jeong, S., Inoue Y., Adachi, H., & Nabeya, K. (2009). A study on the efficiency and effectiveness of integrated health care and social services delivery facilities. *Japanese Association for Health Care Administration, 3*(1).

Kongstvedt, P. R. (1997). *Essentials of managed health care* (2nd ed.). New York: Aspen Publishers.

Korea, S. (2009). Population and Housing. *Statistics Korea*. Retrieved from http://www.kostat.go.kr.

Lawton, R. B., & Mark, V. P. (2002). Integrated delivery networks: A detour on the road to integrated health care? *Health Affairs*, *21*(4), 128–143. doi:10.1377/hlthaff.21.4.128

Lehrman, S., & Shore, K. K. (1998). *Hospitals' vertical integration into skilled nursing: A rational approach to controlling transaction costs*. Blue Cross and Blue Shield of the Rochester Area, Inc.

Long, S. (2000). *Caring for the elderly in Japan and the US: practices and policies*. London, UK: Routledge Publishers. doi:10.4324/9780203464472

Niki, R. (1998). *Health, medical, welfare and care mix*. Tokyo, Japan: Igakushoin.

Niki, R. (2000). *Long- term care insurance and medical insurance reform*. Tokyo, Japan: Keisoshobo.

Pacific Health Summit. (2006). Preparing for the ageing challenge. *Pacific Health Summit*. Retrieved from http://www.pacifichealthsummit.org/downloads/Ageing%20Challenge_Breakout%20Session%20Report.pdf.

Population Statistics of Japan. (2009). National Institute of Population and Social Security Research. *Population Statistics of Japan*. Retrieved from http://www.ipss.go.jp.

Robichon, F. (2004). Robots help Japan care for its elderly. *Popular Mechanics*. Retrieved from http://www.popularmechanics.com/technology/industry/1288241.html.

Shortell, S. M. (1997). Commentary on Physician-hospital integration and the economic theory of the firm. *Medical Care Research and Review*, *54*(1), 25–31. doi:10.1177/107755879705400102

Shortell, S. M., & Kaluzny, A. D. (1994). *Health care management: organization, design, and behavior*. Florence, KY, USA: Delmar Publisher.

Stalldall, E., Caesar, M., & Erickson, R. (2001). Ageing, elderly, and how IT can be used to enhance the quality of care for the elderly. *Vardal Foundation*. Retrieved September 15, 2009, from http://www.vardal.se/japan/SweJapSeminar2.pdf.

Takayama, K. (2000). Health industry complex and hospital in USA. *Research and Study Kyoto University Japan*, *19*, 10–19.

The Technology Research for Independent Living. (2008). Ageing options: An article about independent living. *Technology Research for Independent Living*. Retrieved from http://www.trilcentre.org/news/ageing options: an article about independent living.397.573.news.html.

United Nations. (2008). World Population Prospects. *United Nations*. Retrieved from http://esa.un.org/unpp/.

Chapter 19
Assistive Technologies as Aids to Family Caregivers in Taiwan

Szu-Yao (Zoe) Wang
Australian Catholic University, Australia

ABSTRACT

The social structure in Taiwan has changed dramatically in the last twenty years. An increasing population of people aged over 65, a decreasing birth rate and rising numbers of women entering the workforce have led to the need for more aged care services. Research has demonstrated that nursing home placement of older adults in need of advanced care is the most cost effective option for family caregivers. However, filial piety, which entails looking after older parents at home, is one of the core tenets of Chinese society. Placing older parents into nursing homes can lead to conflicts that are detrimental to adult children psychologically. Moreover, the burden of caregiving does not necessarily end for the family once they have placed their parent(s) into nursing homes. It can continue to evoke deep emotional responses in some former family caregivers. This chapter draws on findings from two case studies to illustrate the dilemmas facing Taiwanese families who must cope with changing social conditions and customary filial expectations. The use of assistive technologies as solutions to these dilemmas is outlined. These technologies are argued to be a cost effective way to assist adult caregivers, their charges, and staff in nursing homes. Their use may apply to other Asian countries with similar cultural beliefs and values.

INTRODUCTION

Cultural beliefs and traditional values impact on all aspects of people's lives. Filial piety is deeply embedded in Chinese society in terms of caregiving to older people. The concept of filial piety means that the adult child, usually the son and especially the eldest son, has the responsibility for looking after his ageing parents.

In practice, the actual caregiver's role is usually undertaken by the wife of the eldest son, that is, the daughter-in-law. It is usually considered "morally wrong" and "unjust" by some Chinese people to think of placing a senior family mem-

DOI: 10.4018/978-1-61520-825-8.ch019

ber into a nursing home. Therefore, keeping the parents at home is the preferable choice. Assistive technologies have the potential to assist caregivers to maintain their filial duty. This chapter will discuss and recommend possible strategies to assist family caregivers in Taiwan.

The first part of this chapter will explain demographic changes occurring in Taiwanese society and consider various care options and their impacts on caregivers. It is worth noting that the rapidly ageing population found in Taiwan is also found in other South-East Asian countries such as China, Japan and Korea (Kim & Lee, 2003; Takeda et al., 2004; Xie, Xia, & Liu, 2007) and assistive technology strategies suggested for Taiwan might also have some application in these countries. The second part of the chapter will discuss specific technologies with reference to two case studies that explain how assistive technologies can be used to reduce the caregiving burden. These cases focused on older people and their family caregivers who live in Taiwan. However, these recommendations may also apply to family caregivers in other Asian societies which have similar cultural beliefs.

DEMOGRAPHIC CHANGES

The island of Taiwan is located in the northwest Pacific Ocean. Like other developed countries, Taiwan has become an ageing society, as illustrated by the following statistics. Since 1990, Taiwan's total population has increased by 9.1%, and by 2000 it had reached more than 22 million people. The percentage of people over the age of 65 increased from 6.4% in 1991 (Directorate-General of Budget Accounting & Statistics (DGBAS) Executive Yuan, 2002) to 9.9% in 2006 (Department-of-Social-Affairs, 2007). Birth rates decreased from 2.6% in 1976 to 1.4% in 2000. The death rate per 1000 decreased from 11.6% in 1971 to 5.6% in 2000 (Department of Health, 2004). Furthermore, the size of the Taiwanese household decreased from 5.7 people per household in 1956 to 3.9 people per household in 2000 (Directorate-General of Budget Accounting & Statistics (DGBAS) Executive Yuan, 2002), highlighting a significant shift in the family structure from large families to small families.

The number of senior people in Taiwan who live with their children has declined in line with the changing social structure and lower fertility rates (Directorate-General of Budget Accounting & Statistics (DGBAS) Executive Yuan, 2002). In 1990, 62.3% of senior people in Taiwan lived with their children; however, by 2000 this had decreased to 57.3%. In 1990, senior people who lived with their spouse accounted for only 17.3% of the total older population. In 2000, this had increased to 20%. The population of people who are 65 years or over and who lived alone increased from 15.9% (168,000 people) in 1990 to 18.3% (298,000 people) in 2000. These statistics demonstrate that there may be a greater need to increase welfare and provide care and assistance for older citizens. Furthermore, in order to provide better care for older people and to maintain the traditional social structure in Taiwan, the government has created a policy to encourage younger generations to live with their parents. In order to protect older people, the policy clearly states that any family members "dumping" their parents will be fined between NTD$30,000 to NTD$150,000 (approximately US$900-US$4500) and have their name published publicly (Department of Social Affairs, 2003). (Dumping refers to the failure of adult children to care for their parents, both financially and physically.)

TRANSFORMATION

Since the 1970s, Chinese society has transformed from an agricultural to an industrial economy. As a consequence, intergenerational power dynamics have also shifted (Thornton & Lin, 1994). More young couples have moved out of the family home for reasons such as insufficient space, friction between family members, or desire for independence. By the early 1990s household patterns were becoming increasingly westernised and nuclear (Thornton, Fricke, Yang, & Chang, 1994). Lan (2002) developed the theory of "a transfer chain of filial care" (p. 813) to determine how children achieve filial duty for elderly care in ethnic Chinese immigrants. There are two relevant concepts in this theory: gender transfer from the son to the daughter-in-law; and market transfer from kin caregivers to home health-care workers. Traditional parental authority and patriarchy in Chinese societies have impacted on the gender transformation from son to daughter-in-law in performing the duty of filial piety. The "patrilineal and patrilocal principle" (Weinstein, Sun, Chang, & Freedom, 1994, p.334) has influenced the pattern of three-generational living in the same household, in traditional Chinese families. The responsibility of the son, especially the eldest son, is to reside with the parents and to take care of them. The actual caregiver role is usually taken on by the daughters-in-law. This situation is influenced by the hierarchical concept of serving rather than caring (Fricke, Chang, & Yang, 1994; Holroyd, 2001; Ngan & Wong, 1995).

Another social structural change is female participation in the labour force. Since the 1970s, women have become significant contributors to the household income by working in the labour force and therefore are not in a position to be care-givers to the parents-in-law in the home (Hermalin, Liu, & Freedman, 1994). In order to fulfil the responsibility of filial piety (and to relieve the daughter-in-law and the son), there is a trend instead to hire healthcare workers to look after parents. In Taiwan, many of these paid caregivers come from the Philippines, Indonesia, Thailand and Vietnam. The monthly wage of a foreign carer in Taiwan is set at NTD$15,840 whereas a Taiwanese carer will cost NTD$30,000-35,000 a month. This means a Taiwanese carer is nearly twice as expensive as a foreign carer (Loveband, 2003). There are two criteria which qualify the family for assistance from foreign carers: firstly, families with either two or more children under the age of six or a dependent person over the age of 75 and, secondly, families with a family member with chronic illness or paralysis (Loveband, 2003). By 2002, there were 120,515 foreign caregivers and domestic helpers in Taiwan (Loveband, 2003). The quality of care provided by foreign caregivers is still not clear.

PATTERNS OF CAREGIVING

Even though social beliefs continue to change, children living in a Chinese society still try to fulfil their filial responsibilities. Lan (2002) identified the reasons for this. Due to societal pressures, the children perceive that fulfilling their filial duty is morally and socially essential. Secondly, the exchange of resources and power in intergenerational relationships, also called social exchange theory, is part of filial duty. Rearing a child, especially a son, is considered to be an investment for the future and the parents expect a delayed pay back. Children are expected to carry out their filial duty of repaying their parents' debts as well as purchasing houses and preparing a bride price for their son (Lan, 2002).

In Taiwan, home care by family caregivers is usually preferred over residential care for older people with a disability or chronic disease (Chiu, Tang, Shyu, & Chang, 1999). This is because home care is believed to promote autonomy, independence and a positive meaning in their lives (Crist, 2005). However, there are occasions when a choice needs to be made by the older person and the family to provide care away from home. In this circumstance, there are a number of other care choices that can be tried before the older person or the family caregivers decide on nursing home placement, such as respite care (short-term care) and employment of a private carer. The decision on the type of care is also dependent on the caregivers' financial status or abilities (Chiu, Shyu, & Liu, 2001).

Making the best choice of care services not only impacts on the health and well-being of the recipient but also has a great impact on family caregivers' general well-being. Using respite care to keep older parents at home is one of the options used by family caregivers in Taiwan (Chiu et al., 2001). Zarit, Stephens, Townsend and Greene (1998) observed that family caregivers of relatives with dementia who used adult day-care (respite care) demonstrated lower levels of caregiver-related stress and better psychological well-being than families who did not use adult day-care. Moreover, this difference was found in both short-term and long-term users of adult day-care. Family caregivers who utilised day-care also demonstrated a significant reduction in feelings of depression and anger.

As further support for day-care services, Adler et al. (1993) found that caregivers of dementia patients reported a reduction in care burden and depression levels when they used day-care services. However, they also found that the care burden returned to pre-respite levels two weeks after cessation of the service. In addition, there was no significant difference found in care recipients' functional abilities and behavioural assessment between pre- and post respite.

In contrast, Gaugler, Jarrott, Zarit, Stephens, and Greene (2003) suggested that utilizing adult day care services reduced the time that the caregiver spent dealing with, and managing behaviour problems in the older persons with dementia. They also showed that adult day-care service utilisation could help reduce the frequency of behaviour problems in older relatives. This research demonstrated that the elderly person who benefitted psychosocially from the adult day-care showed fewer negative behaviours. However, attendance at adult day care did not reduce the number of hours the family caregiver spent in assisting the elders in their Activities of Daily Living (ADL) and Instrumental Activities of Daily Living (IADL). One explanation may be that while programs in day-care can improve mood, they are unable to stop the deterioration due to disease progression (Gaugler et al., 2003).

On the other hand, Pot, Zarit, Twisk & Townsend (2005) found at the initial stages of employment of paid home care, the family reported an increase in anxiety and strain. However, if the family persisted with paid home care, the family caregiver reported a reduction in care burden and depressive symptoms.

Bringing an outsider into the caring role might also be considered a negative caring experience. In some families, paid home care is associated with depressive symptoms because paid home care is perceived as bringing an outsider into the home. There is also anxiety related to the management of outside help. Many families reported a decrease in depressive symptoms after the paid home care ceased (Pot et al., 2005). Therefore, in some cases, utilising other care services in the community setting does not necessarily provide benefits for either the older person or the family caregiver. Family caregivers usually have to evaluate all possible situations before they make a decision of whether to continue looking after the older person at home alone or considering other care choices.

The decision to place older relatives into a nursing home can be emotionally painful and psychologically stressful (Butcher, Holkup, Park, & Maas, 2001). According to Kao and Stuifbergen (1999), Taiwanese family caregivers recognised their filial duties and recognised burdens during the "breaking harmony" phase. The family caregivers recognised that their duty of care was based on either karma, benevolence or obligation (Kao & Stuifbergen, 1999). In addition, the duty of care is influenced by Confucianism to act benevolently. In the cultural context of Taiwan, benevolence requires "extending one's love to the surrounding people especially for those who are older, sick, poor or frail" (Kao & Stuifbergen, 1999, p.1117). One important belief in Chinese society is that when the daughter is identified as the family caregiver, the duty of care stems from benevolence as love. In contrast, when the son is identified as the family caregiver, the duty of care stems from the obligation brought to bear by filial piety. The son is usually the decision maker in the family (Kao & Stuifbergen, 1999). Normally, before the decision is finally reached that there is no option other than nursing home placement for older parents, the family caregivers have come to the realisation that lengthy and heavy burdens have resulted in the deterioration of their general health, family peace, recreation and savings (Kao & Stuifbergen, 1999). It is not clear whether family caregivers feel differently once they have placed the older family member in the nursing home.

Home care by family caregivers of older relatives in Taiwan remains the preferred option. However this option comes with a number of emotional costs to the extended family. The costs are associated with the increasing debility experienced by older persons suffering from chronic illnesses, associated dependency, and disturbing behaviours such as self-harm and wandering.

CAREGIVING IN TAIWAN AND ASSISTIVE TECHNOLOGIES

The second part of this chapter will use two case studies to illustrate a number of difficulties associated with care giving and current social expectations of family caregivers in Taiwan. A number of assistive technology devices will then be briefly explained with reference to their making life for family caregivers easier.

Fictitious names have been used in the following case studies.

Case One

Ms Chang's father has hydrocephalus and for many years her mother had looked after her father at home. The illness increasingly affects the father's memory, and he has a trembling and unsteady gait. Following surgery, he often becomes lost outside the home. Ms Chang's family keeps telling him that he shouldn't go out on his own. If he is to go out, he needs to be accompanied by other family members. Ms Chang's family also asks him to wear an identification tag. However, he is not willing to do that for fear of ridicule and people thinking he has memory problems. As Ms Chang observes: "The only thing we can do is to place an ID card in his wallet. We get phone calls from strangers because he cannot find the way home. In September we couldn't find him and we even turned to the police for help. We searched for him for over 12 hours but it was not until next day that someone called us and said that he's in hospital. He has had a fall which resulted in intracranial haemorrhage. We cannot look after him at home anymore."

The outcome of this case was that the families decided to place Mr. Chang into a nursing home. However, it took a long time for Ms Chang to adjust to that decision and clearly it remains a traumatic event for her and her family. During the interview, Ms Chang was very emotional and expressed a lot of guilt. For cultural reasons she didn't want anyone to know that she had placed her father into a nursing home. She believed it would be considered a disgrace and everyone would think she was unfilial, morally wrong and had failed in her duty as an adult child. Faced with her own feelings of guilt and conflict regarding these traditional cultural beliefs, she has failed to adapt to the inevitable outcome of the family's situation. Now, whenever her father becomes ill, Ms Chang blames herself for placing her father into the nursing home. She believes being in the nursing home resulted in her father's illness. She appears unable to reconcile the fact that illness is part of life.

Case Two

Mrs. Lan has two younger brothers and 3 younger sisters. Mrs. Lan's mother used to live with her sister and brother in the countryside but after she became ill, their family took turns to look after her. Mrs. Lan said that her mother wouldn't sleep at night and would walk around and play with the taps at night.

Mrs Lan observed: "My mother would cook rice on her own when my sister wasn't home and put all the food in the refrigerator into the pot. Taking care includes cooking for her and helping her take a bath and 24 hour monitoring. No one is available to take care of her all the time. We all have other things to do and we all have to go to work"

Mrs. Lan's mother would not sleep at night and instead would wander around incessantly. The family members could not cope with a worsening situation in which someone had to be with her 24 hours a day. Without this constant supervision, there was a danger of the mother wandering off or endangering herself and others by turning on the water or the gas taps and forgetting to turn them off. It was a very dangerous and frustrating situation for the family and in the end they decided to place their mother in a nursing home. The whole family found it difficult to come to terms with this decision, and differing opinions led to family conflicts. Some family members thought that others were not trying hard enough to look after the mother at home. An aunt and uncle thought that Mrs Lan was not filial to her mother. They suggested hiring a private carer. However, Mrs Lan queried the practicality of this suggestion; if they hired a private carer for homecare, who would pay for the cost and in whose home should the mother reside?

These cases highlight different caring dilemmas which were caused by a need for families to balance a cultural expectation of filial piety with the realities of the burden of care and its associated costs. Undoubtedly dilemmas of this kind will continue to confront many families with ageing parents in Taiwan, for many years. The question then is - could technology offer solutions that go at least some of the way towards reconciling the difficulties illustrated in the two case studies?

Assistive Technology Possibilities

Before eventually deciding which services to use, family caregivers must weigh up the cost of various alternatives such as payment for services, and labour costs for care giving and other out of pocket expenses. Chiu et al. (2001) have compared the costs of several care options and concluded that a nursing home option is the most cost effective service for many situations. Eventually, the nursing home option was chosen by both families discussed above.

In Taiwan, little research has been published into the use of assistive technology for addressing social and financial costs associated with looking after older relatives at home. However, research carried out in other countries has demonstrated that using assistive technologies to support the management of chronic illness at home can reduce health expenditure and lower the burden of care (Handley, Shumway, & Schillinger, 2008; Wherton & Monk, 2008).

Wang (2007) highlights the considerable burden placed on informal caregivers of dementia sufferers. As the disease progresses, caregivers must play an increasingly demanding role of assisting with activities of daily living, and supervising and monitoring their charges. Implementation of home care devices can assist with prolonging the independence of dementia sufferers as well as reducing the caregivers' burden. For example, a touch screen has been effectively used to assist demented people to actively direct a conversation without having to rely on caregivers (Astell, Ellis, & Alm, 2004). In fact, Astell (2005) argues that technology can benefit people with dementia perhaps more than it can benefit people without cognitive impairments. Considerable cost savings were reported (Woolham, 2006) when assistive technology was used in supporting the independence of people with dementia in the community.

Implementation of home care devices such as wandering alarms, electronic door locking and monitoring devices, and motion sensors could have assisted both the Chang and Lan families. These quite simple devices could have prevented Ms Chang's father from wandering out of the house in the first place, or notified the family in the event of a fall. Where limited outdoor activity is appropriate, a wandering monitor and alarm can detect movement and produce a verbal message to remind the dementia sufferer of the time and encourage him/her to return home. Should dementia sufferers wander out of the house, an alert is sent to the monitoring centre to notify the carers. The wandering behaviour of loved ones is distressing for family caregivers of dementia sufferers and gives rise to a considerably increased physical and psychological caregiving burden (Wang, 2007). Night time wandering leads to fatigue and can give rise to symptoms of depression among caregivers. However, the use of wandering alarm monitors has been shown to produce greater peace of mind and reduced sleep disturbance patterns among caregivers (Spring, Rowe, & Kelly, 2009).

Furthermore, night-time reminder devices and motion activated lighting could have been installed in the homes to overcome the danger of falls at night and to provide verbal prompts and directions for Mrs Lan and Ms Chang's disorientated parents. This illumination system is activated when older people get out the bed at night. A gentle voice message is also played to encourage the older people to return to bed or go to the toilet (Evans, Orpwood, Adlam, Gibbs, & Faulkner, 2003). Other monitoring systems such as smoke sensors, fall detectors and sensors on kitchen cupboards, the refrigerator and water taps are also recommended for Ms Chang and Mrs Lan as part of the plan to minimise or delay the need for nursing home placement.

Falls by the elderly are common. For example, in Queensland, Australia, one in three older people suffer injury and health problems from falls every year (Queensland-Government, 2002). It has been estimated that in terms of causes of death, hospitalizations and admissions to emergency departments for elderly people, the majority of injuries are from falls (Queensland-Injury-Surveillance-Unit, 1999). Hip fracture is one of the most serious injuries arising from falls. The results of falls adversely affect both the lives of elderly people and their caregivers. Wearing falls detectors can lead to greater peace of mind for both users and their caregivers (Brownsell & Hawley, 2004). The fall of Mrs Chang's father had caused his physical and mental condition to deteriorate. Wearing a falls detector or falls pendant perhaps could have helped Mrs Chang's father to get more speedy assistance or even have diminished the possibility of the fall by providing soothing reminders to be careful when walking.

Even after nursing home placement occurs, the possibility of falls in the nursing home remains an issue for Taiwanese families. In Taiwan, family caregivers are asked to sign a form consenting to the use of restraint as part of the nursing home falls prevention policy. The thought of using restraint on a loved one is stressful, and signing the restraint form evokes deep emotional responses from some family caregivers. However, families know that a nursing home cannot provide one-on-one care. Rather than using restraint as an all-encompassing solution to the possibility of falls, the use of falls detectors and monitoring systems by the nursing home service provider would, in all probability, help to ease the family caregivers' guilt associated with placing older parents in a nursing home.

A final example of the use of assistive technology devices to lessen or delay the likelihood of nursing home placement is relevant to the second case study. Because Mrs Lan's family had work or other commitments outside the home, her mother often cooked when no one was around to supervise. One of Mrs Lan's biggest worries was that her mother would endanger herself when there was no one around; or even endanger the entire family by cooking late at night. She feared the mother would leave the gas cooker on unlit, or leave a pot to boil dry on the cooker, leading to a fire. In cases like this, a cooker control, which automatically turns off the gas supply when extreme high temperatures or the smell of gas is detected, could have been installed. When activated, the control would simultaneously send a message to a control centre who would advise the carer of a potential problem in the home.

CONCLUSION

Nursing home placement of older parents in Taiwan is considered to be morally wrong and a failure of one's filial duties and responsibilities. Guilt associated with the process of placing older parents in nursing homes can be detrimental to caregivers' psychological and physical well-being, which can extend well beyond the period of actual nursing home placement. It is usually considered as the last option for looking after parents in Taiwan society. Family caregivers will often consider other options such as respite care and private carer however these measures can be costly and ineffective. Local governments in Taiwan need to consider utilising assistive technologies of the kind described in this chapter and elsewhere in this book, to assist family caregivers to look after their parents in community settings.

REFERENCES

Adler, G., Ott, L., Jelinski, M., Mortimer, J., & Christensen, R. (1993). Institutional respite care: benefits and risks for dementia patients and caregivers. *International Psychogeriatrics*, *5*(1), 67–77. doi:10.1017/S1041610293001401

Astell, A. J. (2005). Developing technology for people with dementia. *Psychiatric Times*, *22*(13), 28–29.

Astell, A. J., Ellis, M. P., & Alm, N. (2004). Facilitating communication in dementia with multimedia technology. *Brain and Language*, *91*(1), 80–81. doi:10.1016/j.bandl.2004.06.043

Brownsell, S., & Hawley, M. (2004). Fall detectors: Do they work or reduce the fear of falling? *Housing. Care & Support*, *7*(1), 18–24.

Butcher, H. K., Holkup, P. A., Park, M., & Maas, M. (2001). Thematic analysis of the experience of making a decision to place a family member with Alzheimer's disease in a special care unit. *Research in Nursing & Health*, *24*(6), 470–480. doi:10.1002/nur.10005

Chiu, L., Shyu, W. C., & Liu, Y. H. (2001). Comparisons of the cost-effectiveness among hospital chronic care, nursing home placement, home nursing care and family care for severe stroke patients. *Journal of Advanced Nursing*, *33*(3), 380–386. doi:10.1046/j.1365-2648.2001.01703.x

Chiu, L., Tang, K.-Y., Shyu, W.-C., & Chang, T.-P. (1999). The willingness of families caring for victims of stroke to pay for in-home respite care--results of a pilot study in Taiwan. *Health Policy (Amsterdam)*, *46*(3), 239–254. doi:10.1016/S0168-8510(98)00062-1

Crist, J. D. (2005). The meaning for elders of receiving family care. *Journal of Advanced Nursing*, *49*(5), 485–493. doi:10.1111/j.1365-2648.2004.03321.x

Department of Health. E. Y., ROC. (2004). *Health and vital Statistical: Vital statistical*. Taipei: Department of Health, Executive Yuan, ROC.

Department-of-Social-Affairs. (2003). Older People's Welfare and Policy (In Chinese). Retrieved April 13, 2004, from http://volnet.moi.gov.tw/sowf/04/01.htm.

Department-of-Social-Affairs. (2007). Long term care: The ten years plan. Retrieved March 9, 2008, from http://sowf.moi.gov.tw/newpage/tenyearsplan.htm.

Directorate-General of Budget Accounting & Statistics (DGBAS) Executive Yuan. T., R.O.C. (2002, 30/12/2002). 2000 Population and housing census. Retrieved March 31, 2004, from http://www.dgbas.gov.tw/census~n/six/lue5/census_p&h&E.htm.

Evans, N., Orpwood, R., Adlam, T., Gibbs, C., & Faulkner, R. (2003). *Smart house technology: providing practical support for people living with dementia*. College of Occupational Therapists.

Fricke, T., Chang, J. S., & Yang, L. S. (1994). Historical and Ethnographical Perspectives on the Chinese Family. In Thornton, A., & Lin, L.-S. (Eds.), *Social Change and the Family in Taiwan* (pp. 22–48). Chicago: University of Chicago Press.

Gaugler, J. E., Jarrott, S. E., Zarit, S. H., Stephens, M. P., & Greene, R. (2003). Respite for Dementia Caregivers: The effects of adult day service use on caregiving hours and care demands. *International Psychogeriatrics*, *15*(1), 37–58. doi:10.1017/S1041610203008743

Handley, M. A., Shumway, M., & Schillinger, D. (2008). Cost-effectiveness of automated telephone self-management support with nurse care management among patients with diabetes. *Annals of Family Medicine*, *6*(6), 512–518. doi:10.1370/afm.889

Hermalin, A., Liu, P. K. C., & Freedman, D. (1994). The Social and Economic Transformation of Taiwan. In Thornton, A., & Lin, L.-S. (Eds.), *Social Change and the Family in Taiwan* (pp. 49–87). Chicago: University of Chicago Press.

Holroyd, E. (2001). Hong Kong Chinese daughters' intergenerational caregiving obligations: a cultural model approach. *Social Science & Medicine*, *53*, 1125–1134. doi:10.1016/S0277-9536(00)00406-8

Kao, H.-F., & Stuifbergen, A. K. (1999). Family experiences related to the decision to institutionalize an elderly member in Taiwan: an exploratory study. *Social Science & Medicine*, *49*(8), 1115–1123. doi:10.1016/S0277-9536(99)00211-7

Kim, J.-S., & Lee, E.-H. (2003). Cultural and Noncultural Predictors of Health Outcomes in Korean Daughter and Daughter-in-Law Caregivers. *Public Health Nursing (Boston, Mass.)*, *20*(2), 111–119. doi:10.1046/j.1525-1446.2003.20205.x

Lan, P. C. (2002). Subcontracting Filial Piety Elder Care in Ethnic Chinese Immigrant Families in California. *Journal of Family Issues*, *23*(7), 812–835. doi:10.1177/019251302236596

Loveband, A. (2003). Positioning the product: Indonesian Migrant Women Workers in Contemporary Taiwan. Working Papers Series. Retrieved June 10, 2004, from http://www.cityu.edu.hk/searc/WP43_03_Loveband.pdf.

Ngan, R., & Wong, W. (1995). Injustice in family care of the Chinese elderly in Hong Kong. *Journal of Aging & Social Policy*, *7*(2), 77–94. doi:10.1300/J031v07n02_06

Pot, A. M., Zarit, S. H., Twisk, J. W. R., & Townsend, A. L. (2005). Transitions in Caregivers' Use of Paid Home Help: Associations With Stress Appraisals and Well-Being. *Psychology and Aging*, *20*(2), 211–219. doi:10.1037/0882-7974.20.2.211

Queensland-Government. (2002). *Statewide Action Plan Falls Prevention in Older People 2002-2006*. Queensland Government.

Queensland-Injury-Surveillance-Unit. (1999). Falls in older people'. *Injury Bulletin*, *56*, 1–6.

Spring, H. J., Rowe, M. A., & Kelly, A. (2009). Improving caregivers' well-being by using technology to manage nighttime activity in persons with dementia. *Research in Gerontological Nursing*, *2*(1), 39–48. doi:10.3928/19404921-20090101-10

Takeda, Y., Kawachi, I., Yamagata, Z., Hashimoto, S., Matsumura, Y., Oguri, S., et al. (2004). Multigenerational family structure in Japanese society: impacts on stress and health behaviors among women and men. *Social Science & Medicine (1982), 59*(1), 69-81.

Thornton, A., Fricke, T., Yang, L. S., & Chang, J. S. (1994). Theoretical Mechanisms of Family Change. In Thornton, A., & Lin, L.-S. (Eds.), *Social Change and the Family in Taiwan* (pp. 88–51). Chicago: University of Chicago Press.

Thornton, A., & Lin, L.-S. (1994). Introduction. In Thornton, A., & Lin, L.-S. (Eds.), *Social Change and the Family in Taiwan* (*Vol. 1-22*). Chicago: University of Chicago Press.

Wang, S.-Y. (2007). *Nursing home placement in Taiwan an exploration of the experience in adult children.* Unpublished PhD thesis, The University of Queensland, St. Lucia, Queensland, Australia.

Weinstein, M., Sun, T. H., Chang, M. C., & Freedom, D. (1994). Co-Residence and Other Tie Linking Couples and Their Parents. In Thornton, A., & Lin, L.-S. (Eds.), *Social Change and the Family in Taiwan* (pp. 305–334). Chicago: University of Chicago Press.

Wherton, J. P., & Monk, A. F. (2008). Technological opportunities for supporting people with dementia who are living at home. *International Journal of Human-Computer Studies, 66*(8), 571–586. doi:10.1016/j.ijhcs.2008.03.001

Woolham, J. (2006). *Safety at Home. The effectiveness of assistive technology in supporting the independence of people with dementia*. London: Hawker Publication.

Xie, X., Xia, Y., & Liu, X. (2007). Family income and attitudes toward older people in China: comparison of two age cohorts. *Journal of Family and Economic Issues, 28*(1), 171–182. doi:10.1007/s10834-006-9044-5

Zarit, S. H., Stephens, M. A., Townsend, A., & Greene, R. (1998). Stress reduction for family caregivers: effects of adult day care use. *The Journals of Gerontology. Series B, Psychological Sciences and Social Sciences, 53*(5), S267–S277.

Compilation of References

AALIANCE. (2009). *The European Ambient Assisted Living Innovation Alliance Website*. Retrieved December 11, 2009, from http://www.aaliance.eu/public/

AARP. (2005). *Doing the math. Older adults online 2005*. Retrieved from http://www.aarp.org/olderwiserwired/oww-resources/doing_the_math_older_adults_online.html.

Aarts, E., Harwig, R., & Schuurmans, M. (2001). Ambient intelligence. In *The invisible future: The seamless integration of technology into everyday life*. McGraw-Hill.

Abbey, J. (2005). Palliative Care. In R. Nay & S. Garratt (Eds.), *Nursing older people – Issues and innovations* (2nd ed., pp. 259-275). Churchill Livingstone: Elsevier.

Abbott, R., White, L., Ross, W., Masaki, K. H., Curb, J. D., & Petrovitch, H. (2004). Walking and dementia in physically capable elderly men. *Journal of the American Medical Association*, *292*, 1447–1453. doi:10.1001/jama.292.12.1447

ABS. (2008). *3222.0 - Population projections, Australia, 2006 to 2101*. Canberra: Australian Bureau of Statistics.

ABS. (2008). *Population by age and sex, Australian states and territories, Jun 2008. Document 3201.0,* Retrieved September 21 2009, from http://www.abs.gov.au/Ausstats/abs@.nsf/mf/3201.0.

ABS. 2005). Use of information technology by older people. In *1301.0 - Year Book Australia*, 2005. Canberra: Australian Bureau of Statistics.

ACMA. (2009). *Australia in the digital economy: Report 2 Online participation*. Australia Communications and Media Authority Retrieved October, 3, 2009, from http://www.acma.gov.au/WEB/STANDARD/pc=PC_311655

Active Ageing Consortium Asia Pacific (ACAP). Retrieved March 9, 2009 from http://www.wellageing.com.

Adachi, H. (2000). A study on the effectiveness of integrated health care in California USA. *Hospital.*, *59*(10), 872–879.

Adams, A., & Blandford, A. (2005). Digital libraries' support for the user's information journey. *IEEE and ACM Joint conference of digital libraries ACM/IEEE JCDL 2005*.

Adams, A., Blandford, A., & Attfield, S. (2005). Implementing digital resources for clinicians' and patients' varying needs. *BCS Healthcare Computing 2005*.

ADI. (2009). World Alzheimers report 2009. *Alzheimers Disease International*. Retrieved September 2009 from www.alz.co.uk

Adler, G., Ott, L., Jelinski, M., Mortimer, J., & Christensen, R. (1993). Institutional respite care: benefits and risks for dementia patients and caregivers. *International Psychogeriatrics*, *5*(1), 67–77. doi:10.1017/S1041610293001401

Agency for Health Care Research and Quality. (2000). *The characteristics of long-term care users*. Rockville, MD: AHRQ.

Agree, E. M., & Freedman, V. A. (2000). Incorporating assistive devices into community-based long term care. *Journal of Aging and Health, 12*(3), 426–450. doi:10.1177/089826430001200307

AHMC. (2005). *National chronic disease strategy*. Conference communiqué. Australian Health Ministers Council, 18 November 2005.

Aiello, M., & Dustdar, S. (2008). Are our homes ready for services? A domotic infrastructure based on the Web service stack. *Pervasive and Mobile Computing, 4*(4). doi:10.1016/j.pmcj.2008.01.002

AIHW. (2006). *Chronic diseases and associated risk factors in Australia (No. AIHW Cat. No. PHE 81.)*. Canberra: Australian Institute of Health and Welfare.

Alcatel-Lucent. (2008). *Corporate social responsibility report 2008*. Paris: Alcatel-Lucent.

Alciatore, D., & Histand, M. (2003). *Introduction to mechatronics*. USA: McGraw-Hill.

Altinkemer, K., De, P., & Ozdemir, Z. (2006). Toward a Consumer-to-Healthcare Provider (C2H) electronic marketplace. *Communications of the AIS, 18*, 413–430.

Altman, I. (1975). *The environment and social behavior: Privacy, personal space, territoriality and crowding*. Monterey, CA: Brooks/Cole.

Alwan, M., Rajendran, P. J., Kell, S., Mack, D., Dalal, S., Wolfe, M., et al. (2006). *A Smart and Passive Floor-Vibration Based Fall Detector for Elderly.* Paper presented at the 2nd IEEE Information and Communication Technologies.

Alzheimer Nederland. (2009). Cijfers en feiten over dementie, www.alzheimer-nederland.nl.

Aman, E., & Thomas, D. R. (2009). Supervised exercise to reduce agitation in severely cognitively impaired persons. *Journal of the American Medical Directors Association, 10*(4), 271–276. doi:10.1016/j.jamda.2008.12.053

Ambient Assisted Living Joint Programme. (n.d.). "What is AAL?" Retrieved January 20, 2009, from http://www.aal-europe.eu/about-aal

Ambient Assisted Living Joint Programme. (n.d.). AAL: Preparation of a new European Initiative for IT supported solutions. Retrieved January 20, 2009, from http://www.aal169.org/intern/Workpackages/wp0/networking/AALflv2.pdf

American Geriatrics Society, British Geriatrics Society, and American Academy of Orthopaedic Surgeons Panel on Falls Prevention. (in press). Guideline for the prevention of falls in older persons. *Journal of the American Geriatrics Society*.

Amigo (2007). Amigo: Ambient intelligence for the networked home environment. Retrieved August 24, 2009, from http://www.hitech-projects.com/euprojects/amigo/.

Aminian, K., & Najafi, B. (2004). Capturing human motion using body-fixed sensors: outdoor measurement and clinical applications. *Computer Animation and Virtual Worlds, 15*(2), 79–94. doi:10.1002/cav.2

Andel, R., Crowe, M., Pedersen, N. L., Fratiglioni, L., Johansson, B., & Gatz, M. (2008). Physical exercise at midlife and risk of dementia three decades later: a population-based study of Swedish twins. *The Journals of Gerontology. Series A, Biological Sciences and Medical Sciences, 63*(1), 62–66.

Angelo, J. (2000). Factors affecting the use of a single switch with assistive technology devices. *Journal of Rehabilitation Research and Development, 37*(5), 591–598.

Ankem, K. (2005). Types of information needs among cancer patients: A systematic review. *Library & Information Science Research, 15*(2).

Anstey, K. J., Wood, J., Lord, S., & Walker, J. G. (2005). Cognitive, sensory and physical factors enabling driving safety in older adults. *Clinical Psychology Review, 25*(1), 45–65. doi:10.1016/j.cpr.2004.07.008

Antonucci, T. C. (2001). Social relations: An examination of social networks, social support, and sense of control. In Birren, J. E., & Schaie, K. W. (Eds.), *Handbook of the psychology of aging* (5th ed., pp. 427–453). San Diego, CA: Academic Press.

Aphek, E. (2001). Minimizing the digital divide and the inter-generation gap. *Ubiquity: An ACM IT Magazine and Forum*. Retrieved from http://www.acm.org/ubiquity/views/e_aphek_1.html?searchterm=aphek.

Arentze, T., Timmermans, H., Jorritsma, P., Olde-Kalter, M.-J., & Schoemakers, A. (2008). More gray hair—but for whom? Scenario-based simulations of elderly activity travel patterns in 2020. *Transportation*, *35*(5), 613–627. doi:10.1007/s11116-008-9170-z

Armstrong, B. K., Gillespie, J. A., Leeder, S. R., Rubin, G. L., & Russell, L. M. (2007). Challenges in health and health care for Australia. *The Medical Journal of Australia*, *187*(9), 485–489.

Astell, A. J., Ellis, M. P., & Alm, N. (2004). Facilitating communication in dementia with multimedia technology. *Brain and Language*, *91*(1), 80–81. doi:10.1016/j.bandl.2004.06.043

Astell, A. J. (2005). Developing technology for people with dementia. *Psychiatric Times*, *22*(13), 28–29.

Atmel (2007). *ATmega640/1280/1281/2560/2561 datasheet*. Document number 2549LS–AVR 08/07 (p. 37). Retrieved on October 20, 2009, from http://www.atmel.com/dyn/resources/prod_documents/doc2549.pdf.

Australian Bureau of Statistics. (2008). *Population Projections, Australia, 2006–2101*. Canberra: Australian Bureau of Statistics.

Australian Bureau of Statistics. (2004, June 16). *4102.0 - Australian Social Trends, 2004*. Retrieved February 15, 2009, from http://www.abs.gov.au/

Australian Bureau of Statistics. (2004, June 5). *4446.0 - Disability, Australia, 2003*. Retrieved February 10, 2009, from http://www.abs.gov.au/

Australian Government Treasury. (2007). *Intergenerational Report 2007*. Canberra: Commonwealth of Australia.

Australian Intitute of Health and Welfare (AIHW). (2006). *Life Expectancy and Disability in Australia 1988 to 2003*. Canberra: AIHW.

Australian Transport Council. (2008). *National Road Safety Action Plan: 2009 and 2010*.

Austroads. (2004). *Model licence re-assessment procedure for older drivers: Stage 2 research*. Sydney: Austroads Incorporated.

Aware Home. (2008). Aware Home Research Initiative Project, Georgia Institute of Technology. Retrieved August 24, 2009 from http://awarehome.imtc.gatech.edu/.

Ayres, D., Soar, J., & Conrick, M. (2006). Health information systems. In Conrick, M. (Ed.), *Health informatics: Tranforming healthcare with technology* (pp. 197–211). Thomson, Social Science Press.

Azkoitia, J. M. (2004). Mobile monitoring and automatic fall detection device for elderly people living alone. Retrieved February 23rd, 2009, from http://cordis.europa.eu/fetch?CALLER=FP6_PROJ&ACTION=D&DOC=1&CAT=PROJ&QUERY=011fa7ae372c:d909:4196ac8c&RCN=72186.

Bach-y-Rita, P. (2001). Theoretical and practical considerations in the restoration of functions following stroke. *Topics in Stroke Rehabilitation*, *8*(3), 1–15. doi:10.1310/8T1T-ETXU-8PDF-9X7F

Bain, B. K., & Leger, D. (1996). Environmental controls and robotics. In Hammel, J. (Ed.), *Assistive technology and occupational therapy: A link to function*. Bethesda, MD: American Occupational Therapy Association.

Bakaev, M., Ponomarev, V., & Prokhorova, L. (2008). E-learning and elder people: Barriers and benefits. *Computational Technologies in Electrical and Electronics Engineering*, 110-113.

Ball, K. K., Beard, B. L., Roenker, D. L., Miller, R. L., & Griggs, D. S. (1988). Age and visual search: Expanding the useful field of view. *Journal of the Ophthalmological Society of America, Series A*, *5*(12), 2210–2219.

Ball, K. K., Berch, D. B., Helmers, K. F., Jobe, J. B., Leveck, M. D., & Marsiske, M. (2002). Effects of cognitive training interventions with older adults: A randomized controlled trial. *Journal of the American Medical Association*, *288*(18), 2271–2281. doi:10.1001/jama.288.18.2271

Ball, K. K., Edwards, J. D., & Ross, L. A. (2007). The impact of speed of processing training on cognitive and everyday functions. *The Journals of Gerontology. Series B, Psychological Sciences and Social Sciences*, *62*(S1), 19–31.

Ball, K. K., Owsley, C., Sloane, M. E., Roenker, D. L., & Bruni, J. R. (1993). Visual attention problems as a predictor of vehicle crashes in older drivers. *Investigative Ophthalmology & Visual Science*, *34*(11), 3110–3121.

Ball, K. K., Owsley, C., Stalvey, B., Roenker, D. L., Sloane, M. E., & Graves, M. (1998). Driving avoidance and functional impairment in older drivers. *Accident; Analysis and Prevention*, *30*(3), 313–322. doi:10.1016/S0001-4575(97)00102-4

Ball, K. K., Roenker, D. L., Wadley, V. G., Edwards, J. D., Roth, D. L., & McGwin, G. (2006). Can high-risk older drivers be identified through performance-based measures in a Department of Motor Vehicles setting? *Journal of the American Geriatrics Society*, *54*(1), 77–84. doi:10.1111/j.1532-5415.2005.00568.x

Ball, M. M., Whittington, F. J., Perkins, M. M., Patterson, V. L., Hollingsworth, C., King, S. V., & Combs, B. (2000). Quality of life of assisted living residents: Viewpoints of residents. *Journal of Applied Gerontology*, *19*, 304–325. doi:10.1177/073346480001900304

Ball, K. K., Roenker, D. L., & Bruni, J. R. (1990). Developmental changes in attention and visual search throughout adulthood. In Enns, J. T. (Ed.), *The development of attention: Research and theory*. Amsterdam: Elsevier Science Publishers B. V. doi:10.1016/S0166-4115(08)60472-0

Ball, K. K., & Owsley, C. (2000). Increasing mobility and reducing accidents of older drivers. In Schaie, K. W., & Pietrucha, M. (Eds.), *Mobility and transportation in the elderly*. New York: Springer Publishing Company, Inc.

Ball, K. K., Beard, B. L., Miller, R. L., & Roenker, D. L. (1987). Mapping the useful field of view as a function of age. *Gerontologist, 27*(A), 166-167.

Baltes, P. B., & Baltes, M. M. (1990). Psychological perspectives on successful aging: The model of selective optimization with compensation. In Baltes, P. B., & Baltes, M. M. (Eds.), *Successful aging: Perspectives from the behavioral sciences* (pp. 1–34). New York: Cambridge University Press. doi:10.1017/CBO9780511665684.003

Banach, D., Jones, T., & Kalameja, A. (2006). *Autodesk Inventor 11 Essentials Plus*. USA: Autodesk Press.

Banerji, S., & Heng, J. (2009). A unified, neuro-physio platform to facilitate collaborative play in children with learning disabilities. In *Proceedings of the 2009 IEEE 11th International Conference on Rehabilitation Robotics*, 23-26 June 2009, Kyoto, Japan (pp. 912-917).

Banerji, S., Heng, J., & Kangdra, W. (2008). New directions in the creation of upper extremity robotic rehabilitation devices for stroke patients. In *Proceedings of the 2nd International Conference on Assistive Technology and Rehabilitation Engineering iCREATe 2008*, Bangkok, Thailand.

Bank, A. L., Arguelles, S., Rubert, M., Eisdorfer, C., & Czaja, S. J. (2006). The value of telephone support groups among ethnically diverse caregivers of persons with dementia. *The Gerontologist*, *46*, 134–138.

Banquet, J. P. (1973). Spectral analysis of EEG in meditation. *Electroencephalography and Clinical Neurophysiology*, *35*, 143–151. doi:10.1016/0013-4694(73)90170-3

Barbour, R. (1998). Mixing qualitative methods: Quality assurance or qualitative quagmire? *Qualitative Health Research*, *8*(3), 352–361. doi:10.1177/104973239800800306

Bargh, J., & McKenna, K. (2004). The internet and social life. *Annual Review of Psychology*, *55*, 573–590. doi:10.1146/annurev.psych.55.090902.141922

Barlow, J., Singh, D., Bayer, S., & Curry, R. (2007). A systematic review of the benefits of home telecare for frail elderly people and those with long-term conditions. *Journal of Telemedicine and Telecare*, *13*, 172–179. doi:10.1258/135763307780908058

Barry, R. J., Clarke, A. R., Johnstone, S. J., Magee, C. A., & Rushby, J. A. (2007). EEG differences between eyes-closed and eyes-open resting conditions. *Clinical Neurophysiology*, *118*, 2765–2773. doi:10.1016/j.clinph.2007.07.028

Barton, J., & Jung, E. (2009). Distributed, Embedded Sensor and Actuator Platforms. In *Ambient Intelligence with Microsystems* (pp. 105-129).

Bastille, J. V., & Gill-Body, K. M. (2004). A yoga-based exercise program for people with chronic poststroke hemiparesis. *Physical Therapy*, *84*(1), 33–48.

Bayly, M., Young, K. L., & Regen, M. A. (2009). Sources of distraction inside the vehicle and their effects on driving performance. In Regen, M. A., Lee, J. D., & Young, K. L. (Eds.), *Driver Distraction: Theory, Effects, and Mitigation*. Boca Raton, Florida: CRC Press.

Beauchamp, N., Irvine, A. B., Seeley, J., & Johnson, B. (2005). Worksite-based Internet multimedia program for family caregivers of persons with dementia. *The Gerontologist*, *45*, 793–801.

Bechtel, R., & Churchman, A. (Eds.). (2002). *Handbook of environmental psychology*. New York: Wiley.

Beddington, J., Cooper, C., Field, J., Goswami, U., Huppert, F., & Jenkins, R. (2008). The mental wealth of nations. *Nature*, *455*(7216), 1057–1060. doi:10.1038/4551057a

Behringer, R., & Muller, N. (1998). Autonomous road vehicle guidance from autobahnen to narrow curves. *IEEE Transactions on Robotics and Automation*, *14*(5), 810–815. doi:10.1109/70.720356

Belfield, G., & Colin-Thome, D. (2004). *Improving chronic disease management*. Department of Health, UK National Health Service. Retrieved Sept. 12, 2009 from http://www.dh.gov.uk/en/Publicationsandstatistics/Publications/PublicationsPolicyAndGuidance/DH_4075214.

Bell, G., Blythe, M., Gaver, B., Sengers, P., & Wright, P. (2003). Designing culturally situated technologies for the home. In *CHI '03 extended abstracts on human factors in computing systems CHI '03*. Workshops.

Bennett, D. A., Schneider, J. A., Tang, Y., Arnold, S. E., & Wilson, R. S. (2006). The effect of social networks on the relation between Alzheimer's disease pathology and level of cognitive function in old people: a longitudinal cohort study. *The Lancet Neurology*, *5*(5), 406–412. doi:10.1016/S1474-4422(06)70417-3

Bental, D., Cawsey, A., Pearson, J., & Jones, R. (2000). Adapting web-based information to the needs of patients with cancer. In *Proceedings of International Conference on Adaptive Hypermedia and Web-based systems*, Trento, Italy.

Berger, M. L. (2001). *The automobile in American history and culture: A reference guide*. Westport, Connecticut: Greenwood Publishing Group.

Bergstrom, P., Driscoll, K., & Kimball, J. (2001). Making home automation communications secure. *IEEE Computer*, *34*(10), 50–56.

Berthoz, A. (1996). Neural basis of decision in perception and control of movement. *Neurobiology in Decision Making*, 83-100.

Besser, M. P., Selby-Silverstein, L., & Prickett, N. (2001). Predicting Fall Risk in the Elderly Using Temporal-Spatial Parameters of Gait. *Symposium of the International Society for Postural and Gait Research*, 70-73.

Bien, Z., Kim, D., Chung, M., Kwon, D., & Chang, P. (2003). Development of a wheelchair-based rehabilitation robotic syem (KARES 11) with various human-robot interaction interfaces for the disabled. In *Proceedings of the 2003 IEEE/ASME International Conference on Advanced Intelligent Mechatronics 20-24 July 2003* (AIM 2003), 2 (pp. 902-907). Retrieved September 22, 2009, from http://ieeexplore.ieee.org/stamp/stamp.jsp?tp=&arnumber=1225462&isnumber=27509.

Bilney, B., Morris, M., & Webster, K. (2003). Concurrent related validity of the GAITRite® walkway system for quantification of the spatial and temporal parameters of gait. *Gait & Posture*, *17*(1), 68–74. doi:10.1016/S0966-6362(02)00053-X

BioMOBIUS. (2009). Retrieved February 15th, from http://www.biomobius.org.

Birren, J. E., Schaie, K. W., Gatz, M., & Salthouse, T. A. (Eds.). (2006). *Handbook of the Psychology of Aging* (6th ed.). Amsterdam, The Netherlands: Elsevier.

Black, L.-A., McTear, M., Black, N., McMeel, C., Harper, R., & Lemon, M. (2004). Talking telemedicine: Is the interactive voice-logbook evolving into the cornerstone of diabetes healthcare? *AAAI Fall Symposium, Dialogue Systems for Health Communication*, Menlo Park, California.

Blake, D. J., & Bodine, C. (2002). An overview of assistive technology for persons with multiple sclerosis. *Journal of Rehabilitation Research and Development*, *39*(2), 299–312.

Blass, E. (2006). South Korea outfitting elderly disabled with bioshirts. *Engadget.com*. Retrieved September 13, 2009, from http://www.engadget.com/2006/05/15/south-korea-outfitting-elderly-disabled-with-bioshirts/.

Blows, S., Ivers, R. Q., Woodward, M., Connor, J., Ameratunga, S., & Norton, R. (2003). Vehicle year and the risk of car crash injury. *Injury Prevention*, *9*(4), 353–356. doi:10.1136/ip.9.4.353

Blumenthal, D. (2004). New stream from an old cauldron - the physician supply debate. *The New England Journal of Medicine*, *350*(17), 1780–1787. doi:10.1056/NEJMhpr033066

Bodenheimer, T., Wagner, E. H., & Grumbach, K. (2002). Improving primary care for patients with chronic illness. *Journal of the American Medical Association*, *288*(14), 1775–1779. doi:10.1001/jama.288.14.1775

Bosman, E. A., & Charness, N. (1996). Age-related differences in skilled performance and skill acquisition. In Blanchard-Fields, S., & Hess, T. (Eds.), *Perspectives on cognition in adulthood and aging*. New York: McGraw-Hill.

Boult, C., Reider, L., Frey, K., Leff, B., Boyd, C. M., & Wolff, J. L. (2008). Early effects of "Guided Care" on the quality of health care for multimorbid older persons: a cluster-randomized controlled trial. *Biological Sciences & Medical Sciences*, *63*(3), 321–327.

Bowes, A., & McColgan, G. (2006). *Smart technology and community care for older people: innovation in West Lothian, Scotland*. Edinburgh, UK: Age Concern Scotland.

Bowes, A. M., & McColgan, G. M. (2005). *West Lothian interim report*. West Lothian Council and the Department of Applied Social Science, University of Stirling.

Bowes, A. M., & McColgan, G. M. (2003). *Evaluation of home comforts: Smart home technologies initiative*. Final report to South Ayrshire Council. Cited in Tribal - Francesca Richards, Gill Walker, Lorelei Jarvis (2006). Time to Move? A Literature Review of Housing for Older People. Scottish Executive Social Research 2006

Bowling, A., & Farquhar, M. (1991). Associations with social networks, social support, health status and psychiatric morbidity in three samples of elderly people. *Social Psychiatry and Psychiatric Epidemiology*, *26*(3), 15–126. doi:10.1007/BF00782950

Bowling, A. (1994). Social networks and social support among older people and implications for emotional well-being and psychiatric morbidity. *International Review of Psychiatry (Abingdon, England)*, *6*, 41–58. doi:10.3109/09540269409025242

BPEL4People (2007) Specification: WS-BPEL Extension for People, (BPEL4People). Retrieved August 24, 2009, from https://www.sdn.sap.com/irj/sdn/go/portal/prtroot/docs/library/uuid/30c6f5b5-ef02-2a10-c8b5-cc1147f4d58c.

Brabyn, J. A., Shchneck, M. E., Lott, L. A., & Haegerstrom-Portnoy, G. (2005). Night driving self-restriction: Visual function and gender differences. *Optometry and Vision Science*, *82*(8), 755–764. doi:10.1097/01.opx.0000174723.64798.2b

Braga, N. (2002). *Robotics, mechatronics, and artificial intelligence – Experimental circuit blocks for designers*. USA: Newnes.

Braitman, K. A., Kirley, B. B., Ferguson, S., & Chaudhary, N. K. (2007). Factors leading to older drivers' intersection crashes. *Traffic Injury Prevention*, *8*, 267–274. doi:10.1080/15389580701272346

Bronfenbrenner, U. (1979). *The ecology of human development: Experiments by nature and design.* London: Harvard University Press.

Brown, L. B. (2004). Driving and dementia: A review of the literature. *Journal of Geriatric Psychiatry and Neurology*, *17*(4), 232–240. doi:10.1177/0891988704269825

Brownsell, S., & Hawley, M. (2004). Fall detectors: Do they work or reduce the fear of falling? *Housing. Care & Support*, *7*(1), 18–24.

Brubaker, T. H., & Powers, E. A. (1976). The stereotype of 'old': a review and alternative approach. *Journal of Gerontology*, *31*(4), 441–447.

Burns, A., & Rabins, P. (2000). Carer burden in dementia. *International Journal of Geriatric Psychiatry*, *15*(S1), S9–S13. doi:10.1002/1099-1166(200007)15:1+<::AID-GPS160>3.0.CO;2-N

Business Week. (March 26, 2007). *South* Korea*: Video games' crazed capital.* Retrieved from http://www.businessweek.com/globalbiz/content/mar2007/gb20070326_937184.htm.

Butcher, H. K., Holkup, P. A., Park, M., & Maas, M. (2001). Thematic analysis of the experience of making a decision to place a family member with Alzheimer's disease in a special care unit. *Research in Nursing & Health*, *24*(6), 470–480. doi:10.1002/nur.10005

Byles, J. E., Tavener, M., O'Connell, R. L., Nair, B. R., Higginbotham, N. H., & Jackson, C. L. (2004). Randomised controlled trial of health assessments for older Australian veterans and war widows. *The Medical Journal of Australia*, *181*(4), 186–190.

Caird, J., Horrey, W. J., & Edwards, C. J. (2001). Effects of conformal and nonconformal vision enhancement systems on older-driver performance. *Transportation Research Record*, *1759*, 38–45. doi:10.3141/1759-05

Caird, J. (1999). *In-vehicle intelligent transportation systems: Safety and mobility of older drivers.* Paper presented at the Conference on Transportation in an Aging Society: A Decade of Experience, Bethesda, Maryland.

Calkins, E., Boult, C., & Wagner, E. (1999). *New ways to care for older people: Building systems based on evidence*. New York: Springer.

Camberg, L., Woods, P., Ooi, W. L., Hurley, A., Volicer, L., & Ashley, J. (1999). Evaluation of simulated presence: A personalized approach to enhance well-being in persons with Alzheimer's disease. *Journal of the American Geriatrics Society*, *47*(4), 446–452.

Cappozzo, A., Della Croce, U., Leardini, A., & Chiari, L. (2005). Human movement analysis using stereophotogrammetry: Part 1: theoretical background. *Gait & Posture*, *21*(2), 186–196. doi:10.1016/S0966-6362(04)00025-6

Carlile, L. (2007, May). *Active ageing: Theoretical background.* Paper presented at the Namhae Active Ageing Conference in Asia Pacific, Namhae, Korea.

Carnaz, L., Oliveira, A. B., Sato, T. O., Hansson, G. A., & Coury, H. (2008). Effects of sensor, trials and knee joint variables on electrogoniometric gait recordings. *Revista Brasileira de Fisioterapia*, *12*(6), 460–467. doi:10.1590/S1413-35552008005000008

Carpenter, B. D., & Buday, S. (2007). Computer use among older adults in a naturally occurring retirement community. *Computers in Human Behavior*, *23*, 3012–3024. doi:10.1016/j.chb.2006.08.015

Carrasco, E., Epelde, G., Moreno, A., Ortiz, A., García, I., Buiza, C., et al. (2008). Natural interaction between avatars and persons with Alzheimer's disease. In *Computers Helping People with Special Needs* (LNCS 5105, pp. 38-45). Berlin/Heidelberg: Springer-Verlag.

Carroll, D. L., & Rankin, S. H. (2006). Comparing interventions in older unpartnered adults after myocardial infarction. *European Journal of Cardiovascular Nursing*, *5*(1), 83–89. doi:10.1016/j.ejcnurse.2005.09.001

Carstensen, L. L. (1993). Motivation for social contact across the life span: A theory of socioemotional selectivity. In J. E. Jacobs (Ed.), *Nebraska Symposium on Motivation: Developmental perspectives on motivation* (pp. 209-254). Lincoln, NE: University of Nebraska Press.

Carvin, A. (2000). Mending the breach: Overcoming the digital divide. Edutopia. Retrieved from http://www.edutopia.org/mending-breach-overcoming-digital-divide.

CDC. (2009). *Healthy aging: Improving and extending quality of life among older Americans*. Atlanta, GA, USA: Centers for Disease Control.

Cesta, A., Cortellessa, G., Giuliani, M. V., Pecora, F., Rasconi, R., Scopelliti, M., & Tiberio, L. (2007). Proactive assistive technology: An empirical study. *Lecture Notes in Computer Science*, *4662*, 255–268. doi:10.1007/978-3-540-74796-3_25

Chan, M., Estève, D., Escriba, C., & Campo, E. (2008). A review of smart homes - present state and future challenges. *Computer Methods and Programs in Biomedicine*, *91*(1), 55–81. doi:10.1016/j.cmpb.2008.02.001

Chang, B. L., Bakken, S., Brown, S. S., Houston, T. K., Kreps, G. L., & Kukafka, R. (2004). Bridging the digital divide: Reaching vulnerable populations. *Journal of the American Medical Informatics Association*, *11*(6), 448–457. doi:10.1197/jamia.M1535

Chang, B. L., Nitta, S., Carter, P. A., & Markham, Y. K. (2004). Perceived helpfulness of telephone calls. *Journal of Gerontological Nursing*, *30*, 14–21.

Charness, N., Kelly, C. L., Bosman, E. A., & Mottram, M. (2001). Word-processing training and retraining: Effects of adult age, experience, and interface. *Psychology and Aging*, *16*, 110–127. doi:10.1037/0882-7974.16.1.110

Charness, N., Czaja, S., Fisk, A. D., & Rogers, W. (2002). Preview gerontechnology 2002: Creative use of technology for better aging. *Gerontechnology (Valkenswaard)*, *1*, 198–202. doi:10.4017/gt.2001.01.03.008.00

Charnwood Dynamics Ltd. Codamotion. Retrieved February 24, 2009, from http://www.codamotion.com

Cheon, J. S. (2006). Suicide in the Korean elderly. *Journal of Korean Geriatric Psychiatry*, *10*(1), 14–19.

Cheong, H. J., Shin, N. Y., & Joeng, Y. B. (2009). Improving Korean service delivery system in health care: Focusing on National E-health System. *International Conference on eHealth, Telemedicine, and Social Medicine* (pp. 263-268).

Chesbrough, H., Vanhaverbeke, W., & West, J. (Eds.). (2006). *Open innovation: Researching a new paradigm*. Oxford, UK: Oxford University Press.

Chimpan, M. L., Payne, J., & McDonough, P. (1998). To drive or not to drive: The influence of social factors on the decisions of elderly drivers. *Accident; Analysis and Prevention*, *30*(3), 299–304. doi:10.1016/S0001-4575(97)00107-3

Chiu, L., Shyu, W. C., & Liu, Y. H. (2001). Comparisons of the cost-effectiveness among hospital chronic care, nursing home placement, home nursing care and family care for severe stroke patients. *Journal of Advanced Nursing*, *33*(3), 380–386. doi:10.1046/j.1365-2648.2001.01703.x

Chiu, L., Tang, K.-Y., Shyu, W.-C., & Chang, T.-P. (1999). The willingness of families caring for victims of stroke to pay for in-home respite care--results of a pilot study in Taiwan. *Health Policy (Amsterdam)*, *46*(3), 239–254. doi:10.1016/S0168-8510(98)00062-1

Choo, S., & Mokhtarian, P. L. (2004). What type of vehicle do people drive? The role of attitude and lifestyle in influencing vehicle type choice. *Transportation Research Part A, Policy and Practice*, *38*(3), 201–222. doi:10.1016/j.tra.2003.10.005

Clark, D. O., & Stump, D. E. (1998). Predictors of onset of and recovery from mobility difficulty among adults aged 51-61 years. *American Journal of Epidemiology*, *148*(1), 63–71.

Clayton, J. M., Butow, P. N., & Tattersall, M. H. N. (2005). The needs of terminally ill cancer patients versus those of caregivers for information regarding prognosis and end-of-life issues. *Cancer*, *103*(9), 1957–1964. doi:10.1002/cncr.21010

CMU. (2009). *The Pittsburgh Pebbles PDA Project*. Human-Computer Interaction Institute, Carnegie Mellon University. Retrieved February 18, 2009, from http://www.pebbles.hcii.cmu.edu/.

Coddington, D. C., Moore, K. D., & Fischer, E. A. (1996). *Making integrated health care work*. Englewood, Colorado, USA: Center for Research in Ambulatory Health Care Administration.

Cody, M. J., Dunn, D., Hoppin, S., & Wendt, P. (1999). Silver surfers: Training and evaluating Internet use among older adult learners. *Communication Education*, *48*, 269–286. doi:10.1080/03634529909379178

Cohen, J. E. (2003). Human population: The next half century. *Science*, *302*(5648), 1172–1175. doi:10.1126/science.1088665

Cohen, G. (2000). *The creative age*. New York: Harper Collins.

Cohen, G. (2001). Creativity with aging: Four phases of potential in the second half of life. *Geriatrics*, *56*(4), 51–57.

Cohen, G. (2005). *The mature mind: The positive power of the aging brain*. New York: Basic Books.

Colcombe, S. J., Kramer, A. F., Erickson, K. I., Scalf, P., McAuley, E., & Cohen, N. J. (2004). Cardiovascular fitness, cortical plasticity, and aging. *Proceedings of the National Academy of Sciences of the United States of America*, *101*(9), 3316–3321. doi:10.1073/pnas.0400266101

Cole, B. L. (2002). Who's responsible for safe vision on the roads? [Editorial]. *Clinical & Experimental Optometry*, *85*(4), 207–209. doi:10.1111/j.1444-0938.2002.tb03038.x

Coleman, K., Austin, B. T., Brach, C., & Wagner, E. H. (2009). Evidence on the chronic care model in the new millennium. *Health Affairs*, *28*, 75–85. doi:10.1377/hlthaff.28.1.75

Committee on Networked Systems of Embedded Computers, National Research Council. (2001). *Embedded, Everywhere: A research agenda for networked systems of embedded computers*. Washington, DC, USA: National Academy of Sciences.

Connect America. Medical Alarm and Medical Alert Systems. Retrieved February 23, 2009, from http://medicalalarm.com/.

Conrad, D. A., & Shortell, S. M. (1996). Integrated health systems: promise and performance. *Frontiers of Health Services Management*, *13*(1), 3–40.

Consortium, U. R. C. (2009). URC Consortium. Retrieved February 18, 2009, from http://myurc.org/.

Convertino, G., Farooq, U., Rosson, M. B., Carroll, J. M., & Meyer, B. J. F. (2007). Supporting intergenerational groups in computer-supported cooperative work (CSCW). *Behaviour & Information Technology*, *26*, 275–285. doi:10.1080/01449290601173473

Cook, A. M., & Hussey, S. M. (2002). *Assistive technologies: Principles and practice*. St Louis: Mosby.

Cooper, A. (1999). *The inmates are running the asylum*. Indianapolis, IN: Macmillan.

Cooper, R. A., Getzen, T. E., McKee, H. J., & Laud, P. (2002). Economic and demographic trends signal an impeding physician shortage. *Health Affairs*, *21*(1), 140–154. doi:10.1377/hlthaff.21.1.140

COPLINTHO. (2008). COPLINTHO Project, IBBT. Retrieved August 24, 2009, from https://projects.ibbt.be/coplintho/.

Costa-Font, J., Elvira, D., & Mascarilla-Mirò, O. (2008). "Ageing in place"? Exploring elderly people's housing preferences in Spain. *Urban Studies (Edinburgh, Scotland)*, *46*(2), 295–316. doi:10.1177/0042098008099356

Coughlin, J. F. (2005). Not your father's auto industry? Aging, the automobile, and the drive for product innovation. *Generations (San Francisco, Calif.)*, *28*(4), 38–44.

Counsel and Care (2005). *Community care assessment and services*.

Cox, W. (2005). *Robot jacket to help stroke victims*. Retrieved October, 10, 2009 from http://www.gorobotics.net/the-news/latest-news/robot-jacket-to-help-stroke-victims/

Coye, M. J., Haselkorn, A., & DeMello, S. (2009). Remote patient management: technology-enabled innovation and evolving business models for chronic disease care. *Health Affairs*, *28*(1), 126–135. doi:10.1377/hlthaff.28.1.126

Coyle, J. T. (2003). Use it or lose it - Do effortful mental activities protect against dementia? *The New England Journal of Medicine*, *348*, 2489–2490. doi:10.1056/NEJMp030051

Craik, F. I. M. (1994). Memory changes in normal aging. *Current Directions in Psychological Science*, *5*, 155–158. doi:10.1111/1467-8721.ep10770653

Cram, F., & Paton, H. (1993). Personal possessions and self-identity: The experiences of elderly women in three residential settings. *Australasian Journal on Ageing*, *12*, 19–24. doi:10.1111/j.1741-6612.1993.tb00579.x

Crist, J. D. (2005). The meaning for elders of receiving family care. *Journal of Advanced Nursing*, *49*(5), 485–493. doi:10.1111/j.1365-2648.2004.03321.x

Crossen-Sills, J., Toomey, I., & Doherty, M. E. (2009). Technology and home care: implementing systems to enhance aging in place. *The Nursing Clinics of North America*, *44*(2), 239–246. doi:10.1016/j.cnur.2009.03.003

CSCI. (2006). *Time to care? An overview of home care services for older people in England.* Report published by Commission for Social Care Inspection, London, www.csci.org.uk, October 2006.

Cubero, S. N. (1998). *Force, compliance and position control for a pneumatic quadruped robot*, Unpublished PhD dissertation, University of Southern Queensland, Australia.

Cubero, S. N., & Billingsley, J. (1997). Force, compliance and position control for a space frame manipulator. In *Proc 4th International Conference on Mechatronics and Machine Vision in Practice (M^2VIP)*, 22-24th Sep, 1997, Toowoomba, Australia: M2VIP.com.

Cummings, S. M. (2002). Predictors of psychological well-being among assisted living residents. *Health & Social Work*, *27*(4), 293–302.

Cutler, S. J., & Coward, R. T. (1992). Availability of personal transportation in households of elders: Age, gender, and residence differences. *The Gerontologist*, *32*(1), 77–81.

Czaja, S. J., & Rubert, M. P. (2002). Telecommunications technology as an aid to family caregivers of persons with dementia. *Psychosomatic Medicine*, *64*, 469–476.

Damush, T.M., Plue, L., Bakas, T., Schmid, A., & Williams, L.S. (2007). Barriers and facilitators to exercise among stroke survivors. *Rehabilitation Nursing, 32*(6), 253-260+262.

Daniel, K., Cason, C., & Ferrell, S. (2009). Assistive technologies for use in the home to prolong independence. [Corfu, Greece.]. *PETRA*, *09*(June), 9–13.

Daniele, G. (2006). Investigation of fall-risk using a wearable device with accelerometers and rate gyroscopes. *Physiological Measurement*, *27*, 1081–1090. doi:10.1088/0967-3334/27/11/003

Darkins, A., Dearde, C. H., Rocke, L. G., Martin, J. B., Sibson, L., & Wootton, R. (1996). An evaluation of telemedical support for a minor treatment centre. *Journal of Telemedicine and Telecare*, *2*(2), 92–99. doi:10.1258/1357633961929853

Darkins, A., Ryan, P., Kobb, R., Foster, L., Edmonson, E., Wakefield, B., & Lancaster, A. E. (2008). Care coordination / Home telehealth: The systematic implementation of health informatics, home telehealth, and disease management to support the care of veteran patients with chronic conditions. *Telemedicine and e-Health* (10), 1118-1126.

DARPA. (2008). DARPA Urban Challenge. Retrieved 10.02.09, from http://www.darpa.mil/grandchallenge/index.asp.

Davies, E. R. (2005). *Machine vision: Theory, algorithms, practicalities* (3rd ed.). USA: Morgan Kaufmann.

De Jonge, D., & Rodger, S. (2006). Consumer-identified barriers and strategies for optimizing technology use in the workplace. *Disability and Rehabilitation. Assistive Technology*, *1*(1-2), 79–88. doi:10.1080/09638280500167324

Deci, E. L., Eghrari, H., Patrick, B. C., & Leone, D. R. (1994). Facilitating internalization: the self determination theory perspective. *Journal of Personality*, *62*(1). doi:10.1111/j.1467-6494.1994.tb00797.x

Demiris, G., Edison, K., & Vijaykumar, S. (2005). A comparison of communication models of traditional and video-mediated health care delivery. *International Journal of Medical Informatics*, *74*(10), 851–856. doi:10.1016/j.ijmedinf.2005.03.018

Department of Health. E. Y., ROC. (2004). *Health and vital Statistical: Vital statistical*. Taipei: Department of Health, Executive Yuan, ROC.

Department-of-Social-Affairs. (2003). Older People's Welfare and Policy (In Chinese). Retrieved April 13, 2004, from http://volnet.moi.gov.tw/sowf/04/01.htm.

Department-of-Social-Affairs. (2007). Long term care: The ten years plan. Retrieved March 9, 2008, from http://sowf.moi.gov.tw/newpage/tenyearsplan.htm.

DeSilva, H. (1938). Age and highway accidents. *Scientific Monthly, New York*, *47*, 536–545.

Deutsch, J., Lewis, J., & Burdea, G. (2007). Technical and patient performance with a virtual reality-integrated telerehabilitation system. *IEEE Transactions on Neural Systems and Rehabilitation Engineering*, *15*(1), 30–35. doi:10.1109/TNSRE.2007.891384

Dewey, M. E., & Prince, M. J. (2005). Cognitive function. In Börsch-Supan, A., Brugiavini, A., Jürges, H., Mackenbach, J., & Guglielmo Weber, S. (Eds.), *Health, ageing and retirement in Europe*. Mannheim.

Dewsbury, G., Taylor, B., & Edge, M. (2001). Designing safe smart home systems for vulnerable people. *Health Informatics Journal*, *8*, 104–110. doi:10.1177/146045820200800208

Dingus, T. A., Hulse, M. C., Mollenhauer, M. A., Fleischman, R. N., McGehee, D. V., & Manakkal, N. (1997). Effects of age, system experience, and navigation technique on driving with an Advanced Traveller Information System. *Human Factors*, *39*(2), 177–199. doi:10.1518/001872097778543804

Directorate-General of Budget Accounting & Statistics (DGBAS) Executive Yuan. T., R.O.C. (2002, 30/12/2002). 2000 Population and housing census. Retrieved March 31, 2004, from http://www.dgbas.gov.tw/census~n/six/lue5/census_p&h&E.htm.

Dishman, E. (2004). Inventing wellness systems for aging in place. *IEEE Computer Society*, 34-41.

Docherty, A., Owens, A., Asadi-Lari, M., Petchey, R., Williams, J., & Carter, Y. H. (2008). Knowledge and information needs of informal caregivers in paliative care: a qualitative systematic review. *Palliative Medicine*, *22*(2), 153–171. doi:10.1177/0269216307085343

Done, D. J., & Thomas, J. A. (2001). Training in communication skills for informal carers of people suffering from dementia: a cluster randomized clinical trial comparing a therapist led workshop and a booklet. *International Journal of Geriatric Psychiatry*, *16*(8), 816–821. doi:10.1002/gps.436

Doukas, C., & Maglogiannis, I. (2008). *Advanced patient or elder fall detection based on movement and sound data*. Paper presented at the Second International Conference on Pervasive Computing Technologies for Healthcare. Emporia Life Plus. Retrieved 15th January 2010, from http://www2.emporia.at/en/home/.

Drageset, J., Nygaard, H. A., Eide, G. E., Bondevik, M., Nortvedt, M., & Natvig, G. K. (2009). The impact of social support and sense of coherence on health-related quality of life among nursing home residents - a questionnaire survey in Bergen, Norway. *International Journal of Nursing Studies*, *46*, 65–75. doi:10.1016/j.ijnurstu.2008.07.005

Dunbar, J. M., Neufeld, R. R., White, H. C., & Libow, L. S. (1996). Retrain, don't restrain: The educational intervention of the National Nursing Home Restraint Removal Project. *The Gerontologist*, *36*(4), 539–542.

Duras, T. (2007). Raging against the machine: Unions and technological change in Australia 1978-1996. In *Proceedings - Labour Traditions: The 10th National Labour History Conference*, 4-6, July 2007, University of Melbourne.

Dwyer, J., & Eager, K. (2008). *Options for reform of Commonwealth and State governance responsibilities for the Australian health system*. A paper commissioned by the National Health and Hospitals Reform Commission.

Eby, D. W., Molnar, L. J., & Kartje, P. S. (2009). *Maintaining Safe Mobility in an Aging Society*. Boca Raton, Florida: CRC Press.

Edirippulige, S., & Wootton, R. (2006). Telehealth and Communication. In Conrick, M. (Ed.), *Health informatics, transforming health care with technology* (pp. 266–278). Melbourne: Thomson.

Edwards, J. D., Leonard, K. M., Lunsman, M., Dodson, J., Bradley, S., & Myers, C. A. (2008). Acceptability and validity of older driver screening with the Driving Health Reg. Inventory. *Accident; Analysis and Prevention*, *40*(3), 1157–1163. doi:10.1016/j.aap.2007.12.008

Edwards, J. D., Vance, D. E., Wadley, V. G., Cissell, G. M., Roenker, D. L., & Ball, K. K. (2005). Reliability and validity of useful field of view test scores as administered by personal computer. *Journal of Clinical and Experimental Neuropsychology*, *27*, 529–543. doi:10.1080/13803390490515432

Edwards, J. D., Wadley, V. G., Vance, D. E., Wood, K., Roenker, D. L., & Ball, K. K. (2005). The impact of speed of processing training on cognitive and everyday performance. *Aging & Mental Health*, *9*, 262–271. doi:10.1080/13607860412331336788

Eizmendi, G., Aztoika, J., & Craddock, G. (2007). *Challenges for assistive technology*. Netherlands: IOS Press.

Emotiv Systems Inc. (n.d.). Retrieved January 25, 2009 from http://emotiv.com/corporate/3_0/3_1.htm

Enthoven, A., & Vorhaus, C. (2000). *What is a hospital system?*Palo Alto, CA: Graduate School of Business Stanford University.

Epelde, G., Carrasco, E., Zimmermann, G., Bund, J., Dubielzig, M., & Alexandersson, J. (2009). URC based accessible TV. *EuroITV '09: Proceedings of the seventh European conference on European interactive television conference* (pp. 111-114). New York: ACM.

Erke, A. (in press). Red light for red-light cameras? A meta-analysis of the effects of red-light cameras on crashes. [Corrected Proof]. *Accident; Analysis and Prevention.*

Ertel, K., Glymour, M., & Berkman, L. (2008). Effects of social integration on preserving memory function in a nationally representative U.S. elderly population. *American Journal of Public Health*, *98*(7), 1215–1220. doi:10.2105/AJPH.2007.113654

Essen, A., & Conrick, M. (2007). Visions and realities: Developing 'smart' homes for seniors in Sweden, *eJHI - electronic Journal of Health Informatics, 2*(1), e2.

European Commission (2004). *The social situation in the European Union.*

EUROSTAT. (2004.). Retrieved from www.eurostat.com.

Evans, L. (1991). *Traffic safety and the driver*. New York: Van Nostrand Reinhold.

Evans, N., Orpwood, R., Adlam, T., Gibbs, C., & Faulkner, R. (2003). *Smart house technology: providing practical support for people living with dementia.* College of Occupational Therapists.

Eysenbach, G., & Jadad, J. R. (2001). Evidence-based patient choice and consumer health informatics in the Internet age. *Journal of Medical Internet Research*, *3*(2), e19. doi:10.2196/jmir.3.2.e19

Eysenbach, G. (2000). Consumer health informatics. *BMJ (Clinical Research Ed.)*, *320*(7251), 1713–1716. doi:10.1136/bmj.320.7251.1713

Fallon, S. (2009). *Smart wheelchair features a brain-controlled robotic arm.* Gizmodo. Retrieved February 10, 2009, from http://i.gizmodo.com/5150632/smart-wheelchair-features-a-brain+controlled-robotic-arm.

Faulk, L. (1988). Quality of life factors in board and care homes for the elderly: A hierarchical model. *Adult Foster Care Journal*, *2*(2), 100–117.

Fazio, R. H., & Olson, M. A. (2003). Attitudes: Foundations, functions, and consequences. In Hogg, M. A., & Cooper, J. (Eds.), *The Handbook of Social Psychology* (pp. 139–160). London: Sage.

Federal Highway Administration. (1997). *Highway Statistics 1997: Section VIII Nationwide Personal Transportation Survey*: Office of Highway Information Management.

Felkey, B. G., Fox, B., & Thrower, M. R. (2006). *Health care informatics: A skill-based resource*. Washington, D.C.: American Pharmacists Association.

Ferguson, S. A. (2007). The effectiveness of electronic stability control in reducing real-world crashes: A literature review. *Traffic Injury Prevention*, *8*(4), 329–338. doi:10.1080/15389580701588949

Ferguson, T. (1993). What is consumer health informatics? Retrieved May 2008 from http://www.fergusonreport.com/articles/tfr07-03.htm.

Ferri, C. P., Prince, M., Brayne, C., Brodaty, H., Fratiglioni, L., & Ganguli, M. (2005). Global. prevalence of dementia: a Delphi consensus study. *Lancet*, *366*(9503), 2112–2117. doi:10.1016/S0140-6736(05)67889-0

Filan, S. I., & Llewellyn-Jones, R. H. (2006). Animal-assisted therapy for dementia: a review of the literature. *International Psychogeriatrics*, *18*(4), 597–611. doi:10.1017/S1041610206003322

Finapres Medical Systems. *Finometer*. Retrieved January 2010, from http://www.finapres.com/site/page/2/10/Finometer_PRO/.

Findings About the Awareness and Use of Accessible Technology. (n.d.). Retrieved February 10, 2009 from http://www.microsoft.com/enable/research/acctechnology.aspx.

Finland, A. A. L. (2005). *Ambient assisted living*. Country report, Finland.

Finn, J. (2006, June). Fitting cars to their older drivers. *Healthword: Putting Health promotion Back in Motion*.

Fisk, A. D., Rogers, W. A., Charness, N., Czaja, S. J., & Sharit, J. (2004). *Designing for Older Adults: Principles and Creative Human Factors Approaches*. Boca Raton, Florida: CRC Press.

Floeck, M., & Litz, L. (2007). Aging in place: Supporting senior citizens' independence with ambient assistive living technology. *mst / news*.

Forlizzi, J., DiSalvo, C., & Gemperle, F. (2004). Assistive robotics and an ecology of elders living independently in their homes. *Human-Computer Interaction*, *19*, 25–59. doi:10.1207/s15327051hci1901&2_3

Fratiglioni, L., Wang, H. X., Ericsson, K., Maytan, M., & Winblad, B. (2000). Influence of social network on occurrence of dementia: a community-based longitudinal study. *Lancet*, *355*(9212), 1315–1319. doi:10.1016/S0140-6736(00)02113-9

Freedman, V. A., Agree, E. M., & Cornman, J. C. (2005). Development of an assistive technology and environmental assessment instrument for national surveys: Final report. Retrieved February 10, 2009 from http://aspe.hhs.gov/daltcp/reports/ATEAdevI.htm

Freedman, V. A., Martin, L. G., & Schoeni, R. F. (2002). Recent trends in disability and functioning among older adults in the United States. *JAMA*, *288*(24), 3137-3146. Retrieved October 19, 2009, from http://jama.ama-assn.org/cgi/reprint/288/24/3137.

Fricke, T., Chang, J. S., & Yang, L. S. (1994). Historical and Ethnographical Perspectives on the Chinese Family. In Thornton, A., & Lin, L.-S. (Eds.), *Social Change and the Family in Taiwan* (pp. 22–48). Chicago: University of Chicago Press.

Friedman, T. L. (2008). *The world is flat: A brief history of the twenty-first century*. New York: Farrar, Strauss and Giroux.

Friedrich, D. (2003). Personal and societal intervention strategies for successful aging. *Ageing International*, *28*(1), 3–36. doi:10.1007/s12126-003-1014-8

Fries, J. F. (1980). Ageing, natural death, and the compression of morbidity. *The New England Journal of Medicine*, *303*, 130–135. doi:10.1056/NEJM198007173030304

Gagnon, A. J., Schein, C., McVey, L., & Bergman, H. (1999). Randomized controlled trial of nurse case management of frail older people. *Journal of the American Geriatrics Society*, *47*(9), 1118–1124.

Gajos, K., & Weld, D. (2004, January). *SUPPLE: Automatically generating user interfaces.* Paper presented at the international conference on Intelligent User Interfaces (IUI'04), Madeira, Funchal, Portugal. i2home (2009). Intuitive interaction for everyone with home appliances based on industry standards. Retrieved February 18, 2009, from http://www.i2home.org.

Gallant, M. P., Spitze, G. D., & Prohaska, T. R. (2007). Help or hindrance? How family and friends influence chronic illness self-management among older adults. *Journal of Research on Aging*, *29*, 375–409. doi:10.1177/0164027507303169

Gaugler, J. E., Leach, C. R., & Anderson, K. A. (2004). Correlates of resident psychosocial status in long-term care. *International Journal of Geriatric Psychiatry*, *19*(8), 773–780. doi:10.1002/gps.1157

Gaugler, J. E., Roth, D. L., Haley, W. E., & Mittelman, M. S. (2008). Can counseling and support reduce burden and depressive symptoms in caregivers of people with Alzheimer's disease during the transition to institutionalization? Results from the New York University caregiver intervention study. *Journal of the American Geriatrics Society*, *56*(3), 421–428. doi:10.1111/j.1532-5415.2007.01593.x

Gaugler, J. E., Jarrott, S. E., Zarit, S. H., Stephens, M. P., & Greene, R. (2003). Respite for Dementia Caregivers: The effects of adult day service use on caregiving hours and care demands. *International Psychogeriatrics*, *15*(1), 37–58. doi:10.1017/S1041610203008743

Georgantas, N. (2006). Amigo middleware core: Prototype implementation & documentation. *IST Amigo Project Deliverable D3.2.*

Georgeff, M., & Hilton, J. (2009). *The use of a web based chronic disease management service (CDMS) for collaborative care*. Retrieved from www.hisa.org.au/system/files/u2233/hic09-2_MGeorgeffJHilton.pdf.

Giaimo, S. (2002). *Markets and medicine: The politics of health care reform in Britain, Germany, and the United States*. Michigan: University of Michigan Press.

Giannakouris, K. (2008) Ageing characterises the demographic perspectives of the European societies. *Eurostat Statistics in Focus 72/2008* from http://epp.eurostat.ec.europa.eu.

Giansanti, D., Maccioni, G., & Macellari, V. (2005). The development and test of a device for the reconstruction of 3-D position and orientation by means of a kinematic sensor assembly with rate gyroscopes and accelerometers. *IEEE Transactions on Bio-Medical Engineering*, *52*(7), 1271–1277. doi:10.1109/TBME.2005.847404

Giardina, C. W., Fottler, D. F., Shewchuk, R. M., & Hill, D. B. (1990). The case for hospital diversification into long-term care. *Health Care Management Review*, *15*(1), 71–82.

Gill, T. M., & Kurland, B. (2003). The burden and patterns of disability in activities of daily living among community-living older persons. *The Journals of Gerontology. Series A, Biological Sciences and Medical Sciences*, *58A*(1), M70–M75.

Gillespie, L. D., Robertson, M. C., Gillespie, W. J., Lamb, S. E., & Cumming Robert, G, & H, R. B. (2009). Interventions for preventing falls in older people living in the community. *Cochrane Database of Systematic Reviews*, 2.

Gish, K., & Staplin, L. (1995). *Human factors aspects of using head up displays in automobiles: A review of the literature (No. DOT HS 808320)*. Washington, D. C.: U.S. Department of Transportation.

Giuliani, M. V. (1991). Towards an analysis of mental representations of attachment to the home. *Journal of Architectural and Planning Research*, *8*, 133–146.

Giuliani, M. V. (2003). Theory of attachment and place attachment. In Bonnes, M., Lee, T., & Bonaiuto, M. (Eds.), *Psychological theories for environmental issues* (pp. 137–170). Aldershot: Ashgate.

Giuliani, M. V., Scopelliti, M., & Fornara, F. (2005). Elderly people at home: Technological help in everyday activities. *Proceedings of 14th IEEE International Workshop on Robot and Human Interactive Communication* (August 13-15, 2005, Nashville, Tennessee U.S.A.), (pp. 365-370). Helsinki: Omnipress.

Glass, T. A. (2003). Successful aging. In Tallis, R., Fillit, H., & Brocklehurst, J. (Eds.), *Brocklehurst's Textbook of Geriatric Medicine and Gerontology* (6th ed., pp. 173–181). London: Churchill Livingstone.

Goldberg, R. (1984). Psychosocial aspects of stroke. In Kruger, D. W., & Collins, L. B. (Eds.), *Rehabilitation psychology*. Rockville: Aspen Publication.

Goodacre, K., McCreadie, C., Flanagan, S., & Lansley, P. (2007). Enabling older people to stay at home: How adaptable are existing properties? *The British Journal of Occupational Therapy, 70*(1), 5-15(11).

Graham, D. P., Kunick, M. E., Doody, R., & Snow, A. L. (2005). Self-reported awareness of performance in dementia. *Brain Research. Cognitive Brain Research, 25*(1), 144–152. doi:10.1016/j.cogbrainres.2005.05.001

Gray, L. C. (2003). 2020: A vision for aged care in Australia. *Australian Society for Geriatric Medicine Newsletter, 6*(6).

Green, K. E., Walker, I. D., & Brooks, J. (2009). ComforTABLE: a robotic environment for aging in place. *HRI '09: Proceedings of the 4th ACM/IEEE international conference on Human robot interaction*, March 11–13, 2009, La Jolla, California, USA.

Greiner, P. A., Snowdon, D. A., & Schmitt, F. A. (1996). The loss of independence in activities of daily living: the role of low normal cognitive function in elderly nuns. *American Journal of Public Health, 86*, 62–66.

Grossi, F., Matrella, G., De Munrai, I., & Ciampolini, P. (2007). A flexible home automation system applied to elderly care. *International Conference on Consumer Electronics,* 1-2.

Gui, N., Sun, H., De Florio, V., & Blondia, C. (2007). A service oriented infrastructure approach for mutual assistance communities. In *Proceedings of the First IEEE WoWMoM Workshop on Adaptive and DependAble Mission- and bUsiness-critical mobile Systems (ADAMUS 2007), Helsinki, Finland.*

Gupta, R. (2000). A path model of elder caregiver burden in Indian/Pakistani families in the United States. *International Journal of Aging & Human Development, 51*(4), 295–313. doi:10.2190/J9XY-V3E0-NP1B-UNA5

Gutheil, I. (1991). The physical environment and quality of life in residential facilities for frail elderly. *Adult Residential Care Journal, 5*(2), 131–145.

Haas, B. K. (1999). A multidisciplinary concept analysis of quality of life. *Western Journal of Nursing Research, 21*, 728–742. doi:10.1177/01939459922044153

Haigh, K. Z., & Yanco, H. (2002). Automation as caregiver: A survey of issues and technologies. In *Automation as caregiver: The role of intelligent technology in elder care* (pp. 35–53). AAAI Workshop.

Hakamies-Blomqvist, L. (2006). Are there safe and unsafe drivers? *Transportation Research Part F: Traffic Psychology and Behaviour, 9*(5), 347–352. doi:10.1016/j.trf.2006.06.004

Hakamies-Blomqvist, L., & Henriksson, P. (1999). Cohort effects in older drivers' accident type distribution: Are older drivers as old as they used to be? *Transportation Research Part F: Traffic Psychology and Behaviour, 2*(3), 131–138. doi:10.1016/S1369-8478(99)00009-1

Hakamies-Blomqvist, L., Raitanen, T., & O'Neill, D. (2002). Driver ageing does not cause higher accident rates per km. *Transportation Research Part F: Traffic Psychology and Behaviour, 5*, 271–274. doi:10.1016/S1369-8478(03)00005-6

Hakamies-Blomqvist, L., & Siren, A. (2003). Deconstructing a gender difference: Driving cessation and personal driving history of older women. *Journal of Safety Research, 34*(4), 383–388. doi:10.1016/j.jsr.2003.09.008

Hakamies-Blomqvist, L., & Wahlstrom, B. (1998). Why do older drivers give up driving? *Accident; Analysis and Prevention*, *30*(3), 305–312. doi:10.1016/S0001-4575(97)00106-1

Hakamies-Blomqvist, L. (1999). *Safety of older persons in traffic.* Paper presented at the Conference on Transportation in an Aging Society: A Decade of Experience, Bethesda, Maryland.

Halfon, N., & Hochstein, M. (2002). Life course health development: An integrated framework for developing health, policy and research. *The Milbank Quarterly*, *80*, 433–479. doi:10.1111/1468-0009.00019

Han, D. H. (2006). Digital silver for wellageing. [in Korean]. *Journal of Korean Geriatric Psychiatry*, *10*(1), 5–9.

Han, D. H., & Kim, J. O. (1998). Elder abuse: Factors related to Korean elder abuse. *Journal of Asian Regional Association for Home Economics*, *5*(1), 10–16.

Han, D. H. (2007, May). *The new strategy of social integration for older persons through Cyber Family.* Paper presented at the Namhae Active Ageing Conference in Asia Pacific, Namhae, Korea.

Han, D. H. (2008, February). *Perseverance to eradicate abuse of elderly women in Korea.* Paper presented at the Communities Working Together to End Violence against Women Conference, Ontario, Canada.

Handley, M. A., Shumway, M., & Schillinger, D. (2008). Cost-effectiveness of automated telephone self-management support with nurse care management among patients with diabetes. *Annals of Family Medicine*, *6*(6), 512–518. doi:10.1370/afm.889

Hariri, S., Goodyer, L. I., Meyer, J., & Anderson, C. (2000). Assessment of a touch-screen promotion system in independent community pharmacies. *Health Education Journal*, *59*(1), 99–107. doi:10.1177/001789690005900109

Harris, J. E. (1998). *How the brain talks to itself.* USA: The Howarth Press Inc.

Hatherly, C., & Anstey, K. J. (2008). *Extending the Useful Field of View paradigm for screening older drivers.* Paper presented at the ACRS/Qld Travelsafe Committee Joint Conference.

Hawkey, K., Inkpen, M., Rockwood, K., McAllister, M., & Slonim, J. (2005). Requirements gathering with alzheimer's patients and caregivers. *Assets '05: Proceedings of the 7th international ACM SIGACCESS conference on Computers and accessibility.* October 9–12, 2005, Baltimore, Maryland, USA.

Haworth, N., & Bowland, L. (2000). *Serious injury single vehicle crashes (No. 175).* Monash University Accident Research Centre.

Hayashi, K. (2002). Striving for the greatest enjoyment through Collaborative Therapy: The role of the speech therapist in collaborative therapy treatment of patients with communication disorders. *Japanese Journal of Communication Disorders*, *19*(3), 236–241.

Health Resources and Services Administration (HRSA). (2006). *Physician supply and demand: Projections to 2020.* Retrieved September 10, 2009, from http://bhpr.hrsa.gov/healthworkforce/reports/physiciansupplydemand/default.htm.

Hebert, R., Robichaud, L., Roy, P. M., Bravo, G., & Voyer, L. (2001). Efficacy of a nurse-led multidimensional preventive programme for older people at risk of functional decline. A randomized controlled trial. *Age and Ageing*, *30*(2), 147–153. doi:10.1093/ageing/30.2.147

Helal, A., Mokhtari, M., & Abdulrazak, B. (2009). *The engineering handbook on smart technology for aging, disability and independence.* Hoboken, NJ: John Wiley & Sons.

Helander, M., Landauer, T. K., & Prabhu, P. (Eds.). (1997). *Handbook of Human-Computer Interaction* (pp. 813–824). Elsevier Science BV.

Hendrie, D., Hall, S. E., Legge, M., & Arena, G. (2003). *Injury in Western Australia: The Health System Costs of Falls in Older Adults in Western Australia*. Perth, Western Australia: Western Australian Government. Intelesens. Vitalsens. Retrieved January, 2010, from http://www.intelesens.com/.

Heng, J., & Banerji, S. (2010). A step towards multi-level human interface devices: A system that responds to EEG/SEMG triggers. *International Journal of Biorobotics and Biomechatronics, special issue on Rehabilitation Robotics, 1*(2), 93-98.

Hermalin, A., Liu, P. K. C., & Freedman, D. (1994). The Social and Economic Transformation of Taiwan. In Thornton, A., & Lin, L.-S. (Eds.), *Social Change and the Family in Taiwan* (pp. 49–87). Chicago: University of Chicago Press.

Hersey, J. C., Matheson, J., & Lohr, K. N. (1997). *Consumer health informatics and patient decision making* (No. Report NR AHCPR - Publication No.98-N001). Rockville.

Hertzog, C., & Light, L. (2004). Methodological issues in the assessment of technology use for older adults. In Pew, R. W., & Van Hemel, S. B. (Eds.), *Technology for Adaptive Aging*. National Academies Press.

Heyn-Billipp, S. (2001). The psychosocial impact of interactive computer use within a vulnerable elderly population: A report on a randomized prospective trial in a home health care setting. *Public Health Nursing (Boston, Mass.), 18*(2), 138–145. doi:10.1046/j.1525-1446.2001.00138.x

Higgins, S. (2007). *Engineers develop a 'helping hand'*. The Oracle (University of South Florida, USA). Retrieved December 6, 2007, from http://www.usforacle.com/2.6026/1.619334-1.619334.

Hillman, M., Hagan, K., Hagan, S., Jepson, J., & Orpwood, R. (2002). The Weston wheelchair mounted assistive robot - the design story. *Robotica, 20*(2), 125–132. doi:10.1017/S0263574701003897

Hills, B. L. (1980). Vision, visibility and perception in driving. *Perception, 3*, 434–467.

Hiltunen, E. F., Winder, P. A., Rait, M. A., Buselli, E. F., Carroll, D. L., & Rankin, S. H. (2005). Implementation of efficacy enhancement nursing interventions with cardiac elders. *Rehabilitation Nursing, 30*(6), 221–229.

Hocking, C. (1999). Function or feelings: Factors in abandonment of assistive devices. *Technology and Disability, 11*, 3–11.

Hoedemaeker, M., & Brookhuis, K. A. (1998). Behavioural adaptations to driving with an adaptive cruise control (ACC). *Transportation Research Part F: Traffic Psychology and Behaviour, 1*, 95–106. doi:10.1016/S1369-8478(98)00008-4

Hofgren, C., Bjorkdahl, A., Esbjornsson, E., & Stibrant-Sunnerhagen, K. (2007). Recovery after stroke: cognition, ADL function and return to work. *Acta Neurologica Scandinavica, 115*(2), 73–80. doi:10.1111/j.1600-0404.2006.00768.x

Hole, G. (2007). *The psychology of driving*. Mahwah, New Jersey: Lawrence Erlbaum Associates.

Holroyd, E. (2001). Hong Kong Chinese daughters' intergenerational caregiving obligations: a cultural model approach. *Social Science & Medicine, 53*, 1125–1134. doi:10.1016/S0277-9536(00)00406-8

Hooyman, N., & Kiyak, H. A. (2005). *Social Gerontology: A multidisciplinary perspective*. Needham, MA: Allyn & Bacon.

Horner, B., & Boldy, D. P. (2008). The benefit and burden of "ageing-in-place" in an aged care community. *Australian Health Review, 32*(2), 356–365. doi:10.1071/AH080356

Horner, B., Soar, J., & Koch, B. (2009). Assistive technology: Opportunities and implications, gerontic nursing body of knowledge. In Nay, R., & Garratt, S. (Eds.), *Older People: Issues and Innovations in Care* (3rd ed.). Sydney: Elsevier.

Horswill, M. S., Marrington, S. A., McCullough, C. M., Wood, J., Pachana, N. A., & McWilliam, J. (2008). The hazard perception ability of older drivers. *The Journals of Gerontology. Series B, Psychological Sciences and Social Sciences, 63*(4), 212–218.

House, J., Landis, K., & Umberson, D. (1988). Social relationships and health. *Science*, *241*, 540–545. doi:10.1126/science.3399889

How do skin conductance and heart rate rhythms measure stress? (n.d.). Retrieved February 15, 2009 from http://somaticvision.com/measurements.php.

Hsu, C. F., Liao, H. Y. M., Hsiu, P. C., Lin, Y. S., Shin, C. S., Kuo, T. W., & Liu, W. S. (2006). Smart pantries for homes. *IEEE International Conference on Systems, Man and Cybernetics* (pp. 4276-4283).

Huang, T. L., & Charyton, C. (2008). A comprehensive review of the psychological effects of brainwave entrainment. *Alternative Therapies in Health and Medicine*, *14*(5), 38–50.

Hutchison, D., Eastman, C., & Tirrito, T. (1997). Designing user interfaces for older adults. *Educational Gerontology*, *23*, 497–513. doi:10.1080/0360127970230601

Hyer, K., & Rudick, L. (1994). The effectiveness of personal emergency response systems in meeting the safety monitoring needs of home care clients. *The Journal of Nursing Administration*, *24*(6), 39–43. doi:10.1097/00005110-199406000-00010

iHealth Beat (2007). Japan to track elderly health via wireless test zone. *iHealth Beat*. Retrieved from http://www.ihealthbeat.org/articles/2007/5/14/Japan-To-Track-Elderly-Health-Via-Wireless-Test-Zone.aspx.

I-living. (2007). I Assisted Living Project. Retrieved August 24, 2009, from http://lion.cs.uiuc.edu/assistedliving/.

Inada, H., Horio, H., Nakazawa, K., Sekita, Y., Yamanaka, T., & Harasawa, E. (1998). A study on a home health care support information system for health evaluation. *Journal of Medical Systems*, *22*(2), 69–75. doi:10.1023/A:1022639001300

Information Technology Association of America (ITAA) e-Health Committee. (2004*). Chronic care improvement: How Medicare transformation can save lives, save money and stimulate an emerging technology industry.* ITAA May 2004. Retrieved September 10, 2009, from http://www.itaa.org/isec/docs/choniccare.pdf.

Inoue, K., Wada, K., & Ito, Y. (2008). Effective application of Paro: Seal type robots for disabled people in According to Ideas of Occupational Therapists. *Computers Helping People with Special Needs, Springer Berlin/Hiedelberg. 5105*, 1321-1324.

International Telecommunication Union. (2009). Digital Opportunity Index. Retrieved from http://www.itu.int/ITU-D/ict/doi/index.html.

Internet World Stats. (2008). Korea. Retrieved from http://www.internetworldstats.com/asia/kr.htm.

ISO/IEC. (2008). *International Standard ISO/IEC 24752. Information Technology - User Interfaces - Universal Remote Console (5 parts)*. ISO/IEC.

ITTA-eHealth. (2004). *Chronic care improvement: How medicare transformation can save lives, save money, and stimulate an emerging technology industry* (No. An ITAA E-Health White paper): A Product of the ITAA E-Health Committee.

Jackson, L. A., Zhao, Y., Kolenic, A., Fitzgerald, H. E., Harold, R., & Von Eye, A. (2008). Race, gender, and information technology use: The new digital divide. *Cyberpsychology & Behavior*, *11*(4), 437–442. doi:10.1089/cpb.2007.0157

Jacobus, C. (2003). *The billing, cost, and outcome benefits from remote patient monitoring (Whitepaper)*. Cybernet Medical Systems.

Janke, M. K. (1991). Accidents, mileage, and the exaggeration of risk. *Accident; Analysis and Prevention*, *23*(2-3), 183–188. doi:10.1016/0001-4575(91)90048-A

Janse, A., Gemke, R., Uiterwaal, C., van der Tweel, I., Kimpen, J., & Sinnema, G. (2004). Quality of life: Patients and doctors don't always agree: A meta-analysis. *Journal of Clinical Epidemiology*, *57*(7), 653–661. doi:10.1016/j.jclinepi.2003.11.013

Jardón, A., González, J. C., Stoelen, M., Martínez, S., & Balaguer, C. (2009). ASIBOT Assistive robot in a domestic environment. In *Proceedings of the 2nd ACM International Conference on Pervasive Technologies Related to Assistive Environments.* New York: ACM.

Jeong, S. (2008). *A Study on the efficiency and effectiveness of integrated health care and social services delivery facilities: Special focus on integrating facilities of health care and social services on elderly in Japan and S. Korea.* Nagoya, Japan: The Graduate School of Nihon Fukushi University.

Jeong, S., Inoue Y., Adachi, H., & Nabeya, K. (2009). A study on the efficiency and effectiveness of integrated health care and social services delivery facilities. *Japanese Association for Health Care Administration, 3*(1).

Johnson, J. L., & Davenport, R. & Mann. (2007). W. C. Consumer Feedback on Smart Home Applications. *Topics in Geriatric Rehabilitation, 23*(1), 60–72.

Johnson, C. A., & Keltner, J. L. (1983). Incidence of visual field loss in 20,000 eyes and its relationship to driving performance. *Archives of Ophthalmology, 101*(3), 371–375.

Johnson, H. (1946). The detection and treatment of accident-prone drivers. *Psychological Bulletin, 43*(6), 489–532. doi:10.1037/h0061866

Johnson, M. J. (2007). Potential for a suite of robot/computer assisted motivating systems for personalized home based, stroke rehabilitation. *Journal of Neuroengineering and Rehabilitation, 4*(6).

Johnson, M. J., Feng, X., Johnson, L. M., Ramachandran, B., Winters, J. M., & Kosasih, J. B. (2006). Robotic systems that rehabilitate as well as motivate: Three strategies for motivating impaired arm use. In *Proceedings IEEE / RASEMBS Int. Conf. on Biomedical robotics and Biomechatronics*, BioRob 2006, art.no.1639095 (pp. 254-259).

Jones, G. M. (1987). Elderly people and domestic crime: Reflections on ageism, sexism, victimology. *The British Journal of Criminology, 27*(2), 191–201.

Jordan, J., & Osbourne, R. (2007). Chronic disease self-management education programs: challenges ahead. *MJA, 186*(2), 84–87.

Jurjens, J. (2007). Developing secure embedded systems: pitfalls and how to avoid them. *29th International Conference on Software Engineering - ICSE 2007* (pp. 182-183).

Kahn, R. (1994). Social support: Content, causes and consequences. In Abeles, R., Gift, H., & Ory, M. (Eds.), *Aging and quality of life* (pp. 163–184). New York: Springer Publishing Company.

Kane, R. A., Kling, K. C., Bershadsky, B., Kane, R. L., Giles, K., & Degenholtz, H. B. (2003). Measuring quality of life of nursing home residents. *Journal of Gerontology: Medical Sciences, 58*, 240–248.

Kannus, P., Palvanen, M., Niemi, S., & Parkkari, J. (2007). Alarming Rise in the Number and Incidence of Fall-Induced Cervical Spine Injuries among Older Adults. *The Journals of Gerontology. Series A, Biological Sciences and Medical Sciences, 62*(2), 180–183.

Kao, H.-F., & Stuifbergen, A. K. (1999). Family experiences related to the decision to institutionalize an elderly member in Taiwan: an exploratory study. *Social Science & Medicine, 49*(8), 1115–1123. doi:10.1016/S0277-9536(99)00211-7

Karlsson, R. (1996). Cartoon printed in *Helsingin Sanoma, October 18.*

Karp, A., Paillard-Borg, S., Wang, H.-X., Silverstein, M., Winblad, B., & Fratiglioni, L. (2006). Mental, physical and social components in leisure activities equally contribute to decrease dementia risk. *Dementia and Geriatric Cognitive Disorders, 21*(2), 65–73. doi:10.1159/000089919

Kasser, V. G., & Ryan, R. M. (1999). The relation of psychological needs for autonomy and relatedness to vitality, well-being, and mortality in a nursing home. *Journal of Applied Social Psychology, 29*(5), 935–954. doi:10.1111/j.1559-1816.1999.tb00133.x

Kattlove, H., & Winn, R. J. (2003). Ongoing care of patients after primary treatment for their cancer. *CA: a Cancer Journal for Clinicians, 53*(3), 172–196. doi:10.3322/canjclin.53.3.172

Katz, S., Down, T. D., Cash, H. R., & Grotz, R. C. (1970). Progress in the development of the index of ADL. *The Gerontologist, 10*(1), 20–30.

Kaufman, D. R., Patel, V. L., Hilliman, C., Morin, P. C., Pevzner, J., & Weinstock, R. S. (2003). Usability in the real world: Assessing medical information technologies in patients' homes. *Journal of Biomedical Informatics*, *36*(1-2), 45–60. doi:10.1016/S1532-0464(03)00056-X

Kauh, B., Polak, T., Hazelett, S., Hua, K., & Allen, K. (2005). A pilot study: post-acute geriatric rehabilitation versus usual care in skilled nursing facilities. *Journal of the American Medical Directors Association*, *6*(5), 321–326. doi:10.1016/j.jamda.2005.04.008

Keleher, H. (2006). Promoting healthy ageing. In Keleher, H., & Murphy, B. (Eds.), *Understanding health – A determinants approach*. Oxford: Oxford University Press.

Kenny, R. A., Romero-Ortuno, R., & Cogan, L. (2009)... *Falls.*, *37*(2), 84–87.

Kim, J.-S., & Lee, E.-H. (2003). Cultural and Noncultural Predictors of Health Outcomes in Korean Daughter and Daughter-in-Law Caregivers. *Public Health Nursing (Boston, Mass.)*, *20*(2), 111–119. doi:10.1046/j.1525-1446.2003.20205.x

Kim, I. K. (2000, August). *Policy responses to low fertility and population ageing in Korea.* Paper presented at the United Nations Expert Group Meeting on Policy Responses to Population Ageing and Population Decline. Retrieved March 9, 2009 from http://www.un.org/esa/population/publications/popdecline/kim.pdf.

Kinsella, K., & Velkoff, V. A. (2001). *An aging world: 2001 - International population reports. U.S. Department of Health and Human Services, National Institutes of Health, National Institute On Aging and U.S. Department of Commerce, Economics and Statistics Administration, U.* S. Census Bureau.

Kinsella, K., & Phillips, D. (2005). Global ageing: The challenge of success. [Washington, DC: Population Reference Bureau.]. *Population Bulletin*, *60*, 1.

Kitwood, T. (1998). Toward a theory of dementia care: Ethics and interaction. *The Journal of Clinical Ethics*, *9*(1), 23–34.

Klafter, R., Chmielewski, T., & Negin, M. (1989). *Robotic Engineering – An Integrated Approach*. USA: Prentice-Hall International.

Klein, R. (1991). Age-related eye disease, visual impairment, and driving in the elderly. *Human Factors: The Journal of the Human Factors and Ergonomics Society*, *33*, 521–525.

Kleinberger, T., Becker, M., Ras, E., Holzinger, A., & Muller, P. (2007). *Ambient Intelligence in Assisted Living: Enable Elderly People to Handle Future Interfaces. Universal Access in Human-Computer Interaction. Ambient Interaction, Part II.* HCII.

Klusch, M. (2005). Retrieved August 24, 2009, from OWL-MX Matcher. Retrieved from http://projects.semwebcentral.org/frs/?group_id=90.

Koch, S. (2006). Home telehealth - current state and future trends. *International Journal of Medical Informatics*, *75*(8), 565–576. doi:10.1016/j.ijmedinf.2005.09.002

Kolasinski, S. L., Garfinkel, M., Tsai, A. G., Matz, W., Van Dyke, A., & Schumacher, H. R. (2005). Iyengar yoga for treating symptoms of osteoarthritis of the knees: A Pilot Study. *Journal of Alternative and Complementary Medicine (New York, N.Y.)*, *11*(4), 689–693..doi:10.1089/acm.2005.11.689

Kongstvedt, P. R. (1997). *Essentials of managed health care* (2nd ed.). New York: Aspen Publishers.

Koppel, S., Charlton, J. L., & Fildes, B. (2009). Distraction and the older driver. In Regen, M. A., Lee, J. D., & Young, K. L. (Eds.), *Driver distraction: Theory, effects, and mitigation*. Boca Raton: Taylor & Francis Group.

Korea Agency for Digital Opportunity and Promotion. (2008). *2007 Annual report of digital divide for people age 50+ and older.* Seoul, Korea (in Korean).

Korea Agency for Digital Opportunity and Promotion. (2009). About KADO. Retrieved from https://www.kado.or.kr/koil/aboutkado/.

Korea Ministry of Health and Welfare. KIHSA. (2007) *2006 national survey of living status and welfare needs of the elders and needs for the elderly welfare service*. Retrieved March 9, 2009 from http://www.kihasa.re.kr/html/jsp/ (in Korean).

Korea Ministry of Information and Communication. (2006). *U-Korea master plan: To achieve the world's first ubiquitous society*. Retrieved from http://www.ipc.go.kr/servlet/download?pt=/ipceng/public&fn=u-KOREA+Master+Plan+.pdf

Korea National Statistics Office. (2006). *Population prediction for Korea* Retrieved from http://www.nso.go.kr/eng2006/

Korea, S. (2009). Population and Housing. *Statistics Korea.* Retrieved from http://www.kostat.go.kr.

Kosnik, W. D., Sekuler, R., & Kline, D. W. (1990). Self-reported visual problems of older drivers. *Human Factors: The Journal of the Human Factors and Ergonomics Society*, *32*, 597–608.

Kralik, D., Koch, T., Price, K., & Howard, N. (2004). Chronic illness self-management: taking action to create order. *Journal of Clinical Nursing*, *13*(2), 259–267. doi:10.1046/j.1365-2702.2003.00826.x

Krasner, G. E., & Pope, S. T. (1988). A cookbook for using the Model-View-Controller user interface paradigm in Smalltalk-80. *Journal of Object-Oriented Programming*, *1*(3), 26–49.

Krebs, H. I., Ferraro, M., Buerger, S. P., Newbery, M. J., Makiyama, A., & Sandmann, M. (2004). Rehabilitation Robotics- A pilot trial for spatial extension of MIT Manus. *Journal of Neuroengineering and Rehabilitation*, *1*(5). doi:.doi:10.1186/1743-0003-1-5

Kreps, G. L. (2005). Disseminating relevant health information to underserved audiences: Implications for the Digital Divide Pilot Projects. *Journal of the Medical Library Association*, *93*(4Supple), S69–S73.

Kruzich, J., Clinton, J., & Kelber, S. (1992). Personal and environmental influences on nursing home satisfaction. *The Gerontologist*, *32*, 342–350.

Kuttan, A., & Peters, L. (2003). *From digital divide to digital opportunity*. Lanham, MD: Rowman & Littlefield Publications, Inc.

Kwok, T., Lum, C. M., Chan, H. S., Ma, H. M., Lee, D., & Woo, J. (2004). A randomized, controlled trial of an intensive community nurse-supported discharge program in preventing hospital readmissions of older patients with chronic lung disease. *Journal of the American Geriatrics Society*, *52*(8), 1240–1246. doi:10.1111/j.1532-5415.2004.52351.x

Labelle, K. L., & Mihailidis, A. (2006). The use of automated prompting to facilitate hand washing in persons with dementia. *The American Journal of OccupationalT-therapy: Official publication of the American Occupational Therapy Association, 60*, 442-450.

Laguna, K., & Babcock, R. L. (1997). Computer anxiety in young and older adults: Implications for human-computer interactions in older populations. *Computers in Human Behavior*, *13*(3), 317–326. doi:10.1016/S0747-5632(97)00012-5

Lamb, S. E., Hauer, K., & Becker, C. (2007). Manual for the fall prevention classification system. (Publication. Retrieved January 15, 2010 from www.profane.eu.org/profane_documents/Falls_Taxonomy.pdf.

Lan, P. C. (2002). Subcontracting Filial Piety Elder Care in Ethnic Chinese Immigrant Families in California. *Journal of Family Issues*, *23*(7), 812–835. doi:10.1177/019251302236596

Langford, J., & Koppel, S. (2006). Epidemiology of older driver crashes - Identifying older driver risk factors and exposure patterns. *Transportation Research Part F: Traffic Psychology and Behaviour*, *9*(5), 309–321. doi:10.1016/j.trf.2006.03.005

Langford, J., Koppel, S., McCarthy, D., & Srinivasan, S. (2008). In defence of the 'low-mileage bias'. *Accident; Analysis and Prevention*, *40*, 1996–1999. doi:10.1016/j.aap.2008.08.027

Langford, J., Methorst, R., & Hakamies-Blomqvist, L. (2006). Older drivers do not have a high crash risk--A replication of low mileage bias. *Accident; Analysis and Prevention*, *38*(3), 574–578. doi:10.1016/j.aap.2005.12.002

Langford, J., & Oxley, J. (2006). Using the safe system approach to keep older drivers safely mobile. *IATSS Research*, *30*(2), 97–109.

Lautenschlager, N., Cox, K., Flicker, L., Foster, J., van Bockxmeer, F., & Xiao, J. (2008). Effect of physical activity on cognitive function in older adults at risk for Alzheimer disease: a randomized trial. *Journal of the American Medical Association*, *300*(9), 1027–1037. doi:10.1001/jama.300.9.1027

Lawton, M. P. (1989). Three functions of the residential environment. *Journal of Housing for the Elderly*, *5*, 35–50. doi:10.1300/J081V05N01_04

Lawton, M. P. (1994). Quality of life in Alzheimer's disease. *Alzheimer Disease and Associated Disorders*, *8*, 138–150.

Lawton, M. P., & Brody, E. M. (1969). Assessment of older people: Self-maintaining and instrumental activities of daily living. *The Gerontologist*, *9*(3), 179–186.

Lawton, R. B., & Mark, V. P. (2002). Integrated delivery networks: A detour on the road to integrated health care? *Health Affairs*, *21*(4), 128–143. doi:10.1377/hlthaff.21.4.128

Lawton, M. P. (1991). A multidimensional view of quality of life. In Birren, J. E., Lubben, J. E., Rowe, J. C., & Deutchman, D. E. (Eds.), *The concept and measurement of quality of life in the frail elderly* (pp. 3–27). New York: Academic Press.

Leduff, C. (2004, 5 November). Elderly driver to stand trial in deaths of 10. *The New York Times*. Retrieved 19 February, 2009, from http://query.nytimes.com/gst/fullpage.html?res=9B06E7D9143CF936A35752C1A9629C8B63&sec=&spon=&pagewanted=all.

Lee, S. J., & Hidler, J. (2008). Biomechanics of overground vs. treadmill walking in healthy individuals. *Journal of Applied Physiology (Bethesda, Md.)*, *104*(3), 747–755. doi:10.1152/japplphysiol.01380.2006

Lehrman, S., & Shore, K. K. (1998). *Hospitals' vertical integration into skilled nursing: A rational approach to controlling transaction costs*. Blue Cross and Blue Shield of the Rochester Area, Inc.

Leung, A. C., Yau, D. C., Liu, C. P., Yeoh, C. S., Chui, T. Y., & Chi, I. (2004). Reducing utilisation of hospital services by case management: a randomised controlled trial. *Australian Health Review*, *28*, 79–86. doi:10.1071/AH040079

Levy, B. R. (2003). Mind matters: Cognitive and physical effects of aging self-stereotypes. *Journal of Gerontology: Psychological Sciences*, *58*, 203–211.

Levy, B. R., Slade, M. D., Kunkel, S. R., & Kasl, S. V. (2003). Longevity increased by positive self-perceptions of aging. *Journal of Personality and Social Psychology*, *83*, 261–270. doi:10.1037/0022-3514.83.2.261

Lewis, C. B. (1984). Rehabilitation of an older person: a psychosocial focus. *Physical Therapy*, *64*(4), 517–522.

Lewis, D. (1999). Computer-based approaches to patient education: A review of the literature. *Journal of the American Medical Informatics Association*, *6*(4), 272–282.

Li, G., Braver, E. R., & Chen, C.-L. (2003). Fragility versus excessive crash involvement as determinants of high death rates per vehicle-mile of travel among older drivers. *Accident; Analysis and Prevention*, *35*, 227–235. doi:10.1016/S0001-4575(01)00107-5

Liddle, J., March, L., Carfrae, B., Finnegan, T., Druce, J., Schwarz, J., & Brooks, P. (1996). Can occupational therapy intervention play a part in maintaining independence and quality of life in older people? A randomised controlled trial. *Australian and New Zealand Journal of Public Health*, *20*(6), 574–578. doi:10.1111/j.1467-842X.1996.tb01068.x

Lindenberger, J., & Stoltz-Loike, M. (2005). *Why Mentor? Mentoring is a strategic business imperative.* Human Resources, The Lindenberger Group, LLC and SeniorThinking.

Lindenberger, U., Lövdén, M., Schellenbach, M., Li, S.-C., & Krüger, A. (2008). Psychological principles of successful aging technologies: A mini-review. *Gerontology, 54*, 59–68. doi:10.1159/000116114

Litvak, D., Gannot, I., & Zigel, Y. (2008). *Detection of falls at home using floor vibrations and sound.* Paper presented at the IEEE 25th Convention of Electrical and Electronics Engineers in Israel.

Liu, C., Utter, D., & Chen, C.-L. (2007). *Characteristics of crash injuries among young, middle-aged, and older drivers.* National Highway Traffic Safety Administration.

Liu, D., & Castle, N. G. (2009). Health information technology in nursing homes. *Journal of Applied Gerontology, 28*(1), 38–58. doi:10.1177/0733464808321887

Livneh, H. (2009). Denial of chronic illness and disability: Part I. Theoretical, functional, and dynamic perspectives. *Rehabilitation Counseling Bulletin*, (52): 225–236. doi:10.1177/0034355209333689

Lixin, W., Yunfa, L., Kanichi, M., & Shigeo, F. (2007). The psycho-physiological effects of "Taiji sense" in taijiquan exercise. *Japan Journal of Physical Fitness and Sports Medicine, 56*, 131–140.

Loane, D., Flanagan, G., Siun, A., McNamara, E., & Kenny, S. (2004). Nutrition in the community-an exploratory study of oral nutritional supplements in a health board area in Ireland. *Journal of Human Nutrition and Dietetics, 17*(3), 257–266. doi:10.1111/j.1365-277X.2004.00527.x

Lobo A., L. J., Launer, L., Fratiglioni, K., Andersen, A., Di Carlo, M. M. ...A. Hofman. (2000). Prevalence of dementia and major subtypes in Europe: A collaborative study of population-based cohorts. *Neurologic Diseases in the Elderly Research Group*. Neurology 54 (11 Supplement 5), S4-9. Cited after Dewey & Prince 2005.

Logan, R. A., & Tse, T. (2007). A multidiscipline conceptual framework for consumer health informatics. *Studies in Health Technology and Informatics, 29*(Part 2), 1169–1173.

Loges, W. E., & Jung, J. Y. (2001). Exploring the digital divide: Internet connectedness and age. *Communication Research, 28*(4), 536–542. doi:10.1177/009365001028004007

Long, S. (2000). *Caring for the elderly in Japan and the US: practices and policies*. London, UK: Routledge Publishers. doi:10.4324/9780203464472

Lord, S. R., Sherrington, C., Menz, H. B., & Close, J. C. T. (2007). *Falls in Older People: Risk Factors and Strategies for Prevention* (2nd ed.). Cambridge University Press. doi:10.1017/CBO9780511722233

Lord, D., van Schalkwyk, I., Chrysler, S., & Staplin, L. (2007). A strategy to reduce older driver injuries at intersections using more accommodating roundabout design practices. *Accident; Analysis and Prevention, 39*(3), 427–432. doi:10.1016/j.aap.2006.09.011

Lorence, D. P., & Park, H. (2006). New technology and old habits: The role of age as a technology chasm. *Technology and Health Care, 14*(2), 91–96.

Lorincz, K., Kuris, B., Ayer, S. M., Patel, S., Bonato, P., & Welsh, M. (2007). *Wearable wireless sensor network to assess clinical status in patients with neurological disorders*. Paper presented at the Proceedings of the 6th international conference on Information processing in sensor networks.

Louise-Bender Pape, T., Kim, J., & Weiner, B. (2002). The shaping of individual meanings assigned to assistive technology: A review of personal factors. *Disability and Rehabilitation, 24*(1-3), 5–30. doi:10.1080/09638280110066235

Loureiro, R. C. V., Johnson, M. J., & Harwin, W. S. (2006). Collaborative tele-rehabilitation: a strategy for increasing engagement. In *Proceedings of the 1st IEEE Int. Conference on Biomedical Robotics and Biomechatronics,* art. 1639198 (pp. 859-864).

Loveband, A. (2003). Positioning the product: Indonesian Migrant Women Workers in Contemporary Taiwan. Working Papers Series. Retrieved June 10, 2004, from http://www.cityu.edu.hk/searc/WP43_03_Loveband.pdf.

Low Choy, N. L., Brauer, S. G., & Nitz, J. C. (2007). Timed stance performances reflect differences in age, prevalence of comorbidities, medication use, fall history and activity level: Early screening for balance loss is indicated. *Australasian Journal on Ageing*, *26*(1), 29–34. doi:10.1111/j.1741-6612.2007.00202.x

Lutz, R. (2004). Detroit's Mr. Car Guy says driving is dead. *Fortune*, *149*(12), 68.

Lyman, S., Ferguson, S. A., Braver, E. R., & Williams, A. F. (2002). Older driver involvements in police reported and fatal crashes: Trends and projections. *Injury Prevention*, *8*, 116–120. doi:10.1136/ip.8.2.116

Machate, J., & Burmester, M. (2003). *User interface tuning*. Germany: Software and Support.

Maciuszek, D., Aberg, J., & Shahmehri, N. (2005). ASSETS'05, October 9–12, 2005, Baltimore, Maryland, USA.

Maclean, N., & Pound, P. (2000). A critical review of the concept of patient motivation in the literature on physical rehabilitation. *British Medical Journal*, *50*(4), 495–506.

Madden, G., & Savage, S. (2000). Some economic and social aspects of residential Internet use in Australia. *Journal of Media Economics*, *13*(3), 171–185. doi:10.1207/S15327736ME1303_2

Madsen, P. L., Hasselbalch, S. G., Hagemann, L. P., Olsen, K. S., & Bulow, J. (1995). Persistent resetting of cerebral oxygen/glucose uptake ratio by brain activation: evidence obtained by Kety-Schmidt technique. *Journal of Cerebral Blood Flow and Metabolism*, *15*, 485–491.

Mahlke, S., Roesler, D., Seifert, K., Krems, J. F., & Thuering, M. (2007). Evaluation of six night vision enhancement systems: Qualitative and quantitative support for intelligent image processing. *Human Factors: The Journal of the Human Factors and Ergonomics Society*, *49*, 518–531. doi:10.1518/001872007X200148

Mahoney, J. E., Shea, T. A., Przybelski, R., Jaros, L., Gangnon, R., Cech, S., & Schwalbe, A. (2007). Kenosha County falls prevention study: A randomized, controlled trial of an intermediate-intensity, community-based multifactorial falls intervention. *Journal of the American Geriatrics Society*, *55*(4), 489–498. doi:10.1111/j.1532-5415.2007.01144.x

Maltz, M., Sun, H., Wu, Q., & Mourant, R. (2007). In-vehicle alerting system for older and younger drivers: Does experience count? *Transportation Research Record*, *1899*, 64–70. doi:10.3141/1899-08

Mancini, J. (1980). Effects of health and income on control orientation and life satisfaction among aged public housing residents. *International Journal of Aging & Human Development*, *12*, 215–220.

Mann, C. (2001). Assistive technology and older adults. *OT Practice*, *6*(10), 13–15.

Marin, B., Leichsenring, K., Rodrigues, R., & Huber, M. (2009). *Who cares? Care coordination and cooperation to enhance quality in elderly care in the European Union.* European Centre for Social Welfare Policy and Research, Affiliated to the United Nations, Vienna, 24 August 2009.

Maritz, C. A. (2007). Using a model of reciprocal mentorship to develop, implement and sustain a group based exercise program for the frail elderly. *Physical & Occupational Therapy in Geriatrics*, *26*(3), 41–56.

Marottoli, R. A., H., V. P., Araujo, K. L. B., Iannone, L. P., Acampora, D., Charpentier, P., et al. (2007). A randomized trial of an education program to enhance older driver performance. *Journals of Gerontology: Series A: Medical Sciences*, *62*(10), 1113–1119.

Marottoli, R. A., & Richardson, E. D. (1998). Confidence in, and self-rating of, driving ability among older drivers. *Accident; Analysis and Prevention*, *30*(3), 331–336. doi:10.1016/S0001-4575(97)00100-0

Martens, C., Ruchel, N., Lang, O., Ivlev, O., & Graser, A. (2001). A FRIEND for assisting people with disabilities. *IEEE Robotics & Automation Magazine, 8*(1), 57-65, Retrieved September 22, 2009, from http://ieeexplore.ieee.org/stamp/stamp.jsp?tp=&arnumber=924364&isnumber=19982.

Martin, S., Kelly, S., Kernohan, G., McCreight, B., & Nugent, C. (2008). Smart home technologies for health and social care support. *Cochrane Database of System Reviews.* Retrieved January 22, 2009, from http://mrw.interscience.wiley.com/cochrane/clsysrev/articles/CD006412/frame.html.

Martinez, P., Bakardjian, H., & Cichocki, A. (2007). Fully online multicommand brain-computer interface with visual neurofeedback using SSVEP paradigm. *Computational Intelligence and Neuroscience*, 2007: 94561, PubMed Central. doi: 10.1155/2007/94561.

Maslow, A. H. (1971). *The farther reaches of human nature.* New York: Penguin.

May, A., Ross, T., & Osman, Z. (2005). The design of next generation in-vehicle navigation systems for the older driver. *Interacting with Computers, 17*(6), 643–659. doi:10.1016/j.intcom.2005.09.004

Mayagoitia, R. E., Nene, A. V., & Veltink, P. H. (2002). Accelerometer and rate gyroscope measurement of kinematics: an inexpensive alternative to optical motion analysis systems. *Journal of Biomechanics, 35*(4), 537–542. doi:10.1016/S0021-9290(01)00231-7

Mayring, P. (2000). Qualitative content analysis [Electronic version]. *Forum Qualitative Sozial Forschung, 1*(2).

McCarthy, C., Barnes, N., Anstey, K. J., & Horswill, M. S. (2008). *Towards a hazard perception assistance system using visual motion.* Paper presented at the 10th European Conference on Computer Vision.

McCreadie, C., & Tinker, A. (2005). The acceptability of assistive technology to older people. *Ageing and Society, 25*(1), 91–110. doi:10.1017/S0144686X0400248X

McCurry, J. (2006). Video games for the elderly: an answer to dementia or a marketing tool? *The Guardian.* Retrieved 8 February, 2009, from http://www.guardian.co.uk/technology/2006/mar/07/nintendods.games.

McDermott, H. J., & Looi, V. (2004). Perception of complex signals, including musical sounds, with cochlear implants. International Congress Series, Cochlear Implants. In *Proceedings of the VIII International Cochlear Implant Conference, 1273* (pp. 201-204).

McDonald, D. D., Thomas, G. J., Livingston, K. E., & Severson, J. S. (2005). Assisting older adults to communicate their postoperative pain. *Clinical Nursing Research, 14*(2), 109–126, discussion 127–130. doi:10.1177/1054773804271934

McFarland, R., Tune, G., & Welford, A. (1964). On the driving of automobiles by older people. *Journal of Gerontology, 19*, 190–197.

McGrath, M. J., & Dishongh, T. (2009). A Common Personal Health Research Platform - SHIMMER(TM) and BioMOBIUS(TM). *Enabling Healthcare in the Home, 13*(3), 122–147.

McGrath D, Greene B, O'Neill R, & B., C. (2009). *SHIMMER: A new tool for long-term, extra-laboratory gait monitoring.* Paper presented at the European Society for Movement Analysis in Adults and Children 2009.

McKerrow, P. (1991). *Introduction to robotics.* Singapore: Addison-Wesley.

McMurtrey, M. E., McGaughey, R. E., & Downey, J. P. (2009). Seniors and information technology: A potential goldmine of opportunity? *International Journal of Intercultural Information Management., 1*, 300–316.

Medtronic. Reveal® DX Insertable Cardiac Monitor. Retrieved January, 2010, from http://www.medtronic.com/physician/reveal/index.html.

Meinzer, M., Elbert, T., Wienbruch, C., Djundja, D., Barthel, G., & Rockstroh, B. (2004). Intensive language training enhances brain plasticity in chronic aphasia. *BMC Biology, 2*, 20..doi:10.1186/1741-7007-2-20

Menon, V. (2008, 28 October). Scary when GPS voice has it wrong. *Toronto Star*.

Menzel, N. N., Brooks, S. M., Bernard, T. E., & Nelson, A. (2004). The physical workload of nursing personnel: Association with musculoskeletal discomfort. *International Journal of Nursing Studies*, *41*, 859–867. doi:10.1016/j.ijnurstu.2004.03.012

Merrill, D., Kalanithi, J., & Maes, P. (2007). Siftables: towards sensor network user interfaces. In *Proceedings of the 1st international conference on Tangible and embedded interaction* (pp. 75–78).

Metsis, V., Le, Z., Lei, Y., & Makedon, F. (2008). Towards an evaluation framework for assistive environments. *PETRA '08: Proceedings of the 1st international conference on Pervasive Technologies Related to Assistive Environments*. July 15-19, 2008, Athens, Greece.

Meuleners, L. B., Harding, A., Lee, A. H., & Legge, M. (2006). Fragility and crash over-representation among older drivers in Western Australia. *Accident; Analysis and Prevention*, *38*(5), 1006–1010. doi:10.1016/j.aap.2006.04.005

Miller, S. (2003). *Unnecessary and avoidable hospital admissions for older people - A report to the Department of Health and Ageing*. Canberra: COAWG.

Milner, H. V. (2006). The digital divide: The role of political institutions in technology diffusion. *Comparative Political Studies*, *39*(2), 176–199. doi:10.1177/0010414005282983

Mirowsky, J., & Ross, C. E. (1992). Age and depression. *Journal of Health and Social Behavior*, *33*(3), 187–205. doi:10.2307/2137349

Mitchell, J. M., & Kemp, B. (2000). Quality of life in assisted living homes: A multidimensional analysis. *Journal of Gerontology*, *55*, 117–127.

Mittelman, M. S., Roth, D. L., Clay, O. J., & Haley, W. E. (2007). Preserving health of Alzheimer caregivers: Impact of a spouse caregiver intervention. *The American Journal of Geriatric Psychiatry*, *15*(9), 780–789. doi:10.1097/JGP.0b013e31805d858a

Moe-Nilssen, R. (1998). Test-retest reliability of trunk accelerometry during standing and walking. *Archives of Physical Medicine and Rehabilitation*, *79*(11), 1377–1385. doi:10.1016/S0003-9993(98)90231-3

Molnar, L. J., Eby, D. W., St. Louis, R. M., & Neumeyer, A. L. (2007). *Promising Approaches for Promoting Lifelong Community Mobility*. Washington, D.C.: AARP.

Molnar, L. J., & Eby, D. W. (2008). Getting around: Meeting the boomers' mobility needs. In R. Houston (Ed.), *Boomer or Bust? The New Political Economy of Aging*. Westport, Connecticut: Praeger Publishing.

Monaghan, K., Delahunt, E., & Caulfield, B. (2006). Ankle function during gait in patients with chronic ankle instability compared to controls. *Clinical Biomechanics (Bristol, Avon)*, *21*(2), 168–174. doi:10.1016/j.clinbiomech.2005.09.004

Moody, H. (1998). *Aging concepts and controversies*. Thousand Oaks, CA: Pine Forge Press.

Morini, A., & Biocca, L. (2004). Il contributo della domotica. In Micheli, G. A. (Ed.), *La questione anziana. Ridisegnare le coordinate di una società che invecchia* (pp. 166–177). Milano: Franco Angeli.

Morrow-Howell, N., Hinterlong, J., Rozario, P. A., & Tang, F. (2003). Effects of volunteering on the well-being of older adults. *Journal of Gerontology: Social Sciences*, *58*, 137–145.

Mueller, J. (2003). Universal products in the U.S. In Clarkson, J., Coleman, R., Keates, S., & Lebbon, C. (Eds.), *Inclusive Design: Design for the Whole Population*. New York: Springer.

Mueller, S., & Sixsmith, A. (2008). *User requirements for Ambient Assisted Living: Some evidence from the SOPRANO project*. Paper presented at the 6th International Conference of the International Society for Gerontechnology/, Pisa, Tuscany, Italy, June 4-7.

Murray, E., Burns, J., See, T. S., Lai, R., & Nazareth, I. (2005). Interactive health communication applications for people with chronic disease. *Cochrane Database of Systematic Reviews*, (Issue 4), CD004274. doi:. doi:10.1002/14651858.CD004274.pub4

Myers, B. A., Hudson, S. E., & Pausch, R. (2000). Past, present and future of user interface software tools. *ACM Transactions on Computer-Human Interaction*, *7*(1), 3–28. doi:10.1145/344949.344959

Mynatt, E. D., Melenhorst, A.-S., Fisk, A.-D., & Rogers, W. A. (2004). Aware technologies for aging in place: understanding user needs and attitudes. *IEEE Pervasive Computing / IEEE Computer Society [and] IEEE Communications Society*, *3*(2), 36–41. doi:10.1109/MPRV.2004.1316816

Mynatt, E. D., Rowan, J., Craighill, S., & Jacobs, A. (2001). Digital family portraits: Providing peace of mind for extended family members. In *Proceedings of the ACM Conference on Human Factors in Computing Systems* (pp. 333-340). CHI 2001; Seattle, Washington. New York: ACM Press.

Namazi, K. H., & McClintic, M. (2003). Computer use among elderly persons in long term care facilities. *Educational Gerontology*, *29*, 535–550. doi:10.1080/713844391

Nankervis, J., Schofield, H., Herrman, H., & Bloch, S. (1997). Home-based assessment for family carers: a preventative strategy to identify and meet service needs. *International Journal of Geriatric Psychiatry*, *12*(2), 193–201. doi:10.1002/(SICI)1099-1166(199702)12:2<193::AID-GPS580>3.0.CO;2-U

Narayanan, M. R., Lord, S. R., Budge, M. M., & Branko, G. Celler, & Lovell, N. H. (2007). *Falls Management: Detection and Prevention, using a Waistmounted Triaxial Accelerometer.* Paper presented at the 29th Annual International Conference of the IEEE EMBS, Lyon, France.

Nasvardi, G. E., & Vavrik, J. (2007). Crash risk of older drivers after attending a mature driver education program. *Accident; Analysis and Prevention*, *39*, 1073–1079. doi:10.1016/j.aap.2007.02.005

National Health Priority Action Council. (2006). *National chronic disease strategy*. Canberra: Australian Government Department of Health and Ageing.

National Institute for Clinical Excellence (NICE). (2004). *Falls. The Assessment and Prevention of Falls in Older People.* London: National Collaborating Centre for Nursing and Supportive Care.

National Internet Development Agency of Korea. (2009). Internet Usage Statistics. Retrieved from http://isis.nida.or.kr/eng/.

Naumanen, M., & Tukiainen, M. (2007). Seniors' club – Learning and blogging together. In P. Kommers & P. Isaías (Eds.), *Proceedings of the IADIS International Conference Web Based Communities* (pp. 312-316). Salamanca, Spain: IADIS.

Naung, N. (2006). *Robotic arm for electric scooter.* Unpublished B.Eng. Mechatronic Engineering thesis, Curtin University of Technology, Australia.

Nawate, Y., Kaneko, F., Hanaoka, H., & Okamura, H. (2007). Efficacy of a group reminiscence therapy for elderly dementia patients residing at home. *Physical & Occupational Therapy in Geriatrics*, *26*(3), 57–68.

Nay, R., & Garratt, S. (2005). *Nursing older people – Issues and innovations* (2nd ed.). Churchill Livingstone: Elsevier.

Nesselrath, R., Schulz, C., Schehl, J., Pfalzgraph, A., Pfleger, N., Stein, V., & Alexandersson, J. (2009). Homogeneous multimodal access to the digital home for people with cognitive disabilities. In *Proceedings of the second German Congress an Ambient Assisted Living.* Berlin, Germany.

New Zealand Ministry of Social Policy. (2001). *New Zealand positive ageing strategy*. Retrieved from http://www.osc.govt.nz/positive-ageing-strategy/index.html.

Newell, A. F. (1995). Extraordinary human computer operation. In Edwards, A. D. N. (Ed.), *Extraordinary human-computer interactions*. Cambridge University Press.

Newman, S., Steed, L., & Mulligan, K. (2004). Self-management interventions for chronic illness. *Lancet*, *364*(9444), 1523–1537. doi:10.1016/S0140-6736(04)17277-2

Ngan, R., & Wong, W. (1995). Injustice in family care of the Chinese elderly in Hong Kong. *Journal of Aging & Social Policy*, *7*(2), 77–94. doi:10.1300/J031v07n02_06

Nguyen, L., Shanks, G., Vetere, F., & Howard, S. (2008). Information systems and healthcare XXVIII: The information needs of family carers in collaborative healthcare. *Communications of the Association for Information Systems*, *23*(10).

Nguyen, L., & Shanks, G. (2007). Families as carers - Information needs in a cultural context. In *Proceedings of 18th Australasian Conference on Information Systems*, Toowoomba, Australia.

NHHRC. (2009). *A healthier future for all Australians: Final report June 2009*. Australia: National Health and Hospitals Reform Commission.

NHS. (2007). *The expert patients programme*. UK: Department of Health, Chief Medical Officer, National Health Service.

NHTSA. (2006). *Traffic Safety Facts 2006: Older Population*. National Highway Traffic Safety Administration.

Nichols, J., Myers, B. A., Higgins, M., Hughes, J., Harris, T. K., Rosenfeld, R., & Litwack, K. (2003). *Personal universal controllers: controlling complex appliances with GUIs and speech. Extended Abstract CHI'2003: Human Factors in Computing Systems (Demonstration Abstract)* (pp. 624–625). New York: ACM.

Nichols, J., & Myers, B. A. (2003). Studying the use of handhelds to control smart appliances. *International Workshop on Smart Appliances and Wearable Computing (IWSAWC 2003) Proceedings of the 23rd IEEE Conference on Distributed Computing Systems Workshops (ICDCS'03)* (pp. 274-279). Washington: IEEE Computer Society.

Nielsen, J. (1993). *Usability Engineering*. London: Academic Press.

NIH. (2000). *Self- management strategies across chronic diseases*. Bethesda, Maryland, USQ: National Institute of Health.

Niki, R. (1998). *Health, medical, welfare and care mix*. Tokyo, Japan: Igakushoin.

Niki, R. (2000). *Long- term care insurance and medical insurance reform*. Tokyo, Japan: Keisoshobo.

Nurmi, I., & Lüthje, P. (2002). Incidence and costs of falls and fall injuries among elderly in institutional care. *Scandinavian Journal of Primary Health Care*, *20*(2), 118–122.

Nutley, S., & Thomas, C. (1995). Spatial mobility and social change: The mobile and the immobile. *Sociologia Ruralis*, *35*(1), 24–39. doi:10.1111/j.1467-9523.1995.tb00824.x

Nyan, M. N., Tay, F. E. H., & Murugasu, E. (2008). A wearable system for pre-impact fall detection. *Journal of Biomechanics*, *41*(16), 3475–3481. doi:10.1016/j.jbiomech.2008.08.009

O'Donovan, K. J., Greene, B. R., McGrath, D., O'Neill, R., Burns, A., & Caulfield, B. (2009). *SHIMMER: A new tool for temporal gait analysis*. Paper presented at the Engineering in Medicine and Biology Society, 2009. EMBC 2009. Annual International Conference of the IEEE.

O'Donovan, K., Dishongh, T., Foran, T., Leahy, D., & Ni Scanaill, C. (2008). *The Development of a Clinical Gait Analysis System*. Paper presented at the International Conference on Ambulatory Monitoring of Physical Activity and Movement.

OECD. (2001). *Ageing and transport: Mobility needs and safety issues*. Paris, France: Organisation for Economic Co-operation and Development.

Olivier, P., Xu, G., Monk, A., & Hoey, J. (2009). Ambient kitchen: Designing situated services using a high fidelity prototyping environment. *2nd International Conference on Pervasive Technologies Related to Assistive Environments*, Workshop on Affect and Behaviour Related Assistance in Support for the Elderly. June, 2009, Corfu, Greece.

OSGi. (2007). OSGi Service Platform Release 4. Retrieved August 24, 2009, from http://www.osgi.org/Release4/Download.

Osman, L. M., Abdalla, M. I., Beattie, J. A. G., Ross, S. J., Russell, I. T., & Friend, J. A. (1994). Reducing hospital admission through computer supported education for asthma patients. *BMJ (Clinical Research Ed.)*, (308): 568–571.

Ostir, G. V., Markides, K. S., Black, S. A., & Goodwin, J. S. (2000). Emotional well-being predicts subsequent independent functioning and survival. *Journal of the American Geriatrics Society*, *48*, 473–478.

O'Sullivan, M., Blake, C., Cunningham, C., Boyle, G., & Finucane, C. (2009). Correlation of accelerometry with clinical balance tests in older fallers and non-fallers. *Age and Ageing*, •••, afp009.

Oswald, F., Wahl, H.-W., Naumann, D., Mollenkopf, H., & Hieber, A. (2006). The role of the home environment in middle and late adulthood. In Wahl, H.-W., Brenner, H., Mollenkopf, H., Rothenbacher, D., & Rott, C. (Eds.), *The many faces of health, competence and well-being in old age: Integrating Epidemiological, psychological and social perspectives* (pp. 7–24). Heidelberg: Springer. doi:10.1007/1-4020-4138-1_2

OWL-S. (2002). OWL-S Technical Committee (T.C), Web Ontology Language for Web Services (OWL-S), http://www.w3.org/Submission/OWL-S/.

Owsley, C., Ball, K. K., McGwin, G., Sloane, M. E., Roenker, D. L., & White, M. F. (1998). Visual processing impairment and risk of motor vehicle crash among older adults. *Journal of the American Medical Association*, *279*(14), 1083–1088. doi:10.1001/jama.279.14.1083

Owsley, C., Ball, K. K., Sloane, M. E., Roenker, D. L., & Bruni, J. R. (1991). Visual/cognitive correlates of vehicle accidents in older drivers. *Psychology and Aging*, *6*(3), 403–415. doi:10.1037/0882-7974.6.3.403

Owsley, C., McGwin, G., Phillips, J. M., McNeal, S., & Stalvey, B. T. (2004). Impact of an educational program on the safety of high-risk, visually impaired, older drivers. *American Journal of Preventive Medicine*, *26*, 222–229. doi:10.1016/j.amepre.2003.12.005

Oxley, J., Fildes, B., Corben, B., & Langford, J. (2006). Intersection design for older drivers. *Transportation Research Part F: Traffic Psychology and Behaviour*, *9*(5), 335–346. doi:10.1016/j.trf.2006.06.005

Pachana, N. A., & Petriwskyj, A. M. (2006). Assessment of insight and self-awareness in older drivers. *Clinical Gerontologist*, *30*(1), 23–38. doi:10.1300/J018v30n01_03

Pachana, N. A. (2006). Psychogerontology and cognitive disabilities related to ageing. In Morse, C. (Ed.), *The art of ageing in a global context: From theory and research to policy and practice* (pp. 435–452). New York: Baywood Publishers.

Pacific Health Summit. (2006). Preparing for the ageing challenge. *Pacific Health Summit.* Retrieved from http://www.pacifichealthsummit.org/downloads/Ageing%20Challenge_Breakout%20Session%20Report.pdf.

Padgett, D. (2004). *The qualitative research experience.* USA: Wadsworth.

Parette, P., & Scherer, M. (2004). Assistive technology use and stigma. *Education and Training in Developmental Disabilities Journal*, *39*(3), 217–226.

Park, S. H., Won, S. H., Lee, J. B., & Kim, S. W. (2003). Smart home-digitally engineered domestic life. *Personal and Ubiquitous Computing*, *7*(3–4), 189–196. doi:10.1007/s00779-003-0228-9

Parker, M. G., Ahacic, K., & Thorslund, M. (2005). Health changes among Swedish oldest old: Prevalence rates from 1992 and 2002 show increasing health problems. *Journal of Gerontology*, *60A*(10), 1351–1355.

Parker, M. H., & Sabata, D. (2004). Home, safe home: Household and safety assistive technology. In Burdick, D. C., & Kwon, S. (Eds.), *Gerotechnology Research and Practice in Technology and Aging* (pp. 145–160). New York: Springer Publishing Company.

Patel, S., Lorincz, K., Hughes, R., Huggins, N., & Growdon, J. H. Matt Welsh, et al. (2007). *Analysis of Feature Space for Monitoring Persons with Parkinson's Disease With Application to a Wireless Wearable Sensor.* Paper presented at the 29th Annual International Conference of the IEEE EMBS, Lyon, France.

Paulson, L. D. (2008). A New Wi-Fi for Peer-to-Peer Communications. *Computer*, *41*(6), 19–21. doi:10.1109/MC.2008.171

Peden, M., Scurfield, R., Sleet, D., Mohan, D., Hyder, A. A., & Jarawan, E. (Eds.). (2004). *World Report on Road Traffic Injury Prevention.* Geneva, Switzerland: World Health Organization.

Peel, N. M., McClure, R. J., & Bartlett, H. P. (2005). Behavioral determinants of healthy ageing. *American Journal of Preventive Medicine*, *28*(3), 298–304. doi:10.1016/j.amepre.2004.12.002

Peng, W. (2009). Theoretical guidance for using computer and video games for health intervention. *Paper presented at the annual meeting of the International Communication Association*, Sheraton New York.

Perlmutter, L., Monty, R., & Chan, F. (1986). Choice, control and cognitive functioning. In Baltes, M., & Baltes, P. (Eds.), *The psychology of control and aging* (pp. 91–118). Hillsdale, NJ: Lawrence Erlbaum Associates.

Persaud, B. N., Retting, R. A., Garder, P. E., & Lord, D. (2000). *Crash reductions following installation of roundabouts in the United States*. Arlington, VA: Insurance Institute for Highway Safety.

Pfaff, G. E. (1985). *User interface management systems*. Berlin: Springer-Verlag.

Pfurtschellar, G., & Neuper, C. (2001). Motor imagery and direct brain-computer communication. *Proceedings of the IEEE*, *89*(7), 1123–1134. doi:10.1109/5.939829

Philips. (n.d.). Lifeline. Retrieved February 23, 2009, from http://www.lifelinesys.com/.

Philips. (n.d.). Philips Lifeline Tempo Watch. Retrieved February 26, 2009, from http://www.lifelinesys.com/content/lifeline-products/tempo-watch.jsp.

Phillips, B. S. (1957). *A Role Theory Approach to Adjustment in Old Age*. American Sociological Review.

Pierce, J. (2008). World Internet Project International Report (2009). Retrieved September 19, 2009, from http://www.worldinternetproject.net/

Piriyaprasarth, P., Morris, M., Winter, A., & Bialocerkowski, A. (2008). The reliability of knee joint position testing using electrogoniometry. *BMC Musculoskeletal Disorders*, *9*(1), 6. doi:10.1186/1471-2474-9-6

Plainis, S., Murray, I. J., & Pallikaris, I. G. (2006). Road traffic casualties: Understanding the night-time death toll. *Injury Prevention*, *12*(2), 125–138. doi:10.1136/ip.2005.011056

Pohlman, S., & Traenkel, U. (1994). Orientation in road traffic: Age-related differences using an in-vehicle navigation system and a conventional map. *Accident; Analysis and Prevention*, *26*(6), 689–702. doi:10.1016/0001-4575(94)90048-5

Poindexter, K. N. (2003). *Passenger vehicle crash involvement rates by vehicle model year*. Washington, DC: U.S. Department of Transportation.

Pollack, M. E. (2005). Intelligent technology for an aging population: The use of AI to assist elders with cognitive impairment. *AI Magazine*, *26*(2), 9–24.

Pollack, M., Engberg, S., Matthews, J. T., Thrun, S., Brown, L., Colbry, D., et al. & Roy N. (2002) Pearl: A mobile robotic assistant for the elderly. In *Proceedings of Workshop on Automation as Caregiver: the Role of Intelligent Technology in Elder Care (AAAI)*. Edmonton, AB.

Pons, J. L. (2008). *Wearable robots: Biomechatronic exoskeleton*. USA: Wiley. doi:10.1002/9780470987667

Population Statistics of Japan. (2009). National Institute of Population and Social Security Research. *Population Statistics of Japan*. Retrieved from http://www.ipss.go.jp.

Pot, A. M., Zarit, S. H., Twisk, J. W. R., & Townsend, A. L. (2005). Transitions in Caregivers' Use of Paid Home Help: Associations With Stress Appraisals and Well-Being. *Psychology and Aging*, *20*(2), 211–219. doi:10.1037/0882-7974.20.2.211

Powell, J. A., Lowe, P., Griffiths, F. E., & Thorogood, M. (2005). A critical analysis of the literature on the Internet and consumer health information. *Journal of Telemedicine and Telecare, 11 Suppl*(1), 41-43.

Preusser, D. F., Williams, A. F., Ferguson, S. A., Ulmer, R. G., & Weinstein, H. B. (1998). Fatal crash risk for older drivers at intersections. *Accident; Analysis and Prevention*, *30*(2), 151–159. doi:10.1016/S0001-4575(97)00090-0

Prichep, L., John, E., Ferris, S., Reisberg, B., Almas, M., Alper, K., & Cancro, R. (1994). Quantitative EEG correlates of cognitive deterioration in the elderly. *Neurobiology of Aging*, *15*(1), 85–90. doi:10.1016/0197-4580(94)90147-3

Productivity Commission (2008). *Trends in aged care services: Some implications.*

Profane. (n.d.). ProFaNE Clinical Assessment Tool (CAT) Publication. Retrieved January 15 2010 http://www.profane.eu.org/CAT/.

Proshansky, H. M., Fabian, A. K., & Kaminoff, R. (1983). Place-identity: Physical world socialization of the self. *Journal of Environmental Psychology*, *3*, 57–83. doi:10.1016/S0272-4944(83)80021-8

Qassis, S., & Hayden, D. C. (1990). Effects of environment on psychological well-being of elderly persons. *Psychological Reports*, *66*(1), 147–150. doi:10.2466/PR0.66.1.147-150

Queensland Health. (2002). Smart State 2020: A Vision for the Future. *Directions Statement* (pp. 6-11).

Queensland-Government. (2002). *Statewide Action Plan Falls Prevention in Older People 2002-2006*. Queensland Government.

Queensland-Injury-Surveillance-Unit. (1999). Falls in older people'. *Injury Bulletin*, *56*, 1–6.

Raichur, A., Wihardo, G., Banerji, S., & Heng, J. (2009). A step towards home-based robotic rehabilitation: An interface circuit for EEG/SEMG actuated orthosis. In *Proceedings of the 2009 IEEE/ASME International Conference on Advanced Intelligent Mechatronics*, Singapore, 1998-2003.

Rajendran, P., Corcoran, A., Kinosian, B., & Alwan, M. (2008). Falls, Fall Prevention, and Fall Detection Technologies. In *Eldercare Technology for Clinical Practitioners* (pp. 187-202).

Rakowski, W., & Hickey, T. (1992). Mortality and the attribution of health problems to aging among older adults. *American Journal of Public Health, 82*(8), 1139-1141, Retrieved October 19, 2009, from http://www.ajph.org/cgi/reprint/82/8/1139.

Reid, D., & Ziegler, M. (1980). Validity and stability of a new desired control measure pertaining to psychological adjustment of the elderly. *Journal of Gerontology*, *35*, 315–402.

Research Institute of Science for the Better Living of the Elderly. (2007). *Cyber-family program*. Busan, Korea: Author.

Rialle, V., Duchene, F., Noury, N., Bajolle, L., & Demongeot, J. (2002). Health "smart" home: Information technology for patients at home. *Telemedicine Journal and e-Health*, *8*(4), 395–409. doi:10.1089/15305620260507530

Rice, D., & Fineman, N. (2004). Economic implications of increased longevity in the United States. *Annual Review of Public Health*, *25*, 457–473. doi:10.1146/annurev.publhealth.25.101802.123054

Richards, T.F., Walker, G., & Jarvis. L. (2006). Time to move? A literature review of housing for older people. *Scottish Executive Social Research*. UK Audit Commission (2004). Older people: Assistive technology: Independence and well-being No. 4.

Ricklefs, R. (1995). *Aging a natural history*. New York: Scientific American Library.

Robbins, S. (2009). Large print finds its mark. *Publishers Weekly.* Retrieved 17 September 2009 from http://www.publishersweekly.com/article/CA6658685.html?q.

Robertson, I. H., & Murre, J. M. J. (1999). Rehabilitation of brain damage: Brain plasticity and principles of guided recovery. *Psychological Bulletin, 125*(5), 544–547. doi:10.1037/0033-2909.125.5.544

Robichon, F. (2004). Robots help Japan care for its elderly. *Popular Mechanics*. Retrieved from http://www.popularmechanics.com/technology/industry/1288241.html.

Roenker, D. L., Cissell, G. M., Ball, K. K., Wadley, V. G., & Edwards, J. D. (2003). Speed-of-processing and driving simulator training result in improved driving performance. *Human Factors, 45*(2), 218–233. doi:10.1518/hfes.45.2.218.27241

Rogè, J., Pèbayle, T., Aurèlie, C., & Muzet, A. (2005). Useful visual field reduction as a function of age and risk of accident in simulated car driving. *Investigative Ophthalmology & Visual Science, 46*(5), 1774–1779. doi:10.1167/iovs.04-0540

Rogers, W. A., & Fisk, A. D. (1991). Age-related differences in the maintenance and modification of automatic processes: arithmetic stroop interference. *Human Factors, 33*, 45–56.

Rolland, Y., Pillard, F., Klapouszczak, A., Reynish, E., Thomas, D., & Andrieu, S. (2007). Exercise program for nursing home residents with Alzheimer's disease: A 1-Year Randomized, Controlled Trial. *Journal of the American Geriatrics Society, 55*(2), 158–165. doi:10.1111/j.1532-5415.2007.01035.x

Rosel, N. (2003). Aging in place: Knowing where you are. *International Journal of Aging & Human Development, 57*(1), 77–90. doi:10.2190/AMUD-8XVX-9FPK-MR8G

Rosenberg, P. B., Mielke, M. M., Samus, Q. M., Rosenblatt, A., Baker, A., & Brandt, J. (2006). Transition to nursing home from assisted living is not associated with dementia or dementia-related problem behaviors. *Journal of the American Medical Directors Association, 7*(2), 73–78. doi:10.1016/j.jamda.2005.06.003

Ross, A. C., Adam, L. B., Yonghao, P., Paul, M., Kim, B., & Michael, H. (2009). Validity and reliability of the Nintendo Wii Balance Board for assessment of standing balance. *Gait & posture.*

Rosson, M. B., Carroll, J. M., Seals, C., & Lewis, T. (2002). Community design of community simulations. [New York: ACM.]. *Proceedings of Designing Interactive Systems: DIS, 2002*, 74–83.

Row, S., Schagrin, M., & Briggs, V. (2008). [*ITS International, August.*]. *Future*, VII.

Rowe, J., & Kahn, R. (1999). *Successful Aging*. New York: Random House.

Rowe, J. W., & Kahn, R. L. (1998). *Successful ageing*. New York: Pantheon Books.

Rowe, J. W., & Kahn, R. L. (1987). Human aging: usual and successful. *Science, 237*(4811), 143-149. Retrieved October 19, 2009, from http://www.sciencemag.org/cgi/content/abstract/sci;237/4811/143.

Rubin, G. S., Ng, E. S. W., Bandeen-Roche, K., Keyl, P. M., Freeman, E. E., & West, S. K. (2007). A prospective, population-based study of the role of visual impairment in motor vehicle crashes among older drivers: The SEE study. *Investigative Ophthalmology & Visual Science, 48*(4), 1483–1491. doi:10.1167/iovs.06-0474

Rudin-Brown, C. M., & Parker, H. A. (2004). Behavioural adaptation to adaptive cruise control (ACC): implications for preventive strategies. *Transportation Research Part F: Traffic Psychology and Behaviour*, 7(2), 59–76. doi:10.1016/j.trf.2004.02.001

Rumar, K. (2002). *Night vision enhancement systems: What should they do and what more do we need to know? University of Michigan.* Ann Arbor: Transportation Research Institute.

Ryan, G., Legge, M., & Rosman, D. (1998). Age related changes in drivers' crash risk and crash type. *Accident; Analysis and Prevention, 30*(3), 379–387. doi:10.1016/S0001-4575(97)00098-5

Sakamura, K. (2008). *Ubiquitous ID technologies* 2008. Tokyo, Japan: YRP Ubiquitous Networking Laboratory. Retrieved from http://www.uidcenter.org/pdf/UID910-W001-080226_en.pdf.

Sangiovanni-Vincentelli, A., & Di Natale, M. (2007). Embedded system design for automotive applications. *IEEE Computer*, *40*(10), 42–51.

Schehl, J., Pfalzgraf, A., Pfleger, N., & Steigner, J. (2008). The BabbleTunes system - Talk to your iPod! In V. Digalakis, A. Potamianos, M. Turk, R. Pieraccini, & Y. Ivanov (Eds.), *Proceedings of the 10th International Conference on Multimodal Interfaces (ICMI 2008)* (pp. 77-80). New York: ACM.

Schein, C., Gagnon, A. J., Chan, L., Morin, I., & Grondines, J. (2005). The association between specific nurse case management interventions and elder health. *Journal of the American Geriatrics Society*, *53*(4), 597–602. doi:10.1111/j.1532-5415.2005.53206.x

Scherer, M. (2002). The change in emphasis from people to person: Introduction to the special issue on assistive technology. *Disability and Rehabilitation*, *24*(1-3), 1–4. doi:10.1080/09638280110066262

Scherer, M. (1997). The impact of assistive technology on the lives of people with disabilities. In Gray, D. Q. (Ed.), *Designing and using assistive technology: The human perspective*. Baltimore, Maryland: Brookes Publishing Co.

Schulz, C., Neßelrath, R., & Alexandersson, J. (2009). Homogeneous multimodal access to the digital home for people with cognitive disabilities. In *Proceedings of the second German Congress an Ambient Assisted Living*. VDE, Berlin.

Scopelliti, M., Giuliani, M. V., & Fornara, F. (2005). Robots in a domestic setting: A psychological approach. *Universal Access in the Information Society*, *4*(2), 146–155. doi:10.1007/s10209-005-0118-1

Sears, A., & Jacko, J. A. (Eds) (2007). *The Human-Computer Interaction handbook: Fundamentals, evolving technologies and emerging applications* (2nd ed.). New York: CRC Press.

Sekuler, R., & Ball, K. K. (1986). Visual localization: Age and practice. *Journal of the Ophthalmological Society of America, Series A*, *3*(6), 864–867.

Selwyn, N. (2004). The information aged: A qualitative study of older adults' use of information and communication technology. *Journal of Aging Studies*, *18*, 369–384. doi:10.1016/j.jaging.2004.06.008

Setright, L. K. J. (2002). *Drive on!: A social history of the motor car*. London: Palawan Press.

Shaheen, S. A., & Neimeier, D. A. (2001). Integrating vehicle design and human factors: Minimizing elderly driving constraints. *Transportation Research Part C, Emerging Technologies*, *9*, 155–174. doi:10.1016/S0968-090X(99)00027-3

Shapira, N., Barak, A., & Gil, I. (2007). Promoting older adults' well-being through Internet training and use. *Aging & Mental Health*, *11*(5), 477–484. doi:10.1080/13607860601086546

Sherrington, C., & Whitney, J., C., R. Lord, S., Herbert, R., D., Cumming, R., G., & Close, J. C. T. (2008). Effective Exercise for the Prevention of Falls: A Systematic Review and Meta-Analysis. *Journal of the American Geriatrics Society*, *56*(12), 2234–2243. doi:10.1111/j.1532-5415.2008.02014.x

Shortell, S. M. (1997). Commentary on Physician-hospital integration and the economic theory of the firm. *Medical Care Research and Review*, *54*(1), 25–31. doi:10.1177/107755879705400102

Shortell, S. M., & Kaluzny, A. D. (1994). *Health care management: organization, design, and behavior*. Florence, KY, USA: Delmar Publisher.

Silver, S. (2007). "Internet Romance: How Match.com Found Love among Boomers; Dating Site Prospers Targeting Older Singles; The Body Art Question", in *Wall Street Journal. (Eastern edition)*, New York, January 27.

Sims, R. V., McGwin, G. Jr, Allman, R. M., Ball, K., & Owsley, C. (2000). Exploratory study of incident vehicle crashes among older drivers. *The Journals of Gerontology. Series A, Biological Sciences and Medical Sciences, 55A*(1), 22–27.

Sister Theresa-Never too old to help others, (n.d.). Retrieved September 18, 2009 from http://www.hearttoheartservice.org/AboutFounder.htm

Sixsmith, A. (2008). *Ambient technologies: Developing user-driven approaches to research and development.* Paper presented at the Gerontological Society of America 61st Annual Scientific Meeting, Gaylord National Resort and Convention Center. *MD Medical Newsmagazine*, (Nov): 21–25.

Sixsmith, A., & Johnson, N. (2004). A smart sensor to detect the falls of the elderly. *Pervasive Computing, IEEE, 3*(2), 42–47. doi:10.1109/MPRV.2004.1316817

Sixsmith, J. (1990). *Driving experiences and new technology: Evaluations and expectations of older drivers.* London: Occasional Paper 31. Department of Geography, King's College.

Slegers, K., van Boxtel, M. P. J., & Jolles, J. (2008). Effects of computer training and internet usage on the well-being and quality of life of older adults: A randomized, controlled study. *Journal of Gerontology, 63B*, 176–P184.

Small, G., Moody, T., Siddarth, P., & Bookheimer, S. (2009). Your brain on Google: Patterns of cerebral activation during Internet searching. *The American Journal of Geriatric Psychiatry, 17*(2), 116–126. doi:10.1097/JGP.0b013e3181953a02

Small, G. W. (2002). *The memory bible.* New York: Hyperion.

Small, G., Moody, T., Siddarth, P., & Bookheimer, S. (2009). Your brain on Google: Patterns of cerebral activation during Internet searching. *The American Journal of Geriatric Psychiatry, 17*(2), 116–126. doi:10.1097/JGP.0b013e3181953a02

Smiley, A. (1999). *Adaptive strategies of older drivers.* Paper presented at the Conference on Transportation in an Aging Society: A Decade of Experience, Bethesda, Maryland.

Smith, G. E., Housen, P., Yaffe, K., Ruff, R., Kennison, R. F., Mahncke, H. W., & Zelinski, E. M. (2009). A cognitive training program based on principles of brain plasticity: Results from the improvement in memory with plasticity-based adaptive cognitive training (IMPACT) Study. *Journal of the American Geriatrics Society, 57*(4), 594–603. doi:10.1111/j.1532-5415.2008.02167.x

Smith, J. E., & Hall, M. J. (2005). Injuries caused by seatbelts. *Trauma, 7*(4), 211–215. doi:10.1191/1460408605ta348oa

Soar, J., & Seo, Y. (2007). Health and aged care enabled by information technology. *Third international conference on healthy ageing and longevity. Annals of the New York Academy of Sciences, 1114*, 154–161. doi:10.1196/annals.1396.040

Soar, J., & Wang, S. Y. (2009). Information for guided chronic disease self-management in community settings. In Sintchenko, V., & Croll, P. (Eds.), *Frontiers of Health Informatics – Redefining Healthcare, HIC 2009 Proceedings*. Health Informatics Society of Australia.

Soar, J. (2004). Improving health and public safety through knowledge management. *Thailand International Conference on Knowledge Management*, Bangkok, Thailand.

Soar, J. (2008). *Information management in modern healthcare organisations*. Proceedings IBIMA, 4-6 January 2008, Marrakesh, Morocco

Soar, J., & Croll, P. (2007). Assistive technologies for the frail elderly, chronic illness sufferers and people with disabilities - A case study of the development of a smart home. In *Proceedings of 18th Australasian Conference on Information Systems*, Toowoomba, Australia.

Soar, J., Livingstone, A., & Wang, S. Y. (2009). A case study of an ambient living and wellness management health care model in Australia. In M. Mokhtari, I. Khalil, J. Bauchet, D. Zhang & C. Nuget (Eds.) *Ambient Assistive Health and Wellness Management in the Heart of the City*, Refereed Proceedings of the 7th International Conference On Smart Homes and Health Telematics (ICOST2009) 1-3 July, 2009–Tours, France, Springer.

Son, Y. (2005). *KADO 2004 annual report*. Seoul: Korea Agency for Digital Opportunity & Promotion.

Son, Y. (2007, May). Addressing the digital divide within the Korean ageing society. Paper presented at Namhae Active Ageing Conference in Asia Pacific, Namhae, Korea.

Song, R., Lee, E., Lam, P., & Bae, S. C. (2003). Effects of tai chi exercise on pain, balance, muscle strength, and perceived difficulties in physical functioning in older women with osteoarthritis: A randomized clinical trial. *The Journal of Rheumatology*, *30*(9), 2039–2044.

SOPRANO. (2009). *Service-oriented Programmable Smart Environments for Older Europeans*. Retrieved August 31, 2009 from http://www.soprano-ip.org

Spence, C., & Ho, C. (2008). Multisensory warning signals for event perception and safe driving. *Theoretical Issues in Ergonomics Science*, *9*(6), 523–554. doi:10.1080/14639220701816765

Spring, H. J., Rowe, M. A., & Kelly, A. (2009). Improving caregivers' well-being by using technology to manage nighttime activity in persons with dementia. *Research in Gerontological Nursing*, *2*(1), 39–48. doi:10.3928/19404921-20090101-10

Srinivasan, N. OWL-S UDDI Matchmaker (2004). Retrieved August 24, 2009, from http://projects.semwebcentral.org/projects/owl-s-uddi-mm.

Stalldall, E., Caesar, M., & Erickson, R. (2001). Ageing, elderly, and how IT can be used to enhance the quality of care for the elderly. *Vardal Foundation*. Retrieved September 15, 2009, from http://www.vardal.se/japan/SweJapSeminar2.pdf.

Stanton, N. A., & Young, M. S. (1998). Vehicle automation and driving performance. *Ergonomics*, *41*(7), 1014–1028. doi:10.1080/001401398186568

Stanton, N. A., & Young, M. S. (2005). Driver behaviour with adaptive cruise control. *Ergonomics*, *48*, 1294–1313. doi:10.1080/00140130500252990

Staplin, L., Lococo, K., Byington, S., & Harkey, D. (2001). *Highway Design Handbook for Older Drivers and Pedestrians*. McLean, VA: U.S Department of Transportation, Federal Highway Administration.

Stefanov, D. H., Zeungnam, B., & Bang, W.-C. (2004). The smart house for older persons and persons with physical disabilities: structure, technology arrangements, and perspectives. *Neural Systems and Rehabilitation Engineering. IEEE Transactions on Rehabilitation Engineering*, *12*(2), 228–250. doi:10.1109/TNSRE.2004.828423

Steg, H. Strese. H., Loroff, C., Hull, J., & Schmidt, S. (2006). Europe is facing a demographic challenge: Ambient assisted living offers solutions. *Ambient Assisted Living – European overview report. VDI/VDE/IT*, Berlin, Germany.

Stessman, J., Hammerman-Rozenberg, R., Cohen, A., Ein-Mor, E., & Jacobs, J. M. (2009). Physical activity, function and longevity among the very old. *Archives of Internal Medicine*, *169*(16), 1476–1483. doi:10.1001/archinternmed.2009.248

Stevens, M., Holman, C. D., Bennett, N., & de Klerk, N. (2001). Preventing falls in older people: Outcome evaluation of a randomized controlled trial. *Journal of the American Geriatrics Society*, *49*(11), 1448–1455. doi:10.1046/j.1532-5415.2001.4911236.x

Story, M. F. (1998). Maximizing usability: the principles of universal design. *Assistive Technology*, *10*(1), 4–12.

Story, M.F. (1998). Maximising usability: The principles of universal design. *Assistive Technology-The official journal of RESNA, 10*(1), 4-12.

Strandberg, T. E., & Pitkälä, K. H. (2007). Frailty in elderly people. *Lancet*, *369*, 1328–1329. doi:10.1016/S0140-6736(07)60613-8

Street, D., Burge, S., Guadagno, J., & Barrett, A. (2007). The salience of social relationships for resident well-being in assisted living. *The Journals of Gerontology. Series B, Psychological Sciences and Social Sciences*, *62*, 129–134.

Subzwari, S., Desapriya, E., Babul-Wellar, S., Pike, I., Turcotte, K., & Rajabali, F. (2009). *Vision screening of older drivers for preventing road traffic injuries and fatalities*. Chichester, UK: John Wiley & Sons, Ltd.

Sun, H., De Florio, V., & Blondia, C. (2006). A design tool to reason about ambient assisted living systems. In *Proceedings of the International Conference on Intelligent Systems Design and Applications* (ISDA 06), IEEE Computer Society, Jinan, China.

Sung, K. T. (1995). Measures and dimensions of filial piety in Korea. *The Gerontologist*, *35*(2), 240–247.

Sung, K. T. (2001). Family support for the elderly in Korea: continuity, change, future directions, and cross-cultural concerns. *Journal of Aging & Social Policy*, *12*(4), 65–79. doi:10.1300/J031v12n04_04

Sussman, J. M. (2005). *Perspectives on Intelligent Transportation Systems (ITS)*. New York: Springer.

Swindell, R. (in press). Educational initiatives for older learners. *Education Resources Information Center.*

Swindell, R., & Mayhew, C. (1996). Educating the isolated ageing: Improving the quality of life of the housebound elderly through educational teleconferencing. *International Journal of Lifelong Education*, *15*(2), 85–93. doi:10.1080/0260137960150203

Swindell, R., Singer, L., & Singer, G. (1994). Teleconferencing as a medium for providing expert support to the isolated ageing. *Australian Journal on Ageing*, *13*(2), 93–94. doi:10.1111/j.1741-6612.1994.tb00651.x

Swindell, R., & Thompson, J. (1995). An international perspective of the University of the Third Age. *Educational Gerontology*, *21*(5), 429–447. doi:10.1080/0360127950210505

Swindell, R., James, C., & Mann, M. (1992). *A study of teleconferencing as a medium for improving the quality of life of the frail elderly* (ERIC Document Reproduction Service No. ED 346 310.)

Taggart, W., Turale, S., & Kidd, C. D. (2005). An interactive robot in a nursing home: Preliminary remarks. In *Toward Social Mechanisms of Android Science*. Stresa, Italy: Cognitive Science Society.

Takayama, K. (2000). Health industry complex and hospital in USA. *Research and Study Kyoto University Japan*, *19*, 10–19.

Takeda, Y., Kawachi, I., Yamagata, Z., Hashimoto, S., Matsumura, Y., Oguri, S., et al. (2004). Multigenerational family structure in Japanese society: impacts on stress and health behaviors among women and men. *Social Science & Medicine (1982)*, *59*(1), 69-81.

Tang, P., & Venables, T. (2000). Smart Homes and Telecare for independent living. *Journal of Telemedicine and Telecare*, *6*, 8–14. doi:10.1258/1357633001933871

Tang, S., & Liebetruth, C. (2006.). *The TUB OWL-S Matcher*. Retrieved August 24, 2009 from http://owlsm.projects.semwebcentral.org.

Taskforce, A. C. T. G. P. (2009). *Issues and challenges for general practice and primary health care*. A Discussion Paper, Canberra, June 2009.

Taylor, J. B. (2009). *My stroke of insight* (pp. 147–158). UK: Hodder & Stoughton.

Teel, C. S., & Leenerts, M. H. (2005). Developing and testing a self-care intervention for older adults in caregiving roles. *Nursing Research*, *54*(3), 193–201. doi:10.1097/00006199-200505000-00007

The Economist Intelligence Unit. (2009). *Healthcare strategies for an ageing society*.

The Technology Research for Independent Living. (2008). Ageing options: An article about independent living. *Technology Research for Independent Living*. Retrieved from http://www.trilcentre.org/news/ageing options: an article about independent living.397.573.news.html.

The World Health Report. (2006). Retrieved September 10, 2009, from http://www.who.int/whr/2006/en/.

Thompson, L. K., Tonnis, M., & Lange, C. (2006). *Using glance behaviour to evaluate ACC driver controls in a driving simulator*. Paper presented at the Human Factors and Ergonomics Society 50th Annual Meeting.

Thornton, A., Fricke, T., Yang, L. S., & Chang, J. S. (1994). Theoretical Mechanisms of Family Change. In Thornton, A., & Lin, L.-S. (Eds.), *Social Change and the Family in Taiwan* (pp. 88–51). Chicago: University of Chicago Press.

Thornton, A., & Lin, L.-S. (1994). Introduction. In Thornton, A., & Lin, L.-S. (Eds.), *Social Change and the Family in Taiwan* (*Vol. 1-22*). Chicago: University of Chicago Press.

Trewin, S., Zimmermann, G., & Vanderheiden, G. (2004). Abstract representations as a basis for usable user interfaces. *Interacting with Computers*, *16*(3), 477–506. doi:10.1016/j.intcom.2004.04.005

Twigger-Ross, C. L., & Uzzell, D. L. (1996). Place and identity processes. *Journal of Environmental Psychology*, *16*, 205–220. doi:10.1006/jevp.1996.0017

Tyrer, H. W., Alwan, M., Demiris, G., He, Z., Keller, J., Skubic, M., & Rantz, M. (2006). Technology for Successful Aging. In *Proceedings, IEEE 2006 International Conference of the Engineering in Medicine and Biology Society* (pp. 3290-3293). New York.

Tyson, S. F., & Connell, L. A. (2009). How to measure balance in clinical practice. A systematic review of the psychometrics and clinical utility of measures of balance activity for neurological conditions. *Clinical Rehabilitation*, *23*(9), 824–840. doi:10.1177/0269215509335018

U.S. Department of State and Department of Health and Human Services. (2007). *Why population matters: A global perspective*. Washington, DC: Authors.

U.S. Department of State. (2009). South Korea. Retrieved from http://www.state.gov/r/pa/ei/bgn/2800.htm.

Ulfarsson, G., Kim, S., & Lentz, E. (2006). Factors affecting common vehicle-to-vehicle collision types: Road safety priorities in an aging society. *Transportation Research Record: Journal of the Transportation Research Board*, *1980*(1), 70–78. doi:10.3141/1980-12

Ulleberg, P., & Rundmo, T. (2003). Personality, attitudes and risk perception as predictors of risky driving behaviour among young drivers. *Safety Science*, *41*(5), 427–443. doi:10.1016/S0925-7535(01)00077-7

United Nations. (2002). *Population ageing 2002*. Retrieved from www.un.org/esa/population/publications/ageing/Graph.pdf.

United Nations. (2008). World Population Prospects. *United Nations*. Retrieved from http://esa.un.org/unpp/.

United Nations. (2009). *Age-friendly cities*. Retrieved from http://www.who.int/ageing/age_friendly_cities/en/index.html.

Ushering in the second digital revolution, (n.d.). Retrieved February 19, 2009 from http://www.digitaldivide.org/dd/index.html

Utz, R. L., Carr, D. B., Nesse, R., & Wortman, C. B. (2002). The effect of widowhood on older adults' social participation: An evaluation of activity, disengagement, and continuity theories. *The Gerontologist*, *42*(4), 522–533.

Vaa, T., Penttinen, M., & Spyropoulou, I. (2007). Intelligent transport systems and effects on road traffic accidents: State of the art. *IET Intelligent Transport Systems*, *1*(2), 81–88. doi:10.1049/iet-its:20060081

Vaillant, G. E. (2002). *Aging well*. Boston: Little Brown.

Vallerand, R. J., & O'Connor, B. P. (1989). Motivation in the elderly: A theoretical framework and some interesting findings. *Canadian Psychology*, *30*(3). doi:10.1037/h0079828

van Dijk, J. (1999). *The network society: Social aspects of the new media*. Thousand Oaks, CA: Sage Publications.

van Dijk, J. (2005). *The deepening divide: Inequality in the information society*. Thousand Oaks, CA: Sage Publications.

Van Dijk, J. (2005, December). *From digital divide to social opportunities*. Paper presented at the International Conference for Bridging the Digital Divide, Seoul, Korea

Van Mierlo, J., Maggetto, G., & Lataire, P. (2006). Which energy source for road transport in the future? A comparison of battery, hybrid and fuel cell vehicles. *Energy Conversion and Management*, *47*(17), 2748–2760. doi:10.1016/j.enconman.2006.02.004

Van Putten, M. J. A. M., & Tavy, D. L. J. (2004). Continuous quantitative EEG monitoring in hemispheric stroke patients using the brain symmetry index. *Stroke*, *35*, 2489–2492. doi:10.1161/01.STR.0000144649.49861.1d

Vance, D., Dawson, J., Wadley, V., Edwards, J., Roenker, D., & Rizzo, M. (2007). The accelerate study: The longitudinal effect of speed of processing training on cognitive performance of older adults. *Rehabilitation Psychology*, *52*(1), 89–96. doi:10.1037/0090-5550.52.1.89

Vanderheiden, G. (1998). Universal design and assistive technology in communication and information technologies: Alternatives or complements? *Assistive Technology*, *10*(1), 29–36.

Verghese, J., Lipton, R. B., Katz, M. J., Hall, C. B., Derby, C. A., & Kuslansky, G. (2003). Leisure activities and risk of dementia in the elderly. *The New England Journal of Medicine*, *348*, 2508–2516. doi:10.1056/NEJMoa022252

Von Korff, M., Gruman, J., Schaefer, J., Curry, S. J., & Wagner, E. H. (1997). Collaborative Management of Chronic Illness. *Annals of Internal Medicine*, *127*(12), 1097–1102.

Vrkljan, B. H., & Polgar, J. M. (2007). Driving, navigation, and vehicular technology: experiences of older drivers and their co-pilots. *Traffic Injury Prevention*, *8*(4), 403–410. doi:10.1080/15389580701576423

W3C (2007). XForms 1.0 (Third Edition) as W3C Recommendation 29 October 2007. Retrieved February 18, 2009, from http://www.w3.org/TR/2007/REC-xforms-20071029/.

Wadley, V. G., Benz, R. L., Ball, K. K., Roenker, D. L., Edwards, J. D., & Vance, D. E. (2006). Development and evaluation of home-based speed-of-processing training for older adults. *Archives of Physical Medicine and Rehabilitation*, *87*(6), 757–763. doi:10.1016/j.apmr.2006.02.027

Wagner, E., Bennett, S., Austin, B., Greene, S., Schaefer, J., & Vonkorff, M. (2005). Finding common ground: Patient-centeredness and evidence-based chronic illness care. *The Journal of Alternative and Complementary Medicine*, *11*(Supplement 1), S7-0S15.

Walker, L. (2008). Equipment funding schemes — blocking innovation? In *Proceedings ARATA 2008*. Australian Rehabilitation and Assistive Technology Association.

Wallace, B. E., Wagner, A. K., Wagner, E. P., & McDeavitt, J. T. (2001). A history and review of quantitative electroencephalography in traumatic brain injury. *The Journal of Head Trauma Rehabilitation*, *16*(2), 165–190. doi:10.1097/00001199-200104000-00006

Wang, L., Hu, W., & Tan, T. (2003). Recent developments in human motion analysis. *Pattern Recognition*, *36*(3), 585–601. doi:10.1016/S0031-3203(02)00100-0

Wang, C. C., & Carr, D. B. (2004). Older driver safety: A report from the older drivers project. *Journal of the American Geriatrics Society*, *52*(1), 143–149. doi:10.1111/j.1532-5415.2004.52025.x

Wang, S.-Y. (2007). *Nursing home placement in Taiwan an exploration of the experience in adult children*. Unpublished PhD thesis, The University of Queensland, St. Lucia, Queensland, Australia.

Warmerdam, L., van Straten, A., & Cuijpers, P. (2007). Internet-based treatment for adults with depressive symptoms: the protocol of a randomized controlled trial. *BMC Psychiatry*, *7*, 72–78. doi:10.1186/1471-244X-7-72

Weinberger, M., Nagle, B., Hanlon, J. T., Samsa, G. P., Schmader, K., & Landsman, P. B. (1994). Assessing health-related quality of life in elderly outpatients: Telephone versus face-to-face administration. *Journal of the American Geriatrics Society*, *42*(12), 1295–1299.

Weinert, C., Cudney, S., & Hill, W. G. (2008). Rural women, technology, and self-management of chronic illness. *Canadian Journal of Nursing Research*, *40*(3), 114–134.

Weinstein, M., Sun, T. H., Chang, M. C., & Freedom, D. (1994). Co-Residence and Other Tie Linking Couples and Their Parents. In Thornton, A., & Lin, L.-S. (Eds.), *Social Change and the Family in Taiwan* (pp. 305–334). Chicago: University of Chicago Press.

Weiser, M. (1991). The computer for the twenty-first century. *Scientific American*, (September): 94–100. doi:10.1038/scientificamerican0991-94

Wessels, R., Dijcks, B., Soede, M., Gelderblom, G. J., & De Witte, L. (2003)... *Technology and Disability*, *15*(4), 231–238.

Wessels, R. D. (2003). Non-use of provided assistive technology devices: A literature overview. *Technology and Disability*, (15): 231–238.

Whaley, K. C. (2004). America's digital divide: 2000-2003 trends. *Journal of Medical Systems*, *28*(2), 183–195. doi:10.1023/B:JOMS.0000023301.09308.d9

What is our special technology? (n.d.). Retrieved February 2, 2009 from http://www.jaipurfoot.org/03_Technology_ourspecialtech.asp

Wherton, J. P., & Monk, A. F. (2008). Technological opportunities for supporting people with dementia who are living at home. *International Journal of Human-Computer Studies*, *66*(8), 571–586. doi:10.1016/j.ijhcs.2008.03.001

Wherton, J., & Prendergast, D. (2009). Involving Older Adults in the Design of a Communication Technology to Support Peer-to-Peer Social Engagement. In *HCI and Usability for e-Inclusion* (pp. 111–134). The Building Bridges Project. doi:10.1007/978-3-642-10308-7_8

Wherton, J. P., & Monk, A. F. (2008). Technological opportunities for supporting people with dementia who are living at home. *International Journal of Human-Computer Studies*, *66*(8), 571–586. doi:10.1016/j.ijhcs.2008.03.001

Whetton, S. (2005). *Health informatics: a socio-technical perspective*. South Melbourne: Oxford University Press.

White, H., McConnell, E., Clipp, E., Branch, L. G., Sloane, R., Pieper, C., & Box, T. L. (2002). A randomized controlled trial of the psychosocial impact of providing internet training and access to older adults. *Aging & Mental Health*, *6*(3), 213–221. doi:10.1080/13607860220142422

White, H., McConnell, E., Clipp, E., Louise, B., Teague, C., & Navas, L. (1999). Surfing the net in later life: A review of the literature and a pilot study of computer use and quality of life. *Journal of Applied Gerontology*, *18*(3), 358–378. doi:10.1177/073346489901800306

WHO (2002). *Innovative care for chronic conditions: Building blocks for action* (No. WHO/MNC/CCH/02.01 - NLM classification: WT 31).

Wielandt, T. A. (2000). Compliance with prescribed adaptive equipment: A literature review. *British Journal of Occupational Therapy*, *63*(2), 65–75.

Wiener, J. M., & Tilly, J. (2002). Population ageing in the United States of America: Implications for public programmes. *International Journal of Epidemiology*, *31*, 776–781. doi:10.1093/ije/31.4.776

Williams, J., Ramaswamy, D., & Oulhaji, A. (2006). 10Hz flicker improves recognition memory in older people. *BMC Neuroscience, 7*(21), 1471-2202/7/21.

Williamson, K., & Asla, T. (2009). Information behaviour of people in the fouth age: Implications for the conceptualisation of information literacy. *Library & Information Science Research*, *31*, 76–83. doi:10.1016/j.lisr.2009.01.002

Wilson, J. (1999). Acknowledging the expertise of patients and their organisations. *BMJ (Clinical Research Ed.)*, *319*(7212), 771–774.

Wilson, T. (2000). Human Information Behaviors. *Informing Science, Special Issue on Information Science Research, 3*(2).

Windsor, T. D., & Anstey, K. J. (2006). Interventions to reduce the adverse psychosocial impact of driving cessation in older adults. *Clinical Interventions in Aging*, *1*(3), 205–211. doi:10.2147/ciia.2006.1.3.205

Witkowski, J. M., & Buick, T. R. (1985). Travel behavior of residents of retirement communities. *Transportation Research Record*, *1018*, 13–22.

Witte, R. (1998). Shrinkage, neuron and synapse loss: aging takes its toll on the brain. *Geriatrics & Aging*, *1*(1), 14–15.

Wood, J. M., Anstey, K. J., Kerr, G. K., Lacherez, P. F., & Lord, S. (2008). A multidomain approach for predicting older driver safety under in-traffic road conditions. *Journal of the American Geriatrics Society*, *56*(6), 986–993. doi:10.1111/j.1532-5415.2008.01709.x

Wood, J. M., & Owens, A. D. (2005). Standard measures of visual acuity do not predict drivers' recognition performance under day or night conditions. *Optometry and Vision Science*, *82*(8), 698–705. doi:10.1097/01.opx.0000175562.27101.51

Woolham, J. (2006). *Safety at Home. The effectiveness of assistive technology in supporting the independence of people with dementia.* London: Hawker Publication.

Wootton, R., Kvedar, J., & Dimmick, S. L. (2006). *Home telehealth: Connecting care within community*. London: Royal Society of Medicine Press.

World Health Organization (WHO). (2002). Active ageing: A policy framework. Retrieved from http://whqlibdoc.who.int/hq/2002/WHO_NMH_NPH_02.8.pdf.

World Health Organization. (2008). *WHO global report on falls prevention in older age*. Geneva.

Wright, K. (2000). Computer-mediated social support, older adults, and coping. *The Journal of Communication*, *50*, 100–118. doi:10.1111/j.1460-2466.2000.tb02855.x

Wrosch, C., & Schulz, R. (2008). Health-engagement control strategies and 2-year changes in older adults' physical health. *Psychological Science*, *19*(6), 537–541. doi:10.1111/j.1467-9280.2008.02120.x

WS-HumanTask. (2007). *Specification: Web Services for Human Task (WS-HumanTask), version 1.0.* Retrieved August 24, 2009 from https://www.sdn.sap.com/irj/sdn/go/portal/prtroot/docs/library/uuid/a0c9ce4c-ee02-2a10-4b96-cb205464aa02

Xie, X., Xia, Y., & Liu, X. (2007). Family income and attitudes toward older people in China: comparison of two age cohorts. *Journal of Family and Economic Issues*, *28*(1), 171–182. doi:10.1007/s10834-006-9044-5

Yagil, D. (1998). Instrumental and normative motives for compliance with traffic laws among young and older drivers. *Accident; Analysis and Prevention*, *40*(4), 417–424.

Yamada, K., & Kuchar, J. K. (2006). Preliminary study of behavioural and safety effects of driver dependence on a warning system in a driving simulator. *IEEE Transactions on Systems, Man, and Cybernetics. Part A, Systems and Humans*, *36*(3), 602–610. doi:10.1109/TSMCA.2006.871646

Yamaguchi, A., Ogawa, M., Tamura, T., & Togata, T. (1998). Monitoring behavior in the home using positioning sensors. In *Proceedings of the 20th annual IEEE Conference on Engineering in Medicine and Biology*.

Yang, J. W. (1996). *Tai chi theory and martial power* (pp. 27–32). Boston: YMAA Publications.

Yunfa, L., Kanichi, M., Lixin, W., & Komei, I. (2003). Physiological benefits of 24-style taijiquan exercise in middle-aged women. *Journal of Physiological Anthropology and Applied Human Science*, *22*, 219–225. doi:10.2114/jpa.22.219

Zarit, S. H., Stephens, M. A., Townsend, A., & Greene, R. (1998). Stress reduction for family caregivers: effects of adult day care use. *The Journals of Gerontology. Series B, Psychological Sciences and Social Sciences*, *53*(5), S267–S277.

Zedlewski, S., & Butrica, B. (2007). Are we taking full advantage of older adults' potential? Perspectives on productive aging, *The Urban Institute. Number 9, December.* Retrieved September 19, 2009, from http://www.urban.org/UploadedPDF/411581_adult_potential.pdf

Zhang, D., & Nunamaker, J. (2004). Powering e-learning in the new millennium: An overview of e-learning and enabling technology. *Information Systems Frontiers*, *5*(2), 207–218. doi:10.1023/A:1022609809036

Zijlstra, G. A. R., van Haastregt, J. C. M., van Eijk, J. T. M., van Rossum, E., Stalenhoef, P. A., & Kempen, G. I. J. M. (2007). Prevalence and correlates of fear of falling, and associated avoidance of activity in the general population of community-living older people. *Age and Ageing*, *36*(3), 304–309. doi:10.1093/ageing/afm021

Zijlstra, W., & Aminian, K. (2007). Mobility assessment in older people: new possibilities and challenges. *European Journal of Ageing*, *4*, 3–12. doi:10.1007/s10433-007-0041-9

Zimmerman, S., Gruber-Baldini, A., Sloane, P. D., Eckert, J. K., Hebel, J. R., & Morgan, L. A. (2003). Assisted living and nursing homes: Apples and oranges? *The Gerontologist*, *43*, 107–117.

Zimmermann, G. (2007, September). *Open user interface standards - towards coherent, task-oriented and scalable user interfaces in the home environments*. Paper published at the Proceedings of 3rd IET International Conference on Intelligent Environments (IE07), Ulm University, Germany.

Zimmermann, G., & Vanderheiden, G. (2007). The universal control hub: an open platform for remote user interfaces in the digital home. In *Human-Computer Interaction. Interaction Platforms and Techniques* (L NCS 4551, pp. 1040-1049). Berlin/Heidelberg: Springer.

Zurawski, R. (Ed.). (2006). *Embedded systems handbook*. Boca Raton: Taylor & Francis.

About the Contributors

Jeffrey Soar is a researcher in ehealth and specifically in informatics for ageing and independent living. He is holds the Chair in Intelligent Domestic Healthcare Infrastructure, a joint initiative of the University of Queensland and the University of Southern Queensland. He is the Founding Director of the Collaboration for Ageing & Aged-care Informatics Research (CAAIR); Convener of the Queensland Smart Home Initiative (QSHI) and founder of Aged Care Informatics Australia, a Special Interest Group of the Health Informatics Society of Australia. Dr Soar came into academia from a senior executive-level career in health and community service government departments in Australia and New Zealand. This included national and state-wide strategy development, large-scale facilities management, consulting, research and education. In academia Dr Soar built lasting research consortia involving care provider organisations, government, consumers and technology companies. He has published over 100 research papers in peer-reviewed journals and conference proceedings, attracted national and international competitive research funding and commissions for research by national and overseas governments. He has been a key-note presenter at leading international conferences, has taught ICT management and Health Informatics courses at four Australian universities and has been an invited guest lecturer at overseas universities. Dr Soar has been engaged to advise governments on information strategy particularly by international agencies for developing countries.

Richard Swindell received his PhD in inorganic chemistry from the University of Idaho. In 2005 he retired from the paid workforce and continues his research and development activities through Griffith University in Brisbane. In 1998 he was a cofounder of the first virtual U3A, U3AOnline, and subsequently its president for five years. He has played a leading role in many organisations for the ageing including Australian Council on the Ageing. In 2008 he was appointed to the Queensland Seniors Council. He has been on the management team of the Queensland Smart Home Initiative from its earliest days. Throughout his university life he won several awards for innovative teaching including an Australian Award for University Teaching. In 2004 he was awarded an Order of Australia for services to education.

Philip Tsang was a senior academic member of staff at the Open University of Hong Kong (OUHK). He was conferred the OUHK President's Award for Excellent Teaching and Research in 2006, 2007 and in 2009. He is a senior member of the Institute of Electrical and Electronics Engineers, IEEE. Prof. Tsang has published widely in SCI journals. He is author of eight ICT and education books. He was a graduate of Washington University, USA. Dr Tsang has been the conference chair of the Int'l ICT conference series: Enhancing Healthcare Education, Research and Practice since 2006. He is editor of five international journals in the areas of Teaching & Learning, Mobile Communications, Education, Finance and

Health. Dr Tsang is an advisor of the Hong Kong Doctors' Union. Dr Tsang is Chair Professor and Vice President (Academic and Research) of the Caritas Francis Hsu College, and Caritas College of Careers. One of his current projects is to amalgamate Caritas' 4-year and 2-year colleges to lay the foundation for the first Catholic University in Hong Kong, SAR, China. Philip would like to give special thanks to his wife Dr Sandy Tse for her support during the project activities in the past 12 months. This project has also benefited from the research grants (27/QEGS/A-08-09) from the Quality Enhancement Grant Scheme of the Education Bureau; (6/21)(R189-2)(ST-08/09-2) from The Open University of Hong Kong; and (HK-R1209) from Johnson & Johnson. For these, Philip wants to thank the Education Bureau, Caritas-HK, and Diabetes Team of the United Christian Hospital, The Open University of Hong Kong, and Johnson & Johnson research committees.

* * *

Jan Alexandersson is a senior researcher at the Intelligent User Interfaces lab at the German Research Institute of Artificial Intelligence, DFKI GmbH. He received his Master of Science from the University of Linköping in 1993 and has published over 50 peer-reviewed papers, book chapters etc. He has been a member of the scientific advisory board of the ACL Special Interest Group of Dialogue - SIGDial. He has been working since 1993 at DFKI on topics like spoken language translation, multimodal human-computer interaction and recently, assistive and accessible technology for the elderly and persons with disabilities. He defended his PhD in 2003 at the University of the Saarland. Recently, he became head of the DFKI Competence Center for Ambient Assisted Living and is the coordinator of the i2home project.

Elena Avatangelou is a senior project manager at the Research Department of Exodus S.A., one of the leading IT companies in Greece. She has obtained a Bachelor degree in Informatics and an MBA from the Athens University of Economics and Business. She has been working at EXODUS since 2002. She has long experience in the technical and administrative coordination of research projects, and in designing, developing and evaluating software solutions. She has worked in research projects of various sectors including information portals (for tourism, employment, digital publishing), educational systems (e-learning), web-conferencing applications, and lately ambient assisted living systems focusing on older people.

Subhasis Banerji is a Research Associate at the Robotics Research Centre, School of Mechanical and Aerospace Engineering, Nanyang Technological University, Singapore. After graduating in Production Engineering in 1987, he worked in industry for 18 years, specializing in the design of machinery and robotics/mechatronics application in the pharma and aerated beverages industries. In the past several years, he has devoted his energies and time studying the natural functional recovery in human beings after trauma, which led to his completing his MSc in Biomedical Engineering in Singapore. His current research interests include brain plasticity, study of bio-signals, and the application of robotics, mechatronics, yoga and martial art to accelerated learning and functional recovery in the aged and elderly disabled. He is pursuing his PhD in this field of study. His practice of yoga and martial art spans 30 years.

James Barrientos is the Chief Executive Officer of LifeTec Queensland, a statewide professional advisory organisation that provides people with assistive technology solutions. James has a combined background in the management and organisational development of several health service organisations, as well as being a health professional. He has held senior positions which have seen him establish and diversify a number of companies and organisations ranging from prosthetics and orthotics to health retail. James has also worked as a medical prosthetist-orthotist within the public and private sector in Queensland. He is also an active director of private companies in the corporate communications and investment sectors. James has tertiary qualifications in Prosthetics and Orthotics as well as Management. He lives with his wife and two young sons in Brisbane, Australia.

Michele Barry is the former CEO of LifeTec Queensland, an organisation that promotes assistive technology for people with health conditions or disabilities. Previous to this Michele has held various senior roles in the sector including that of Service Director at Vision Australia, the Victorian Office of the Public Advocate and various roles in the health and aged care services within local government. Michele has a Master of Public Health from LaTrobe University, a Post Graduate Diploma in Health Promotion from Curtin University of Technology and Bachelor of Applied Science from RMIT. She has written and presented numerous articles and papers in Australia and internationally including the Association for Advancement of Assistive Technology Europe (AAATE) Conference in 2007. Michele is currently the Business Operations Manager for the Centre for Palliative Care; part of St Vincent's health as well as a Collaborative Centre of the University of Melbourne.

Neil Bergmann is Professor of Embedded Systems in the School of ITEE, the University of Queensland. He is relatively new to the research domain of health informatics, although he has substantial research expertise in computer systems, where he has worked for more than 25 years. During his PhD at University of Edinburgh, UK (1984) he worked in the area of integrated circuit CAD tools, including a specialist silicon compiler for signal processing algorithms. Prof. Bergmann's current research projects are based around the most efficient uses of various types of computing system, especially embedded computer systems. Topics of interest wireless sensor networks, smart house technology, computer-based diagnostics, industrial automation, and networked computing systems.

Ilse Bierhoff is a research project manager at Smart Homes. She studied at the technical university of Eindhoven at the faculty Technical Innovation Science, department Human Computer Interaction. In 2002 she joined Smart Homes and her main activities are in the field of the use of smart home technology in the care and cure sector. Her research activities can be divided into three main areas. The first area is the implementation of the user centred design approach with a focus on the gathering of user requirements with innovative methods that allow an equal and creative interaction between user and experts. The second area is on a more practical level and focuses on giving guidance to the process of actually installing smart home technology and the evaluation of those projects with all the stakeholders. The third area focuses on the development of educational material on ambient assisted living for multidisciplinary teams of students.

Chris Blondia obtained his Master in Science and PhD in Mathematics, both from the University of Ghent (Belgium) in 1977 and 1982 respectively. In 1983 he joined Philips Belgium, where he was a researcher in the Philips Research Laboratory Belgium (PRLB). From 1991-1994 he was an Associate Professor in the Computer Science Department of the University of Nijmegen (The Netherlands). In 1995 he joined the Department of Mathematics and Computer Science of the University of Antwerp (UA), where he is currently a Full Professor and head of the research group "Performance Analysis of

Telecommunication Systems" (PATS - www.pats.ua.ac.be). The group is a member of the Flemish Interdisciplinary institute for Broad Band Technology (IBBT) (www.ibbt.be). His main research interests are related to performance evaluation of communication systems. He is editor of the Journal of Network and Computer Applications and of the International Journal of Electronics and Communications. He is co-founder of the spin-off company Wishbone (www.wishbone.be).

Kathryn L. Braun is Professor of Public Health and Social Work and chair of the Doctor of Public Health (DrPH) program at the University of Hawaii, from which she holds a Board of Regent's Medal for Excellence in Teaching. She also is Research Director of Imi Hale—Native Hawaiian Cancer Network and Co-Director of Ha Kupuna—National Resource Center for Native Hawaiian Elders, both in Honolulu, Hawaii. Dr. Braun is known for her work in community-based participatory research in cancer and gerontology, and she has published more than 120 peer-reviewed journal articles on these topics. In 2008, she completed a Fulbright at Kosin University in Busan. She is a fellow in the Gerontological Society of America and the Association for Gerontology in Higher Education, and she is the 2009-2011 President of the Active Ageing Consortium Asia Pacific (ACAP).

Cristina Buiza holds a Bachelor's degree in Psychology from Universidad Complutense de Madrid. Holds a Master's degree in Clinical Gerontology from Universidad del País Vasco and in Neuropsychology from the Universidad Autonoma de Barcelona and is finishing her doctoral dissertation on Severe Cognitive Impairment. She is currently Senior Researcher at Ingema and also takes part in the Matia Foundation Memory and Alzheimer Unit. She has participated in several research multi-partner projects within the local, national and European levels. As a member of the Spanish Society of Gerontology and Geriatrics, and of the International Neuropsychological Society, has presented numerous papers to different international conferences in the field of attention to elderly people, and the interaction of the elderly with the technology. She has received a number of awards from national public and private institutions.

Paula Byrne is a lecturer within the Medical School at the University of Liverpool in the UK with a background in psychology and sociology. Her research interests are within Science and Technology Studies and include: the making of a diagnosis between medical clinicians and patients; the use of technology in a number of arenas; and sickness absence. She is involved in a number of research projects and is associate editor of Medical Sociology Online.

Eduardo Carrasco is a graduate of the San Sebastián Higher School of Industrial Engineers where he read Electronic and Control Systems Engineering. From 1998 until 2000 Eduardo held the position of Assistant Researcher at Centro de Estudios e Investigaciones Técnicas de Gipuzkoa (CEIT). During the same period Eduardo was an Assistant Lecturer at the San Sebastian Higher School of Industrial Engineers. In 2001, he held the position of Visitor Researcher at the Fraunhofer Institüt fur Graphische Datenverarbeitung (Fraunhofer IGD). From 2003 onwards Eduardo has been a Staff Researcher at VICOMTech participating in several national and European projects on Human Computer Interaction and e-Accessibility. He is the author of several scientific publications for relevant international events.

Samuel N. Cubero was born in the Philippines and has lived in Australia since 1974. He graduated with Honours after completing a Bachelors degree in Mechanical Engineering at The University of Queensland in 1993. During 1994-1998, Sam Cubero completed a PhD in Mechatronic Engineering at the University of Southern Queensland. Since 1998, he has researched and lectured at Curtin University and USQ in the areas of mobile robots, UAVs, robotics, automation, machine vision and object recognition, sensor design, 3D scanning, 3D simulation programming, CAD/CAM design, mechanical design, stress analysis and manufacturing. Some videos of his past projects are at: www.samcubero.com

Vincenzo De Florio was researcher for six years in Tecnopolis/SASIAM (School for Advanced Studies in Industrial and Applied Mathematics), Italy, where he served as a researcher, lecturer, and tutor. He then was researcher for eight years with the Catholic University of Leuven (Belgium). He is currently a post-doctoral researcher with the Performance Analysis of Telecommunication Systems (PATS) research group at the University of Antwerp, where he is responsible for PATS' branch on adaptive and dependable software systems. Vincenzo has published 84 reviewed research papers, 20 of which appeared in international research journals, and the book "Application-layer Software Fault-Tolerance", published by IGI-Global. He is founding editor and editor-in-chief of the International Journal of Adaptive, Resilient and Autonomic Systems (IJARAS), also published by IGI-Global. He is a member of various conference program committees. He was co-chair of workshop ADAMUS-09 (the third Workshop on Adaptive and DependAble Mobile Ubiquitous Systems, http://www.adamus.ua.ac.be).

Sarah Delaney is a Senior Research Consultant at the Work Research Centre with extensive experience in health and social services research. She holds a BA in Social Anthropology and MSc in Applied Social Research and is currently studying for a PhD in Health Services Research. Key areas of interest include health services for older people and family carers, health informatics and gerontechnology, and service delivery models for health and social care.

Unai Díaz has a PhD in Psychology from the Deusto University in 2006, (Bilbao, Spain). He worked as a clinical psychologist in different healthcare settings: 1 year at the Crownsville Hospital Center, Crownsville, Maryland, USA (2000-2001) and 6 months at the Bermeo Hospital, belonging to the Basque Country Public Health System –Osakidetza (2001-2002). Between 2003 and 2005 he worked as a psychologist at the La Loma residence for elderly people (Castro Urdiales, Spain), implementing a group-based cognitive stimulation program specifically developed for residentialized elderly people, which led to his dissertation "Effects of Psychological Intervention in Cognitive Decline of Residentialized Elderly People" (Ann Arbor, MI, UMI Dissertation Publishing). In 2007, he developed memory intervention groups at diverse elderly associations under the financial support of IPACE S.L. (Vitoria, Spain). Currently, he works at the R&D department of the Matia Gerontological Institute (INGEMA) as a researcher in topics related to ageing and disability.

Sisira Edirippulige is the coordinator of undergraduate and graduate courses in e-Healthcare at The University of Queensland Centre for Online Health, Brisbane, Australia. He is also responsible for coordinating continuing professional development courses in telehealth at the Centre. His research interests include the development, promotion and integration of telehealth education and telemedicine applications into the healthcare sector. Before joining The University of Queensland he held teaching positions at Kobe Gakuin University in Japan and at the University of Auckland in New Zealand. He has extensive experience in development studies and education; and he has worked in a number of countries including Russia, Sri Lanka, South Africa, Japan and New Zealand.

Maria Vittoria Giuliani is currently associated researcher at the Institute of Cognitive Sciences and Technologies (ISTC) of the Italian National Research Council (CNR) in Roma. She has been involved in environmental psychology for the last twenty years and is responsible of many research projects. She is affiliated lecturer and member of the doctoral programme in environmental psychology at the University of Rome "La Sapienza". Two main lines of research characterised her work, the first concerning users' residential needs and satisfaction across the lifespan; the second focusing on the concept of attachment to place and psychological consequences of displacement. Recently, this perspective has been widened to assistive technology for the elderly, in accordance with the aging in place concept. She published chapters and articles in international journals, organised international workshops on housing, and has been member of the scientific committee of many international conferences.

Peter Grimbeek is a specialist research methodologist who has worked at Griffith University, Queensland University of Technology, University of New England, University of Tasmania, and EIDOS. His research interests include perception and imagery, language and culture, and the interpretation of human response data.

Ning Gui received his BS degree in information engineering from Central South University (China) in 1999, and his Master's in Computer Science from the same University in 2002. From 2002 to 2006, he worked as lecturer in the Central South University. He is currently a PhD candidate of University of Antwerp, PATS Research Group and a research assistant for the IBBT (Institute of Broad Band Technology). His research interests include adaptive software architecture, service component models especially on embedded systems. Ning Gui has published more than 20 reviewed research papers. He also serves as program committee member for several international conferences and reviewer for several journals.

Donghee Han is Director of Busan Health Family Support Center and President of the Research Institute of Science for the Better Living of the Elderly (RISBLE) in Busan, Korea. She oversees the delivery of a variety of programs to empower older adults and strengthen family. She has won Korean government awards for RISBLE programs, including prizes for "Information and Culture in Cyberspaces for Older Persons" and "Re-design for Dementia Patients and their Families." She also is an invited professor at Kosin University, where she teaches courses on Active Ageing. She serves on the National Unification Advisory Council in Korea and is founder of the Korean Information Network for the Prevention of Elder Abuse (KINPEA). She represents Korea in the International Network for the Prevention of Elder Abuse (INPEA) and the Active Ageing Consortium Asia Pacific (ACAP).

Chris Hatherly is currently studying for a PhD in cognitive psychology at the Australian National University, in Canberra, Australia. His research focuses on the development and evaluation of computerised screening measures for older drivers, and the development of cognitive training interventions for this population targeting visual processing speed. He holds a Bachelor of Science (Psychology) with honours from the Australian National University.

Jan Heffernan teaches in tertiary preparation and first year business programs at Queensland University of Technology. Her research interests include the first year experience, academic and professional literacies, and communication technologies in education.

John Heng is a Teaching Fellow at Nanyang Technological University, School of Mechanical and Aerospace Engineering, Division of Mechatronics and Design, Singapore. He obtained his PhD in Design, Manufacture and Engineering Management from Strathclyde University, Glasgow, UK in September, 1995. He is a member of the Institution of Mechanical Engineers (IMechE), Institution of Engineering and Technology (IET) and is a Chartered Engineer registered with the UK Engineering Council since 1996. His current research interests are in rehabilitation engineering and assistive technologies. In particular, he is working with active accelerated rehabilitation in stroke patients, extending to multi-level haptic interface devices for enhanced man-machine interaction. His teaching responsibilities currently include subjects on mechanical and mechatronics system design and analysis.

Claire Huijnen is project manager at Smart Homes (Dutch expertise centre for smart homes and smart living). She has a MSc in Cognitive Psychology (Human factors, Cognitive Ergonomics at the University of Maastricht) and a second Masters in user system interaction at the Technical University of Eindhoven. Her main driver is to optimally fit technology to the capabilities and needs of the end user. At the moment she is working on projects related to Ambient Intelligence, on Ambient Assisted Living in particular. This is done in the context of several European projects. Her main contribution and expertise is on aspects such as user requirements, conceptualization, HCI/RI matters, user centered design, user experience and evaluation. A number of the projects strive to enable people to live longer independently in their own homes. This will be done by means of supporting (smart/intelligent) technologies applications/services in their smart homes.

Yusuke Inoue was born in Nagoya, Japan. He graduated with a Bachelor's of Social Welfare from Kansai Fukushi Kagaku University in Japan; and an M.A. Social Welfare Management (Marketing) degree in Nihon Fukushi University. He is currently a Social Worker and a PhD candidate in Social Welfare Administration at Nihon Fukushi University. His major is Social Welfare Administration and Accounting. Yusuke Inoue is a member of the Japanese Society for the Study of Social Welfare.

Seungwon Jeong graduated with a Bachelor of Sociology from Yeoungnam University in Korea and subsequently worked for a hospital as a member of an establishment committee for 3 years. In 2005, she returned to university and obtained a M.A. Health Care Administration degree from Yonsei University in Korea. Later, in Japan, she learned about healthcare and social services for the elderly, especially about policy, economics and administration for long-term care services. Seungwon received a PhD in Nihon Fukushi University Japan in 2008 and is currently a researcher in the Center for Well-being and Society, Nihon Fukushi University Japan. Seungwon Jeong is a member of the Japan Society for Health care Administration, the Japanese Society for the Study of Social Welfare, and the Japanese Society of Public Health.

Rose Anne Kenny is Head of the academic Department of Medical Gerontology at Trinity College Dublin and Director of the Centre for Successful Ageing at St. James's Hospital. Her research interests are in neurocardiovascular function in ageing and involves collaborative partnership with disciplines from basic science through to health service development and implementation. She has conducted longitudinal cohort studies of vascular factors in cognitive impairment and stroke and is now lead Principal Investigor for the Irish Longitudinal Study of Ageing (TILDA). Other major research programs include assistive technologies in ageing (Technology Research for Independent Living - TRIL) in collaboration with INTEL and IDA; Health Research Board translational program of cardiovascular risk factors for conversion of cognitive impairment to dementia and new treatment strategies for dementia sub types. Professor Kenny has published in excess of 200 papers, 40 book chapters and 3 text books. She has represented her field on international groups for heart failure, syncope and falls.

Michael Klein studied computer science at the University of Karlsruhe and received his PhD in 2006. His main research interests are semantic descriptions of e-services, context-awareness and the interoperability of systems, which he has applied both to business applications and to ambient assisted living applications. Since joining CAS Software AG in 2006, he has been involved in European research projects in this area and has authored and co-authored national and international publications.

Martin Klima is a researcher and a lecturer at the CTU in Prague, Department of Computer Graphics and Interaction. He received his PhD in 2009 at the same university. His research interests include mobile user interaction, data adaptation for mobile environment, computer supported collaborative work in mobile environment, and user interfaces for users with special needs like elderly or people with disabilities. Between 2001 and 2002 he was working on adaptation of multimedia documents on PDA at ZGDV Darmstadt, Germany (analysis, design, prototype implementation). After his return to Prague he became involved in number of EU funded projects including Mummy, ELU, i2home, Vital, Vital Mind, Aegis and others. He is an author or a co-author of more than twenty publications on various international events in HCI.

Felicitas Lull holds a Master degree in Geography and Urban Development from the University of Bonn (2004). Until 2005 she was involved within several adult education training initatives in the field of development cooperation. As research consultant for empirica (2006 to 2009) her special subjects were the European Information Society, its regional development and policies, eInclusion and eAccessbility. Within the SOPRANO project she started working in the field of AAL and independent living.

Rohana B. Marasinghe is a Senior Lecturer at the Department of Medical Education and Health Sciences, Faculty of Medical Sciences, University of Sri Jayewardenepura (USJP) Sri Lanka. He has obtained his M.B.B.S. (Colombo) and MPhil degrees in Medical Education from USJP. Rohana Marasinghe is currently undertaking his PhD research at the Centre for Online Health, University of Queensland, Australia. His PhD study investigates telemedicine applications for developing countries (distantly delivered psychological training using web/mobile networks to address suicidal behaviour in Sri Lanka). He is also interested in Medical Education as well as ICT/Innovative technology use in education and teaching.

José Luis Jorge Marrasé has worked in areas of design, project management, and engineering department management; and is currently Director of the Alcatel-Lucent Multimedia Competence Centre in Barcelona. He has an Electrical Engineering degree with a post grade MBA and more than 20 years of experience in the Telecommunications Industry. He is managing a competence centre that develops multimedia applications for different sectors such as health and social care, TV, advertising, with responsibilities in Project Implementation, Product Development and R and D activities. Nowadays one of the main areas of activity is innovation management. Since 1988 has been working in applications for Telecommunications Networks starting with IN systems.

Michael McGrath is senior technologist in Intel's Digital Health Group. He is also a principal investigator in the TRIL Centre focusing on the development technologies to support independent living research. His areas of interest include sensors, wireless communications, assisted living technologies, intelligent user interfaces, data fusion and data management techniques. Michael co-authored the 2009 book Wireless Sensor Networks for Healthcare Applications. Michael received his B.Sc. in Analytical Science from Dublin City University in 1992, a PhD in sensors and instrumentation from Dublin City University in 1995. In 1999 Michael received a graduate diploma in Information Technology from Dublin City University and a Graduate Diploma in Computing from ITB in 2004. Michael received his Master's Degree in Computing for ITB in 2007. Michael is a Charted Chemist (CChem) and a Charted Scientist (CSi).

Sonja Müller is research consultant at empirica. She holds a degree in geography, urban development, and economic sociology from Bonn University. Main fields of her research activity are ICT applications and their usage patterns amongst older people and people with special needs and the way ICTs impact on societal participation and inclusion of disadvantaged population groups. Since joining empirica in 2005 she has been involved in a number of projects focusing on the development and evaluation of technical systems in the area of Independent Living/Ambient Assisted Living and policy analysis in the area of eInclusion. Sonja Müller has authored and co-authored national and international publications.

Rhonda Nay is Foundation Professor of Interdisciplinary Aged Care and Director of the Institute for Social Participation (ISP); TIME –the Victorian and Tasmanian Dementia Training Studies Centre; the Australian Centre for Evidence Based Aged Care (ACEBAC) and the Australian Institute for Primary Care (AIPC) at La Trobe University. She also leads the Victorian hub of the Dementia Collaborative Research Centre. Rhonda has chaired the Minister's Awards for Excellence in Aged Care and has been a judge for the Aged and Community Services Awards. Her research is focused on getting evidence based, interdisciplinary, person-centred care into practice. Rhonda is a Director of the Aged Care Standards and Accreditation Agency Ltd.

Lemai Nguyen is a Senior Lecturer at Deakin University. Her research interests include health informatics, creative problem solving and requirements engineering, and socio-technical issues in Information Systems. In health informatics, her research focuses on analysing and supporting information needs and information behaviours of patients, their family carers, and healthcare professionals as well as developing innovative technology-enabled solutions for chronic illness care and aged care. Lemai's research has been widely published in international scholarly journals, book chapters and at high quality international conferences. She is a member of the Steering Committee of Australian Workshop on Requirements Engineering (AWRE) and a member of Health Informatics Society of Australia, Special Interest Group in Aged Care Informatics. Lemai is also Program Chair to AWRE for many years and Member of Editorial Board of various international journals.

Nancy A. Pachana is a clinical psychologist and neuropsychologist and Associate Professor in the School of Psychology at The University of Queensland, Brisbane, Australia. Dr Pachana is the national chair of the Australian Psychological Society's Psychology and Ageing Interest Group. She is on the Board of Directors of the International Psychogeriatric Association, and is the editor of the Australian Psychologist, the flagship applied journal of the Australian Psychological Society. She was recently awarded the Clinical College of the Australian Psychological Society's inaugural Alastair Heron Prize for Research in Dementia.

Alexander Pfalzgraf holds a bachelor's degree in computer science from the University of Lübeck and a master's degree in computer science from Saarland University. In 2006 he joined the German Research Center for Artificial Intelligence (DFKI GmbH) in Saarbrücken where he worked as a researcher in the fields of multimodal dialog and semantic technologies for notable national and international research and industry projects. In 2008, Alexander Pfalzgraf was a co-founder of SemVox GmbH which develops and markets commercial-grade and feature-rich multimodal dialog systems for mobile and in-home solutions. Since then he has been a managing director and head of development of this company.

Emma Poulsen holds a bachelor degree in Leisure Management, a bachelor degree in Science majoring in psychology and a bachelor degree in Arts (Psychology) with 1st class Honours from The University of Queensland (UQ). Ms Poulsen is currently completing her Doctorate of Clinical Psychology and working with the Ageing Mind Initiative at UQ. Her speciality areas of study include Health Psychology and Geropsychology and her main research interests are positive ageing and mindfulness.

Cliodhna Ni Scanaill is a Health Research Technologist in the Intel Health Research and Innovation team in Leixlip, Ireland. She is also a co-principal investigator on the Falls Prevention Strand in the TRIL Centre. Her current research interests include falls, gait analysis, wireless sensor networks, telemonitoring, and smart home technology. Prior to joining Intel in 2006, she studied for her PhD on "Remote Mobility Monitoring of the Elderly using SMS messaging" in the Biomedical Electronics Laboratory, University of Limerick, Ireland. Dr. Ni Scanaill holds a B.Eng in Computer Engineering and a PhD in Biomedical Electronics from the University of Limerick.

Robert Savage is an M.A. candidate in the Department of Gerontology at Simon Fraser University in Vancouver British Columbia Canada. His research interests are within the realm of gerontechnology, and the research he is completing as part of his M.A. degree concerns itself with the potential impact ambient assisted living systems may have upon the meaning of home in systems users. He is additionally involved with education and knowledge transfer activities for seniors across Canada as CEO of the consulting firm Campo, Savage, & Associates.

Massimiliano Scopelliti is a researcher in Social and Environmental Psychology at the Libera Università Maria Ss. Assunta (LUMSA) in Rome, Italy. He is author or co-author of many scientific manuscripts including articles, book chapters and conference proceedings. His main research interests concern the evaluation of the restorative potential of natural and built environments; the evaluation of urban quality, place attachment and residential satisfaction; the use/acceptability of new technologies by elderly people in the domestic environment; the assessment of environmental humanization and legibility in the hospital environment; the perception of environmental quality and satisfaction in the workplace.

Andrew Sixsmith is professor and Director of the Gerontology Research Centre at Simon Fraser University in Canada. Andrew's research examines the quality of life of older people and particularly how information and communication technologies can be used to enable active ageing and social participation. He has been involved in numerous international collaborative research projects and is working on a new collaborative team grant in British Columbia to look at how new technologies can help detect and protect against falls amongst older people in nursing homes. Andrew is vice-president of the International Society of Gerontechnology and is the chair of the ISG2010 World Conference on Gerontechnology in Vancouver.

Sandra Sproll is a research associate in the field of human-computer interaction at the Fraunhofer Institute for Industrial Engineering in Stuttgart Germany. She holds a degree in Psychology and Economics. Her research interests are within the realm of Usability Engineering and User Experience focusing the overarching experience a person has as a result of interactions with a technical product or service. In several research and industrial projects she works on human-centered design, user-driven innovation and technology acceptance. In the area of ambient assisted living her research activities focus on methods for the development and evaluation of technical systems according to the special needs of elderly people.

Hong Sun received his degree in information engineering from Southeast University (China) in 2004, and his Master's in electronics from University of York (UK) in 2006. He is currently a PhD candidate of University of Antwerp, PATS Research Group and a research assistant for the IBBT (Institute of Broad Band Technology). His research interests include ambient assisted living, adaptive systems, service oriented architecture and semantic service matching. Hong Sun has published more than 20 reviewed research papers. He received the 'IBM PhD Fellowship 2009-2010'; and was also the winner of "FITCE.be Young ICT Personality 2008' competition'. He is a board member of the IEEE CIS Society, Benelux Chapter Board, and he also serves as program committee member for several international conferences. Hong Sun is expected to receive his PhD degree in May, 2010, and will join AGFA Healthcare from June, 2010.

Lorenza Tiberio currently works at the Institute of Cognitive Science and Technology (ISTC) of the Italian National Research Council (CNR) in Rome. She graduated in clinical psychology from the University of Padua and has recently started her PhD in cognitive psychology on topics related to innovative ICT technologies and their use by elderly people at home. Her main research interests concern the environmental psychology and cognitive and psychological aspects of ageing and human-technology interaction. She has been involved in several research projects on place attachment, community involvement in urban planning and assessment of environmental humanization and legibility in the hospital environment. She is currently involved in the research projects on investigation of human-technology aspects like perceived usefulness and acceptability of new technologies by elderly people in the domestic environment.

Elena Urdaneta has a PhD in Pharmacy. She is Professor of Physiology at Public University of Navarra (Spain) and Deputy Head of the R&D Department at Ingema. Her main areas of research are Successful Aging and Health. She has a long-lasting experience in Physiology, human and animal longitudinal studies, and ageing-related research. She has been Principal Investigator in numerous European and Spanish research project. Her skills and knowledge of ethical issues related to biomedical and clinical research have allowed her to be appointed ICT and Ageing Expert for some European funded initiatives and part of the University of Cornell-Ingema Agreement to further both institution's research on ageing. She also peer-reviews scientific articles for international journals and is author or co-author of more than 25 publications (articles, books and book chapters).

Zoe Wang originally came from Taiwan and has been in Australia for 13 year. She completed her PhD in 2008 and currently she is a nursing lecturer in Australian Catholic University, Banyo Campus in Brisbane. Zoe is passionate about aged care. She is a gerontic nursing practitioner, educator and researcher; and was a state executive member of the Australian Association of Gerontology. Her contribution to nursing practice and gerontology nursing is supported by her clinical work in various health care settings in Australia. Her research interests include culture, aged care and Information technology in health care. Zoe is involved in Queensland Smart Home Initiatives and believes technologies will enhance the lives of elderly people and their caregivers, allowing them to have a longer and more fulfilling place in society.

Gottfried Zimmermann is an expert on IT usability and accessibility, software engineering and quality management. He received a PhD degree in computer science from the University of Stuttgart, Germany, in 1999. As a software architect and consultant at debis (now T-Systems) from 1996-2000, he was involved in large commercial software development projects. In 2000, he joined the Trace Center of the University of Wisconsin-Madison, USA, where he focused on research and development in the area of Universal Design in current and next-generation information and communication technologies. In 2003, he founded Access Technologies Group, a consulting company for ICT accessibility. Recently, he became junior professor of Media Informatics at the University of Tübingen, Germany. He has also been the technical coordinator of the European i2home project since 2006.

Index

G

H

I

J

K

L

S

T

U

V

W

X